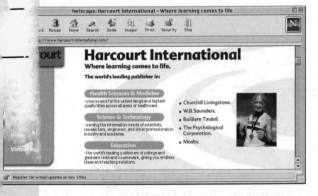
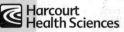

Commissioning Editor: Laurence Hunter
Project Development Manager: Fiona Conn
Project Manager: Frances Affleck
Designer: Erik Bigland

CONTENTS

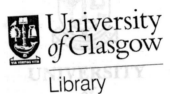

Churchill's Pocketbook of
Medicine

Peter C. Hayes BMSc MB ChB MD PhD FRCP (Edin)
Professor of Hepatology
Department of Medicine
Royal Infirmary
Edinburgh, UK

Thomas W. Mackay BSc (Hons) MBChB FRCPE
Consultant Physician
Department of Respiratory Medicine
Royal Infirmary
Edinburgh, UK

Ewan H. Forrest BMedBiol (Hons) MD MRCP
Consultant Physician
Victorian Infirmary
Glasgow, UK

Roger A. Fisken MA DPhil MD FRCP
Consultant Physician
Friarage Hospital
Northallerton, UK

THIRD EDITION

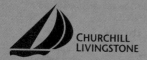

CHURCHILL
LIVINGSTONE

EDINBURGH LONDON NEW YORK PHILADELPHIA ST LOUIS
SYDNEY TORONTO 2002

CHURCHILL LIVINGSTONE
An imprint of Harcourt Publishers Limited

© Harcourt Publishers Limited 2002

 is a registered trademark of Harcourt Publishers Limited

The right of Peter C Hayes, Thomas W Mackay, Ewan H Forrest and
Roger A Fisken to be identified as authors of this work has been asserted by
them in accordance with the Copyright, Designs and Patents Act 1988

First published 1992
Second edition 1996
Third edition 2002
This edition incorporates *Churchill's House Physician's Survival Guide*
First published 1994

ISBN 0443064989
International Student Edition ISBN 0443064970

British Library Cataloguing in Publication Data
A catalogue record for this book is available from the British Library

Library of Congress Cataloging in Publication Data
A catalog record for this book is available from the Library of Congress

Note
Medical knowledge is constantly changing. As new information becomes
available, changes in treatment, procedures, equipment and the use of drugs
become necessary. The editors/authors/contributors and the publishers have,
as far as it is possible, taken care to ensure that the information given in this
text is accurate and up to date. However, readers are strongly advised to
confirm that the information, especially with regard to drug usage, complies
with the latest legislation and standards of practice.

Third edition

Four years have now passed since the publication of the second edition of this *Pocketbook* and a lot can change in four years. As usual new tests and aetiologies have been identified in medicine which need to be included in any textbook, and in most medical schools in the UK a fundamental change is taking place in the medical curriculum, reducing the separation of clinical from preclinical years.

In recognition of this, we have been fairly ambitious in this new edition. We have included more basic science into the introductory sections of text, which we hope will benefit both junior and senior students; we have included colour illustrations of clinical signs and symptoms; and have added Dr Roger Fisken to the author team, incorporating a lot of information from his companion text *Churchill's House Physician's Survival Guide*. We hope you will agree that inclusion of this new material will increase the usefulness of *Churchill's Pocketbook of Medicine* in the early years of medical school right the way through to registration and perhaps beyond. As before we are very grateful to many colleagues for their help in reviewing different sections. Any mistakes or errors that may have crept into the text, however, are entirely the responsibility of the authors, but we do hope that these are few and far between.

P.C.H.
T.W.M.
E.H.F.
R.A.F.
2002

ABBREVIATIONS

AAFB	acid and alcohol fast bacilli
ABG	arterial blood gases
ACE	angiotensin converting enzyme
ACTH	adrenocorticotrophic hormone
ADH	antidiuretic hormone
AF	atrial fibrillation
AIDS	acquired immunodeficiency syndrome
ALL	acute lymphoblastic leukaemia
ALT	alanine transaminase
AML	acute myeloid leukaemia
ANF	antinuclear factor
APUD	amine precursor uptake and decarboxylation
ARDS	adult respiratory distress syndrome
ASD	atrial septal defect
ASO	antistreptolysin O
AST	aspartate transaminase
ATN	acute tubular necrosis
AXR	abdominal X-ray
BBB	bundle branch block
BMT	bone marrow transplant
BTS	blood transfusion service
CABG	coronary artery bypass graft
CAH	chronic active hepatitis
CAPD	chronic ambulatory peritoneal dialysis
CCF	congestive cardiac failure
CCU	coronary care unit
CEA	carcinoembryonic antigen
CLL	chronic lymphatic leukaemia
CML	chronic myeloid leukaemia
CMV	cytomegalovirus
CNS	central nervous system
COPD	chronic obstructive pulmonary disease
CRF	chronic renal failure
CSF	cerebrospinal fluid
CSM	Committee for Safety in Medicine
CT	computerized tomography
CVA	cerebrovascular accident
CVP	central venous pressure
CVS	cardiovascular system
CXR	chest X-ray
DIC	disseminated intravascular coagulation
DIP	distal interphalangeal
DM	diabetes mellitus

DU	duodenal ulcer
DVT	deep venous thrombosis
EBV	Epstein-Barr virus
ECG	electrocardiogram
EEG	electroencephalogram
ELISA	enzyme-linked immunosorbent assay
EMG	electromyography
EMU	early morning urine
ERCP	endoscopic retrograde cholangiopancreatography
ESR	erythrocyte sedimentation rate
FBC	full blood count
FDP	fibrin degradation product
FEV_1	forced expiratory volume in 1 second
FFP	fresh frozen plasma
FSH	follicle stimulating hormone
FTA	fluorescent treponemal antibody test
FVC	forced vital capacity
GABA	gamma-aminobutyric acid
GFR	glomerular filtration rate
GGTP	gamma glutamyl transpeptidase
GH	growth hormone
GN	glomerulonephritis
GVH	graft versus host disease
HBV	hepatitis B virus
HCV	hepatitis C virus
HDV	hepatitis delta virus
HIV	human immunodeficiency virus
HLA	human leucocyte antigen
HOCM	hypertrophic obstructive cardiomyopathy
HR	heart rate
HSV	herpes simplex virus
IBD	inflammatory bowel disease
IBS	irritable bowel syndrome
ICP	intracranial pressure
IDL	intermediate density lipoprotein
IHD	ischaemic heart disease
IM	infectious mononucleosis
INR	International normalised ratio
ITP	idiopathic thrombocytopenia purpura
IVC	inferior vena cava
IVU	intravenous urography
JVP	jugular venous pressure
KCO	transfer factor for carbon monoxide

LA	left atrium
LAD	left axis deviation
LBBB	left bundle branch block
LDH	lactate dehydrogenase
LDL	low density lipoprotein
LFT	liver function test
LH	luteinizing hormone
LVF	left ventricular failure
MCHC	mean cell haemoglobin concentration
MCV	mean cell volume
MEN	multiple endocrine neoplasia
MHC	major histocompatability complex
MI	myocardial infarction
MND	motor neurone disease
MSU	midstream urine
MTP	metatarsophalangeal
NANB	non-A non-B hepatitis
NAP	neutrophil alkaline phosphatase
NMR	nuclear magnetic resonance
NSAID	non-steroidal anti-inflammatory drugs
OCP	oral contraceptive pill
OGTT	oral glucose tolerance test
PA	pulmonary artery
PABA	para-aminobenzoic acid
PAS	p-aminosalicylic acid
PBC	primary biliary cirrhosis
PCH	paroxysmal cold haemoglobinuria
PCP	pneumocystis carinii pneumonia
PCV	packed cell volume
PDA	patent ductus arteriosus
PEEP	positive end-expiratory pressure
PEFR	peak expiratory flow rate
PEG	percutaneous endoscopic gastrostomy
PIP	proximal interphalangeal
PNH	paraoxysmal nocturnal haemoglobin
PPD	purified protein derivative
PPS	plasma protein solution
PR	per rectum
PRV	polycythaemia rubra vera
PT	prothrombin time
PTH	parathyroid hormone
PTT	partial thromboplastin time
PTTK	partial thromboplastin time with kaolin

PUO	pyrexia of unknown origin
PUVA	psoralen ultraviolet A
PV	per vagina
RA	rheumatoid arthritis
RAD	right axis deviation
RAG	R antigen
RAST	radio-allergosorbent test
RBBB	right bundle branch block
RBC	red blood cells
RCC	red cell concentrate
RF	rheumatoid factor
RIF	right iliac fossa
RTA	renal tubular acidosis
RUQ	right upper quadrant
RVF	right ventricular failure
SACD	subacute combined degeneration
SBE	subacute bacterial endocarditis
SLE	systemic lupus erythematosus
SVC	superior vena cava
SVT	supraventricular tachycardia
TB	tuberculosis
TIA	transient ischaemic attack
TIP	terminal interphalangeal
TPHA	treponema pallidum haemaglutination assay
TPN	total parenteral nutrition
TRH	thyroid releasing hormone
TSH	thyroid stimulating hormone
TURP	transurethral resection of the prostate
U&E	urea and electrolytes
UC	ulcerative colitis
URTI	upper respiratory tract infection
US	ultrasound
UTI	urinary tract infection
VDRL	venereal diseases research laboratory
VF	ventricular fibrillation
VLDL	very low density lipoproteins
VSD	ventricular septal defect
VT	ventricular tachycardia
VWF	von Willebrand factor
WBC	white blood count
WPW	Wolff-Parkinson-White

Addison's disease   Primary adrenocortical insufficiency
Alzheimer's disease   Senile dementia
Berger's disease   IgA nephropathy
Bornholm disease   Epidemic myalgia
Budd-Chiari syndrome   Hepatic venous outflow obstruction
Buerger's disease   Thromboangitis obliterans
Caisson disease   Decompression sickness
Chagas' disease   American trypanosomiasis
Charcot-Marie-Tooth syndrome   Peroneal muscular atrophy
Christmas disease   Factor IX deficiency
Churg-Strauss syndrome   Eosinophilic granulomatous vasculitis
Conn's syndrome   Primary aldosteronism
Crohn's disease   Regional enteritis
Cushing's disease   Pituitary dependent adrenocortical
hyperplasia
Devic's disease   Neuromyelitis optica
Dressler's syndrome   Post myocardial infarction syndrome
Eaton-Lambert syndrome   Paraneoplastic myasthenia
Erb's paralysis   Upper root branchial plexus injury
Fabry's disease   Galactosidase-A deficiency
Friedreich's ataxia   Spinocerebellar ataxia
Gardner's syndrome   Variant of familial adenomatous polyposis
Gelineau's syndrome   Narcolepsy
Graves' disease   Autoimmune thyrotoxicosis
Guillain-Barré syndrome   Acute post-infection polyneuritis
Hanot's disease   Primary biliary cirrhosis
Kallman's syndrome   Hypogonadotrophic hypogonadism
Klumpke's paralysis   Lower root brachial plexus injury
Loeffler's syndrome   Simple pulmonary eosinophilia
McArdle's syndrome   Type V glycogen storage disease
Marchiafava-Michell syndrome   Paroxysmal nocturnal
haemoglobinuria
Meyer-Betz syndrome   Paroxysmal myoglobinuria
Osler-Weber-Rendu syndrome   Hereditary haemorrhagic
telangiectasia
Pickwickian syndrome   Obstructive sleep apnoea syndrome
Pott's disease   Spinal tuberculosis
Sheehan's syndrome   Postpartum hypopituitarism
Sjögren's syndrome   Keratoconjunctivitis sicca
Tietze's syndrome   Idiopathic costochondritis
Von Recklinghausen's disease   Neurofibromatosis
Wilson's disease   Hepato-lenticular degeneration

Genetic

Allele Alternate forms of a specific gene within the population that are found at a particular chromosomal location.

Clone A unique segment of DNA (which contains a particular gene) that is generated in vitro, usually through the use of restriction enzymes, and reproduced in vivo (in *E.coli*).

Gene A sequence of chromosomal DNA that codes for single protein.

Hybridization The process whereby fragments of DNA bind specifically to their complementary DNA sequences.

In-situ-hybridization A technique used where DNA probes are used to identify the presence of gene messages in cells or tissue.

Northern blotting A method to identify and quantify the amount of mRNA encoding a particular protein through the hybridization between a radiolabelled DNA clone and immobilised RNA. The method is similar to Southern blotting but does not involve digestion with restriction endonucleases.

PCR Polymerase chain reaction. A method that allows the amplification of genes through the use of heat resistant DNA polymerase and oligonucleotide primers specific to either end of the gene that is to be amplified.

Probe A gene probe is a clone specific sequence of DNA in which nucleotides are radiolabelled.

RFLP Restriction fragment length polymorphism. This is a means of identifying abnormal alleles, by cleaving DNA into sequences using bacterial restriction endonucleases. Abnormal DNA sequences may be digested into different sized lengths if alterations in the nucleotide sequence occur within the regions recognized by the endonucleases.

Southern blotting A method whereby a gene sequence can be identified within a mixture of DNA fragments (that have been separated by electrophoresis and transferred to nitrocellulose paper) by hybridization to a radiolabelled DNA probe and visualization by autoradiography.

Imaging

Digital subtraction Computer assisted radiology whereby a background image can be removed, principally during angiography, to enhance the angiographic appearance.

Doppler Usually used in connection with ultrasonography, using the phenomenon of Doppler shift to identify velocity of flow.

MRI Magnetic Resonance Imaging – provides imaging which depends upon the magnetic spin properties of molecules under a powerful magnetic field. The density of protons, in particular, provides image contrast.

PET scan   Positron emission tomography images positrons emitted from radioactive substances incorporated in tissues. It can be used to measure metabolic activity.

SPECT scanning   Single positron emission computerized tomography. This is a computerized imaging technique dependent upon positron emission tomography following the injection of a radioisotope.

Laboratory

Electrophoresis   Methods used to separate compounds by means of their movement across an electric field.

Enzyme immunoassay   An assay using antibodies to measure the concentration of a specific substance in biological fluids by means of an enzymatic reaction. The method normally requires the use of two antibodies; one raised against the substance to be measured; the second, to which an enzyme is linked, recognizes the first antibody.

HPLC   High performance liquid chromatography. A chromatographic method where compounds are pumped down various columns containing small pore silica and separated depending upon their physical properties.

Immunohistochemistry   The use of antibodies labelled to visible substances to allow identification of proteins during histology.

Monoclonal antibody   Identical antibodies produced by hybridizing plasma cells with malignant cells thereby allowing large amounts of a unique antibody with a known specificity to be produced.

Radioimmunoassay   An assay using radiolabelled biochemical (hormone, protein) to quantify the same substance in blood. The method involves competition for binding to an antibody between the radiolabelled substance and an unknown amount of the same compound in blood.

Ultra centrifugation   High speed centrifugation used to spin down small intracellular particles.

Western blotting   Use of antibodies to identify specific proteins after their separation by gel electrophoresis and transfer to nitrocellulose paper.

CONTENTS

CONTENTS

CONTENTS

Section 3: Problem Solving and Medical Emergencies 343

16. Clinical problem solving 345

Section 1:
Introduction to
clinical medicine

1

Introductory notes

INTRODUCTORY NOTES

Medicine in the 21st century is technically very different from that of 100, or even 50 years ago. However, a doctor of the early 1900s would still recognize much of what his or her successors do, as the doctor's field of work is still human health and disease. Underlying the work of the doctor there should still be the mottoes, 'common things occur commonly' and 'first, do no harm' (or, at least, do your very best to balance the risks of a treatment against its potential benefits), as well as the principles of treating the patient with respect and recognizing clearly the limits of your own abilities. Besides being technically advanced, the medicine of the modern era is highly complex, so that the successful doctor needs to build up a mosaic of academic knowledge, scientific and clinical skills and communication skills. Society has also become much more complex and traditional hierarchies have either fallen down or been forced to undergo major changes: this means that patients' expectations are very different from what they used to be and it is essential that one should involve each patient in decisions about his/her medical care as fully as possible.

The doctor must also work as a member of a clinical team which will include nurses, physiotherapists, social workers, occupational therapists, pharmacists and doctors from other specialties. At the same time, it is important that one person takes overall responsibility for the care of a particular patient and, most importantly, for ensuring that the patient is kept informed as to what is going on at every stage. Perhaps most important of all, every patient should be treated humanely and with dignity and respect at all times.

CONFIDENTIALITY

Hospital medical records are confidential and are the property of the Secretary of State for Health in England and Wales, or a similarly ranking minister in other areas of the UK. Right of access to the medical records is usually granted automatically to members of the medical and nursing staff, allied professions (dietitian, physiotherapist, social worker) and to students in those professions. Patients do not have a right of immediate access but, since 1 November 1991, they have been able to apply to the hospital to see the case notes and such access can only be refused if the consultant in charge of the case considers that disclosure would harm a patient's health. If patients ask to see their notes, the most appropriate response is to ask, 'What is it that you want to know?'. You can then answer the questions as fully and frankly as you think fit – often a patient just wants to see an X-ray or pathology report. If the patient insists, it is best to hedge (politely) and to refer the question to your consultant.

Certain simple rules will help you to avoid any embarrassing breaches of confidentiality:

- Do not leave notes lying around in public areas of the hospital (eg the canteen).
- Do not discuss patients by name in lifts, corridors or stairways where the next-door-neighbour might happen to pass by.
- Do not give information over the telephone to someone claiming to be a relative or close friend unless you have telephoned them to establish identity: confine your remarks to generalities – 'he's a bit better today'.
- When interviewing relatives, be wary of giving sensitive information (eg a diagnosis of cancer, poor prognosis or sexually transmitted disease) unless you are sure that the patient is agreeable to your disclosure or that the patient is mentally or physically too enfeebled to give or withhold consent. Remember that your ethical responsibility is to the patient in the first instance, not to the relatives. If the relatives say, 'If it's cancer, I don't want Mother to know', you should, politely but firmly, point out that you tell the patients whatever they wish to know and, in particular, that you do not propose to tell the patient a direct lie such as falsely answering the question, 'Is it cancer?'.

CONSENT FORMS

The purpose of asking a patient to sign a consent form is not simply to cover the legal niceties of medical treatment; rather it is to ensure that you explain to the patient in clear and simple language what is to happen to him/her and that you satisfy yourself that the patient understands and feels comfortable with what is to be done. If you, yourself, do not understand the procedure sufficiently well to explain it to the patient or to answer his/her questions, ask a more senior colleague to obtain consent.

When is written consent required?

Technically, anything done to a patient (including tapping with a reflex hammer or taking blood) is an assault if performed without the patient's consent. However, implicit consent is assumed for most of these day-to-day, minor interventions. Written consent is required:

- for any operation, even a minor one
- for any investigation or treatment which carries a risk of complications (eg endoscopy, liver biopsy, cardioversion, arteriography)
- for any form of research.

> **Table 1.1**
> **The consent form – summary of information required**
>
> - Patient's name and address
> - A statement that the patient (or the parent or guardian) agrees that the patient will undergo the procedure or operation
> - The exact name of the procedure (with side, if appropriate)
> - A statement by the patient confirming that the effects of the procedure have been explained to him/her and the name of the doctor who explained them
> - A statement by the patient (if he or she so wishes) that certain measures are not consented to (eg blood transfusion)
> - The patient's signature and the date of signing
> - A statement by the doctor confirming that he/she has explained the procedure to the patient
> - The doctor's signature and the date of signing

When you go to explain the procedure to the patient and to obtain his/her signature on the consent form, try to pick a time when you will not have to rush. A summary of what the consent form contains is shown in Table 1.1. You should be prepared to mention possible complications of the procedure (such as haematoma after arterial puncture for angiography) but how fully you explore the subject of complications will obviously vary from patient to patient. If the patient appears at all unhappy about the prospect of complications, or the procedure is moderate to high risk (eg cerebral angiography), it is wise to:

- ask a more senior person to speak to the patient
- write a full description in the notes of what you have said to the patient.

You cannot obtain valid consent from a patient who:

- has been given a sedative or other drug which interferes with higher mental function
- is under 16 years of age
- is demented.

Note also that the law provides ways in which treatment for psychiatric disease can be given to a mentally incompetent patient without his/her consent; *it does not do the same in respect of treatment for physical disease.* You cannot, therefore, simply ask a relative to sign the consent form. In practice, emergency treatment (such as direct current (DC) cardioversion or laparotomy for appendicitis) is unlikely to result in a prosecution for assault, but in the case of non-emergency procedures you should consult a more senior colleague.

The patient who refuses treatment

Patients have a full legal right to refuse consent to treatment and to take their own discharge from hospital, unless they are deemed to be of such unsound mind that they cannot be allowed to do so (see below: 'Sectioning'). If patients wish to discharge themselves you should:

- try to persuade the patient to stay and explain to him/her why the investigation or treatment is necessary
- tell the patient that leaving is against medical advice
- ask the patient to sign a self-discharge form (discharge against medical advice form).

Legally, patients are not obliged to sign a self-discharge form and a few refuse to do so. In any case of self-discharge, and especially if the patient refuses to sign the form, you must write a full account of events in the notes. You should also, wherever possible, ask a registered nurse to sign the notes as a witness to the truth of your account.

'Sectioning' Occasionally patients become so mentally disturbed that they behave in bizarre and dangerous ways and/or try to discharge themselves when clearly of unsound mind. The Mental Health Act of 1983 provides powers, under Section 5(2), to detain a patient in hospital if he/she is a danger to himself/herself or others and if the condition is urgent. The application must be made on the correct form and requires the signature of a doctor who has seen the patient in the preceding 24 hours, and of the nearest relative or a social worker. Normally the medical signature is that of a member of the medical team looking after the patient; the first time you find yourself in this situation, however, you should ask for help from a more senior colleague.

Once you have decided to 'section' a patient, consult the duty psychiatrist for advice about further treatment.

Refusal of specific treatments

Jehovah's Witnesses, Christian Scientists and members of other minority sects may refuse specific treatments such as blood transfusion. You should explain the nature of the treatment to such patients, but if it is refused the patients should sign a declaration to that effect. The patients' wishes must then dictate what treatment they receive.

THE NIGHT-ROUND CHECK LIST

To avoid being woken unnecessarily at night you should try, some time between 10 pm and midnight, to go round the wards for which you are responsible, checking the following:

- Intravenous cannulae (Venflons, etc): are they working satisfactorily or are they likely to pack up before morning? If in doubt, put in a new one.
- Intravenous infusions: are the iv prescriptions written up, with sufficient fluid to last through to the following morning? In the case of small-volume infusions given via syringe drivers (eg insulin, heparin), make sure that syringes are loaded, correctly labelled with the patient's name, name of the drug and date and stored in the ward refrigerator.

It is not reasonable for you to be expected to get up at 3 am to make up drug infusions simply because the nurses on the ward are 'not allowed' or 'not certified' to do it or are not permitted to connect up a solution which you have already made up. If this problem affects you, contact your consultant or BMA representative.

- Night sedation and analgesia: are all those patients who might need these drugs written up for them?
- Beds: does the receiving ward have enough empty beds for emergency admissions? If not, contact your SHO or registrar to arrange transfers of convalescent patients to other wards.
- Sick patients: make sure you have visited all of the very ill patients under your care and done whatever is necessary in the way of either tests or treatment.

DISCHARGING A PATIENT

Ideally, a plan for discharge should be sketched out as soon as a patient is admitted to hospital, so you and the nursing staff should try to assess the likely length of stay and make some provisional plans for discharge. When discharge is imminent, follow the check list below.

- Write your standard letter to the general practitioner: make sure that it includes the name of the consultant, *all* important diagnoses (including chronic conditions like hypertension or diabetes), date of discharge, drugs to be taken after discharge, special home arrangements (eg district nurse, home help, discharge to nursing home) and whether the patient will be seen in the out-patient clinic. In special cases, it should also indicate what the patient and/or relatives have been told.
- Where the patient needs a visit from the general practitioner (GP) shortly after discharge or if there have been any special problems it is wise to telephone the GP before discharge.
- Write the prescription for drugs to be taken home, commonly known as TTOs (To Take Out) or TTAs (To Take Away).

Whenever possible, try to do this at least 24 hours before discharge. Ensure that the supply is sufficient, particularly if the patient brought in a supply of tablets on admission. Make sure that a copy of this TTO prescription goes to the GP, either on its own or as part of the standard letter.

- Check that the patient knows when and how to take tablets and how to use other devices such as inhalers (usually the nursing staff will do this, but you may need to check yourself, especially where inhalers are concerned).
- Check that any support services have been arranged (district nurse, meals-on-wheels, home help, domiciliary oxygen).
- Check that an out-patient clinic appointment is being arranged.
- Write out request forms for any tests to be done after discharge (eg a barium meal or an ultrasound scan).

CERTIFYING DEATH

CONFIRMING DEATH

Check that the patient has no palpable pulse and no audible heart sounds or breath sounds. With patients who have suffered from neurological disease it is wise to check that the pupils are fixed and dilated. Write your observations in the notes and add your signature, the time and the date.

> Do not get involved in confirming brainstem death in a comatose patient. This is a very delicate matter medico-legally and must be done by a senior doctor.

INFORMING THE RELATIVES

There is no easy way to do this. Try and take a nurse in with you when you meet the relatives, particularly if the patient was relatively young or death was sudden. Try to mention the peaceful nature of the demise or the release from suffering. It is best not to ask for permission for an autopsy immediately after death. If the relatives are not present when death occurs they will usually be telephoned by a senior nurse.

DEATH CERTIFICATE

The death certificate asks you to give your opinion of the cause of death and of any contributory causes. It also asks whether a post-mortem has been or will be held.

Can you issue a death certificate?
You can do so if:

- you have seen the patient alive within 14 days of death *and*
- you are quite satisfied that death was due to natural causes *and*
- you are reasonably sure of the cause of death *and*
- there was nothing about the death which requires referral to HM Coroner or the Procurator fiscal (see below).

It is generally good practice to see the body after death, though this is not absolutely necessary if another doctor has confirmed the death. If you work in a hospital where a senior nurse is allowed to confirm expected deaths during the night, you should still visit the mortuary the next morning to see the body before issuing the death certificate.

If you are not sure about the death being a natural one or if you cannot make a reasonable, educated guess at the cause of death, ask a more senior colleague for advice.

If you can issue a death certificate, fill in the appropriate sections, sign and date it; do not forget to fill in the counterfoil in the book.

A few points to remember about filling in death certificates
'Cause of death' means the disease or pathological disorder leading to death: it does not mean the mode of dying. Thus coma, cardiac arrest, uraemia, etc, are not causes of death, whereas cerebral haemorrhage, myocardial infarction and hypertensive nephrosclerosis are. Similarly, septicaemia is a contentious term and is only acceptable as a cause of death if it can be ascribed to an underlying disease process. The underlying condition leading to death should be on the last line (usually Ib or Ic).

Section II is used for disease or conditions which may have contributed to the death, although they were not the primary cause, eg diabetes in someone who died of septicaemia due to perforated cholecystitis. Section II should not be a ragbag of any old conditions from which the patient might have suffered.

You do not have to be 100% cast-iron certain of the diagnosis in order to enter it as the cause of death on a death certificate. Thus, if you are reasonably confident that a patient died of left ventricular failure due to ischaemic heart disease (IHD), and there is no question of any unnatural cause contributing to death, you can put this down as the cause.

Do not use abbreviations on the death certificate.

In complex cases filling in the death certificate may be difficult. Do not hesitate to discuss any problems with more senior colleagues. Remember that an incorrectly completed death certificate will be picked up by the Registrar of Births, Marriages and Deaths and any uncertainty may delay the funeral arrangements.

If you cannot issue a certificate

If you did not see the patient before death, another member of the hospital staff may be able to issue. If no one in the hospital can, the general practitioner may be able to issue a certificate. If you cannot issue a certificate because there is doubt about the nature or cause of death you should discuss the case with the Procurator fiscal or coroner's officer (a police officer – see below). Often, after discussion, the coroner will advise you to go ahead and issue a death certificate; if this is not possible a post-mortem examination or an inquest may be ordered by the Procurator fiscal or the coroner. There is space on the back of the death certificate to notify the registrar that you have discussed the case with the coroner but in practice you will hardly ever have to fill this in. In particular, it is *not* wise to do so if you have discussed the case with the coroner and have been advised to issue a certificate, as filling in the box will delay the funeral arrangements.

REFERRAL OF A DEATH TO HM CORONER OR PROCURATOR FISCAL

If you do not feel able to issue a death certificate and no one else can, it is wise to discuss the death with the coroner's officer or procurator fiscal. The key issue here is whether death was due to natural causes; if it is beyond doubt that it was, then a certificate can generally be issued. Coroner's referral is recommended in certain specific circumstances, namely if:

- the deceased was not seen by a doctor within the 14 days prior to death
- there is any element of suspicious circumstances
- there is any history of violence connected with the death
- the death occurred in police custody or while in prison
- the death may be linked with an accident (whenever it occurred)
- the death was due, or could be related, to an industrial disease or to the deceased's occupation
- the actions of the deceased may have contributed to the death, eg self-neglect, drug abuse or overdose, solvent abuse
- there is any history of neglect either by the deceased or by others
- the deceased was detained under the Mental Health Act
- the death is linked with an abortion

- the deceased was receiving a war pension or industrial disability pension
- the death occurred during an operation or before full recovery from the anaesthetic or was possibly related to anaesthesia or a medical procedure
- the death might be related to lack of medical care.

Some coroners/procurators fiscal are keen to enforce a 24-hour rule, whereby any death which occurs in hospital within 24 hours of a patient's admission is automatically notified to them. There is, however, no legal basis for this and it seems pointless to refer deaths of, for example, people with massive strokes, myocardial infarctions or known disseminated malignancy. It is wise, however, to check with your local pathology department as to what the local practice is.

CONSENT FOR A HOSPITAL POST-MORTEM

Doctors often wish to have a hospital autopsy for their own education and interest; this is quite separate from an autopsy ordered by the coroner. You may ask permission of the relatives for a hospital post-mortem only if you have already decided to issue a death certificate: what you cannot legally do is to ask the relatives' permission and then, if they refuse, refer the case to the coroner. Try to obtain consent on the morning after the patient's death, not immediately they have died, and emphasize the educational value to yourself and colleagues. Stress that the body will be treated respectfully and that the relatives can, if they wish, state that they do not wish for a particular part (usually the head and neck) to be examined. If organs are to be retained for more detailed study you must say so clearly to the next of kin. You will then need to ask the next of kin to sign a consent form for the autopsy. If you are filling in the death certificate before you have spoken to the relatives and you intend to ask for permission, but are subsequently refused, the registrar will get to know about it eventually, so no harm is done.

WHOM TO INFORM ABOUT A DEATH

Poor communications in this area can lead to long-lasting bitterness and resentment, so make sure that the following are informed as soon as possible:

- the relatives
- the GP (it is quite in order for the ward clerk or a nurse to do this, so long as it is done)
- the team looking after the patient (if not your own team)
- your consultant (if it is one of your own team's patients).

MEDICO-LEGAL PROBLEMS

It is as well to be aware right at the outset that medical practice has become increasingly hedged in with legal problems and dangers. You must understand that *no one is immune* – however good a doctor you are and no matter how much your actions may have been in good faith, you may still find yourself hauled before a court if you are unlucky or make a simple (though under-standable) mistake. The commonest legal pitfalls can be considered under several headings (see also Confidentiality (→ p 4) and Prescribing controlled drugs (→ p 530)).

Note-keeping

Medical defence societies will tell you that they are often unable to defend an action against a doctor, not because he/she has done wrong but because they cannot establish from the notes that the right things were done at the right time. You must, therefore:

- write legible, complete notes, preferably using an ink that will not fade and which will photocopy well
- sign and date your entries in the notes and make sure that your signature is legible or is accompanied by a printed rendering of your name
- avoid slang and any abusive or sarcastic remarks, either relating to the patient or to any other doctors involved in the case.

It is also advisable to state in the notes what the plan of management is, so that it is clear that you have thought about the problems and are trying to do the best for the patient.

Disclosure of information to third parties

You must not discuss details of a patient's illness or treatment with anyone without his/her permission. If a close relative asks about the patient there is usually no problem over providing simple information, especially face to face (see below). However, if the information is in any way sensitive you may need to withhold it, at least until you are sure that the patient is willing for it to be disclosed: remember that, ethically, your 'contract' is with the patient, not the relatives.

Telephone enquiries If you receive a telephone call from someone who is apparently the relative of a patient, do not say anything specific but confine your remarks to generalities such as, 'He's had a better day today,' or, 'She's quite comfortable at the moment'. If the caller is very anxious to know more (eg if he/she is a long way away and wants to know if an urgent trip to the hospital is necessary) offer to ring the caller back and, in the mean-time, ask the patient's permission to discuss details of his/her condition with the caller. In general, full discussions about a person's illness are much better conducted by asking the relative to come into the ward at a mutually convenient time.

Press and media enquiries It is extremely easy to say the wrong thing under questioning from an experienced journalist. In almost all cases it is best to say nothing to the media but to refer all enquiries to your boss or to an official hospital spokesperson.

Police enquiries The police may ask you to give them information about a patient in connection with the investigation of a crime or a potential prosecution. You should tactfully point out that you cannot release privileged information to them except with the patient's permission: ethically it is much better to say nothing, even if that means that the patient escapes prosecution for a minor offence. Where the offence in question is a serious one, however (such as murder, rape, arson or terrorism), you may feel that your duty as a citizen overrides your duty as a doctor. Certainly, in such a case a court is unlikely to rule against you if you find yourself being sued for breach of confidence.

Communication

Failure on the part of doctors to keep each other informed is a major cause of ill-feeling between colleagues and also of medico-legal hazards. When you go off duty, make sure that you have told your colleague who is on-call about any seriously ill patients under your care. Similarly, when you have been on-call you must tell other firms about any of their patients who have been admitted during the night or to whom you have been called.

Communication with nursing staff is also important; your life can be made a misery if you ignore this principle. Do not go off for your half-day without telling the nurses and do not turn your bleep off when on-call. Make sure that any instructions you write for them (such as iv fluid prescriptions) are clear, sensible and will last through the night. Finally, remember communication with the GP: tell him/her immediately if a patient dies ($\rightarrow$ p 12) and make sure that the note you write for the GP when a patient is discharged is legible and clear, especially in relation to take-home drugs.

Prescribing

The prescribing of controlled drugs is dealt with on page 530. Many of the cases which occupy the energies of the medical defence societies are, however, related to the prescribing of ordinary, everyday drugs. Be especially careful with:

- drugs which commonly cause allergy (eg penicillin)
- drug interactions, especially with chemically promiscuous substances such as warfarin

- drugs with similar names, eg aminophylline and amitriptyline, chlorpropamide and chlorpromazine
- dilutions, eg of cardiovascular drugs like dopamine/dobutamine – check your arithmetic carefully (with an experienced nurse or colleague), especially in the middle of the night.

Fitness to drive

People with certain medical conditions may be partially or completely unfit to drive: such restrictions can apply to people with epilepsy, diabetes, angina, strokes, syncopal attacks, etc. The regulations are especially severe for holders of vocational licences (Large Goods Vehicles and Passenger Carrying Vehicles). Full details of these regulations can be found in the 'red book', *Medical Aspects of Fitness to Drive*, which should be available in your hospital library. A brief summary of the most important regulations is given in Table 1.2.

Table 1.2
Regulations for fitness to drive

Condition	Regulation
Epilepsy	Cannot drive unless he/she has been free of fits for 1 year or has had a fit only during sleep, together with a history of sleep-only fits for 3 years or more. Note that a fit which occurs *for any reason* (including missed medication) will result in a driving ban. Vocational driving is forbidden unless the person has been free of fits for 10 years or more and does not require any medication to treat epilepsy
Myocardial infarction (MI) or CABG	May not drive for 4 weeks after the event
Angina	Should not drive if angina occurs at rest or while driving. *Note:* people with ischaemic heart disease of any kind are almost always banned from holding a vocational licence
Complete heart block	Driving is forbidden until 1 month after the fitting of a pacemaker. Vocational licence holders may not drive for 3 months after a pacemaker has been fitted

Table 1.2
Regulations for fitness to drive *(cont'd)*

Condition	Regulation
Syncopal attacks	May not drive for at least a year, patient must be free of attacks during that time. Resumption of driving may be possible if a cause is identified and treated
Diabetes	No restriction if treated by diet alone, or diet/tablets and has normal vision. Treatment with insulin restricts licence to a 3-year term, and prohibits holding of vocational licence. Hypoglycaemic loss of awareness leads to automatic ban.
Stroke	Should not drive for at least a month, longer in more severe cases (eg those with a hemianopia). Rules for vocational driving depend on individual case, but ban of at least 5 years is usual

Note that the responsibility for informing the Driving and Vehicle Licensing Agency (DVLA) about a medical condition which may affect driving rests with the patient, not the doctor. Patients should be warned, however, that they risk prosecution if they knowingly withhold information about a serious medical disorder.

HUMAN IMMUNODEFICIENCY VIRUS (HIV) TESTING

People at risk of HIV infection

The HIV virus is of relatively low infectivity and is, therefore, transmitted by intimate contact or by blood-borne transmission; it cannot be passed on by casual non-intimate contact such as shaking hands, sharing towels, crockery, etc, social kissing or being in a confined space with an infected person. There is a risk of infection from:

- penetrative sexual intercourse (vaginal, anal or oral if the recipient partner has an open lesion in the mouth or on the lips)

- sharing needles or syringes to inject drugs
- receiving contaminated blood products via a transfusion (now a very rare cause of infection in the UK but may be a risk for those travelling abroad, eg to East Africa)
- vertical transmission from mother to baby.

Testing patients

If a patient asks for an HIV test you should try to establish:

1. Why has a test been asked for? Has there been true at-risk behaviour or does the patient have a misconception about how HIV is transmitted?
2. When did the at-risk behaviour take place? Remember that it can take up to 3 months for the HIV antibody to become detectable after infection has occurred, so a negative test within that time does not rule out infection.
3. What does the patient hope to learn from the test? The test does not detect acquired immunodeficiency syndrome (AIDS) nor does it predict, for those who are positive, who will develop AIDS or how long it will be before they do so.
4. What will the patient do if the result is positive? Try to ask a specific question such as, 'What support will you have,' or, 'What will be your greatest concern,' rather than a very general one such as, 'How will you feel?'.

If you are unhappy with the responses to any of these questions ask someone more senior to see the patient. You should also explain that, if the test is positive, there are organizations which will provide counselling and support, often on an urgent basis. On the negative side, having an HIV test can have certain disadvantages. For example, most life-assurance companies ask if a proposer has been HIV tested or has sought counselling in relation to HIV. If the answer to the question is yes, insurance (and therefore such things as mortgages) may be refused, or granted only at increased premium, even if the result of the HIV test was negative.

Surgical or other invasive treatment

There are very few circumstances in which it is necessary to obtain the result of an HIV test as an emergency. If the at-risk patient needs elective surgery the question of HIV status should have been sorted out well in advance. If, on the other hand, emergency surgery is needed, then it should be assumed that the patient is HIV-positive and management should be on that basis. If one of your seniors objects, try pointing out that a negative test would not in any way be reassuring: if the person has been indulging in high-risk behaviour within the last 3 months, he/she might be infected and yet test negative. The only safe thing to do is to assume that people with a history of high-risk behaviour are HIV-positive.

Transplant donors

An ethical difficulty arises in relation to persons who are brain-dead and are suitable to be organ donors for transplantation. Most transplant centres require that donors be tested for various infections, including HIV. You should, ideally, explain this to the relatives when permission is being sought for the use of the brain-dead person's organs. It is worth spending a moment thinking about what will be said if the HIV test proves to be positive. If there are no implications for the health of others (for example if the donor is unmarried or has not had a sexual partner for many years) then the relatives may not wish to know the result of the test and you should not force it upon them. If, however, there are potential health hazards involving other people then someone needs to discuss this with the family once the result is known. This job is best delegated to one of your superiors.

Positive test results

Patients who have a positive test need to be interviewed (not necessarily by you) so that the significance of the result can be explained. Point out again that the test is not a test for AIDS and that it cannot predict when (if ever) the person will develop AIDS, though the great majority of HIV-positive individuals do eventually develop the disease. Try to put patients in touch with a counsellor, either locally via an AIDS helpline or via one of the national charities such as the Terence Higgins Trust.

Negative test results

You should again emphasize that the result does not definitely exclude infection and that it certainly does not sanction unsafe behaviour such as unprotected sex or sharing needles. If the patient is in doubt, most hospitals now have a counselling service which can provide leaflets to educate patients about safe behaviour.

Nursing HIV-positive patients

HIV is of low infectivity and there is no need for these patients to be isolated unless they have some other indication such as diarrhoea. Staff with cuts or open wounds on the hands should not handle vomitus, urine, faeces, etc, from HIV-infected patients – indeed, anyone handling such material should wear gloves. You should also wear gloves when taking blood from an HIV-positive patient and take extreme care over sharps disposal.

Needlestick injuries

If you prick yourself with a needle after taking blood from

someone who is, or might be, HIV-positive, contact the micro-biology department, the A&E department, genitourinary medicine department, or the Consultant in Communicable Disease Control immediately. The hospital should make available to you a cocktail of anti-retroviral drugs which will prevent infection even if virus transmission has occurred. These drugs need, however, to be taken within an hour of the injury.

POTENTIAL ORGAN DONORS

Many patients in the UK die or suffer prolonged dependency because of a lack of organs for transplantation. Therefore, all doctors should consider organ donation in any young or middle-aged patient with a fatal condition whose kidneys, liver, heart or corneas are healthy.

Suitable organ donors
- Victims of severe head injury
- Severe subarachnoid or intracerebral haemorrhage
- In the case of corneal donation, any young patient with healthy eyes and a rapidly fatal illness.

Unsuitable organ donors
- Where brain-death is uncertain (see below)
- Those over 60
- Where there has been significant hypotension or hypoxia during the final illness
- Where there is a history of previous disease affecting the potential donor organ (eg hypertension or diabetes in the case of kidneys or hepatitis B or alcohol abuse in the case of the liver)
- Where the patient has received drug or other treatment which might have affected the organs to be transplanted
- In the case of kidneys, where there is persistent oliguria.

Diagnosis of brain-death
This is a complex area and you should not attempt to make this diagnosis yourself – it requires the involvement of a senior doctor. However, there is no point in even considering brain-death if the following apply:

- the patient is able to breathe spontaneously
- the coma might be due to drugs, poisoning or a metabolic disorder such as uraemia
- the patient has easily-elicitable brain-stem reflexes, such as pupil reactions or gag reflex.

Potential organ donors
- Talk to the relatives (UK law does not allow the removal of organs without the consent of the next of kin, even if the patient was carrying a donor card). It is best to interview the relatives in the company of a senior nurse and, preferably, not in the middle of the night. Try to put across the point that a tragedy has already occurred and that one way for some good to come out of it is for the organs to be used for transplantation.

Many families are helped by being told that they can receive information later about the person who has received their loved one's organs, a practice which many transplant surgeons will undertake.

- You will need to explain to the family that, as a matter of routine, all potential organ donors are tested for the presence of infections, including HIV. Ask the family whether they wish to be told the results of the HIV test and *write their reply in the notes.*
- Talk to a senior member of your firm; raise the question of establishing the diagnosis of brain-stem death.
- Discuss with your senior colleagues the question of contacting your local transplant coordinator or the nearest transplant centre.
- While waiting for a decision about organ donation or for the organs to be removed, make sure that the potential donor is kept supplied with adequate fluid and that blood pressure is maintained.
- The transplant centre will ask you to carry out tests on the potential donor such as hepatitis B and HIV testing and HLA determination. As regards HIV tests, you should ask the family if they wish to be told the result (see above). If a potential donor is found to be HIV-positive, this will have implications for spouse, children and sexual partners, so tell your consultant and leave it to him/her to take the matter further.

2

History and examination

CLINICAL HISTORY

Introduction   Introduce yourself and ask permission to interview and examine the patient. Developing a rapport with patients is essential for a good interview and this skill comes only with practice • Ask name and age • Ask about presenting complaint • Ask the questions relevant to the system suspected of being involved (see below).

Past medical and surgical history   Specifically ask about jaundice, epilepsy, rheumatic fever, tuberculosis, diabetes mellitus and operations.

Drugs   Obtain as much information as possible including any bought over the counter. Allergies to drugs must be sought and any reaction understood.

Smoking history and alcohol consumption   Past and present.

Social and family history   • Ask about marital status, occupation, home conditions and social circumstances, health of immediate family and causes of death of parents or siblings • Any information about illnesses that appear to run in families should be elicited • Any recent overseas travel should be discussed.

Systemic enquiry   (excluding that discussed under history of presenting complaint):

CVS: • chest pain – site, character, duration, severity, radiation, exacerbating factors, relieving factors, associated features • breathlessness – onset, eg worse on exertion, at night – and relieving factors, eg sitting upright, fresh air and any associated wheeze • palpitations – ask patient to tap out a rhythm • intermittent claudication • ankle swelling.

RS: breathlessness • cough (whether productive and what colour the sputum) • haemoptysis • night sweats • wheeze.

GI: weight (whether increasing, steady or falling) • appetite • dysphagia • dyspepsia (including exacerbating and relieving features) • abdominal pain • bowel habit, noting any change from normal • stool consistency and colour, tendency to float • faecal incontinence • rectal bleeding.

GUS: • urinary frequency • dysuria • hesitancy and dribbling • incontinence • haematuria or altered colour • menstrual cycle, noting any change from usual • post-menopausal bleeding • impotence • sexual orientation (if appropriate).

MS: • mobility • arthralgia • joint stiffness or swelling.

CNS: • headache • eyesight including diplopia • dizzy spells, faints and falls • weakness • numbness • tremor or involuntary movement • dysarthria and dysphasia • sense of taste and smell.

EXAMINATION

GENERAL FEATURES

Well/ill-looking, orientation in time, place and person, agitation, state of hydration, cyanosis (central/peripheral), jaundice, pallor, state of nutrition, lymphadenopathy, breast examination, distribution of body hair, skin, hands and nails (joints, palmar erythema, Dupuytren's contracture, clubbing, splinter haemorrhages), tongue, throat, goitre.

CARDIOVASCULAR SYSTEM

- Pulse (radial) – rate, rhythm, volume, character (normal, slowly rising, collapsing, bisferiens), compare both radial pulses simultaneously to assess synchronicity and check for radial-femoral delay. Tabulate the presence/absence of each radial, brachial, carotid, femoral, popliteal, posterior tibial and dorsalis pedis pulse.
- Assess height and character of jugular venous pulse (JVP) with patient sitting comfortably at 45°. Palpate precordium for apex beat (usually in the 5th intercostal space medial to the mid-clavicular line) heaves or thrills.
- Auscultate at the apex (bell), left sternal edge (diaphragm), aortic and pulmonary areas (2nd right and left intercostal spaces respectively using the diaphragm) before listening at the apex with the patient rolled onto their left side (mitral stenosis) and at the lower left sternal edge with the patient sitting forward and the breath held in expiration (aortic incompetence). Pay attention to the character of the first and second heart sounds (normal/fixed/reversed, splitting) and for the presence of any additional heart sounds (III or IV) or for any pericardial rubs.
- Listen for any murmurs and assess their quality, site of origin and maximal intensity and direction of radiation (→ Fig. 2.1, p 24).
  Check for the presence of dependent oedema (ankles/sacrum). Always measure the BP (erect and supine if possible) and check for pulsus paradoxus. Auscultate the chest for crackles in LVF.

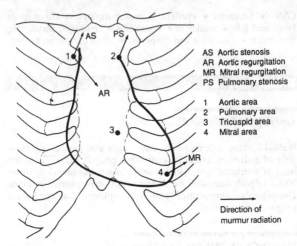

AS Aortic stenosis
AR Aortic regurgitation
MR Mitral regurgitation
PS Pulmonary stenosis

1 Aortic area
2 Pulmonary area
3 Tricuspid area
4 Mitral area

→ Direction of murmur radiation

Fig. 2.1 Sites of cardiac auscultation.

RESPIRATORY SYSTEM

- Central and peripheral cyanosis, dyspnoea at rest, digital clubbing, tar staining of fingers, wasting of 1st dorsal interossei muscles in the hand (sign of possible apical lung tumour), signs of carbon dioxide retention (coarse flapping tremor, warm peripheries, bounding pulse, confusion, papilloedema).
- Record respiratory rate (normally 12–14 breaths/min) and breathing pattern (normal/Cheyne-Stokes/Kussmaul).
- Always compare both sides of the chest during the examination.
- Observe chest wall movement during both quiet breathing and deep inspiration and expiration. Measure chest expansion in both lateral and anteroposterior directions (should be at least 5 cm). Note presence of intercostal indrawing and the use of accessory muscles of respiration.
- Palpate for subcutaneous emphysema.
- Palpate the position of the trachea.
- Palpate for tactile fremitus.
- Percuss, auscultate and assess vocal resonance/whispering pectoriloquy of both the anterior and posterior aspects of the chest, including the apices and in both axillae. Listen to the quality of the breath sounds (normal/absent/bronchial) and for any additional sounds (crackles/wheezes/pleural rubs).
- Always examine any sputum (pink, frothy/purulent/mucoid/haemoptysis).

GASTROINTESTINAL SYSTEM

- Stigmata of chronic liver disease (leuconychia, palmar erythema, spider telangiectasiae, flapping tremor, lack of secondary sexual hair, jaundice, testicular atrophy, gynaecomastia, caput medusae, ascites, scratch marks).
- Check the appearance of dentition, tongue and fauces.
- Inspect the abdomen (scars, movement with respiration, peristalsis, swellings, cough impulses, herniae).
- Palpate gently and superficially with a warm hand having asked first about any particularly tender areas. Then palpate each area of the abdomen a little deeper. Feel for the liver, spleen and kidneys specifically, and check size by percussion (always percussing in the direction of resonant to dull).
- Differentiate spleen from kidney by identifying the anterior notch of the spleen, the dullness to percussion over the spleen, and the inability to 'get above' the spleen.
- Percuss gently throughout the abdomen and demonstrate any shifting dullness (ascites).
- Auscultate paying attention to the character of the bowel sounds (normal/diminished/increased in intensity/tinkling in obstruction/absent), and the presence of any bruits.
- Examine genitalia.
- Perform a PR and PV examination.

NERVOUS SYSTEM

- Level of consciousness; (see Table 17.1)
- Assess speech:
  Cerebellar dysarthria: slow, staccato, scanning
  Pseudobulbar palsy: 'Donald Duck' speech
  Bulbar palsy: nasal slurring
  Expressive dysphasia: difficulty word finding, retains comprehension
  Receptive dysphasia: fluent but unintelligible, no comprehension
  Nominal dysphasia: unable to name specific objects
- Assess gait:
  Cerebellar: wide-based gait, Romberg sign negative
  Spastic paraplegia: stiff, scissor-like gait
  Parkinson's disease: hesitant, shuffling gait, no arm swing
  Sensory ataxia: wide-based, stamping gait, Romberg sign positive
  Foot drop: high-stepping gait
- Cranial nerves:
  I – smell; test each nostril separately
  II – fundi, visual fields, acuity, direct and consensual pupillary response

III, IV, VI – external ocular movements ('Any double vision?'), ptosis, nystagmus

V – sensation in all three divisions, corneal reflex, muscles of mastication

VII – facial movements ('Raise your eyebrows', 'Show me your teeth'), taste on anterior $\frac{1}{3}$ of tongue

VIII – hearing (Rinne and Weber tests)

IX, X – palatal movement, gag reflex, taste on posterior $\frac{2}{3}$ of tongue

XI – trapezius and sternocleidomastoid ('Shrug your shoulders')

XII – tongue movements

- Limb tone: move limbs passively; compare each side
  Normal, decreased, flaccid, increased (spasticity: 'clasp knife'; rigidity: 'lead pipe')
- Limb power: grade 1 (flaccid paralysis) to grade 5 (normal)
  Upper limbs
  > Shoulder abduction (C5)
  > Elbow flexion (C5,6)
  > Elbow extension (C7)
  > Finger grip (C8, T1)
  > Finger spread (dorsal interossei, ulnar nerve)
  > Opposition of thumb and little finger (median nerve)

  Lower limbs
  > Hip flexion (L1,2)
  > Knee flexion (L5,S1,2)
  > Knee extension (L3,4)
  > Plantar flexion (S1)
  > Dorsiflexion (L4,5).
- Limb reflexes: compare each side, use reinforcement if necessary
  > Biceps (C5,6)
  > Triceps (C7,8)
  > Supinator (C6)
  > Quadriceps (L3,4)
  > Ankle (S1)
  > Plantar response
- Coordination: 'finger – nose' test, tap back of hand, 'heel – shin' test
- Limb sensation: test dermatomes for soft-touch, pinprick, temperature
  Upper limbs
  > Lateral upper arm (C5)
  > Lateral forearm (C6)
  > 2nd, 3rd digits (C7)
  > Distal medial forearm (C8)
  > Proximal medial forearm (T1)
  > Medial upper arm (T2)

Lower limbs
    Outer thigh (L2)
    Inner thigh (L3,5)
    Inner calf (L4)
    Outer calf (L5)
    Lateral foot (S1)
Test for proprioception and vibration

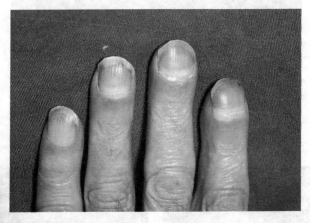

Fig. 2.2 Finger clubbing
Associated tenderness of the wrists is characteristic of hypertrophic
pulmonary osteoarthropathy, which is accompanied by periosteal
elevation and new bone formation.
Aetiology can be divided into four groups:
Thoracic: bronchial carcinoma, mesothelioma, thymoma,
neurofibroma, lymphoma, asbestosis, fibrosing alveolitis, abscess,
bronchiectasis, empyema and cystic fibrosis
Cardiovascular: infective endocarditis, pulmonary a–v
malformation, cyanotic heart disease, eg atrial or ventricular septal
defect with R–L shunt, Fallot's tetralogy
Gastrointestinal: cirrhosis, eg PBC or CAH, Crohn's disease,
ulcerative colitis, coeliac disease
Miscellaneous: thyrotoxicosis, brachial a–v malformation, familial.
Clubbing may regress if the underlying disorder, eg bronchial
carcinoma, is treated.

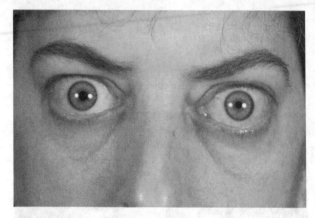

Fig. 2.3   Thyrotoxic exophthalmos (Courtesy of Dr Pierre-Marc Bouloux)

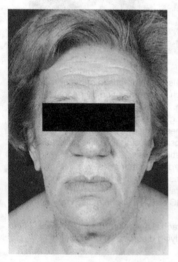

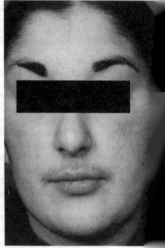

Fig. 2.4   Acromegaly (Courtesy of Dr Pierre-Marc Bouloux)

Fig. 2.5   Cushingoid facial appearance (Courtesy of Dr Pierre-Marc Bouloux)

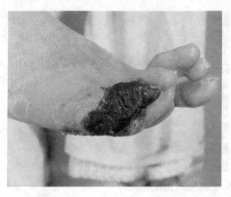

Fig. 2.6 Gangrene

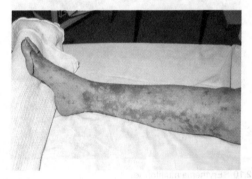

Fig. 2.7 Meningococcal purpura

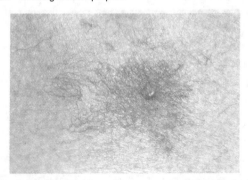

Fig. 2.8 Spider naevus

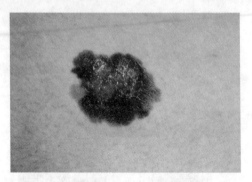

Fig. 2.9 Malignant melanoma

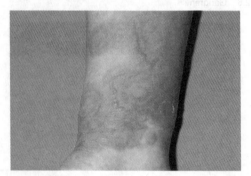

Fig. 2.10 Erythema multiforme

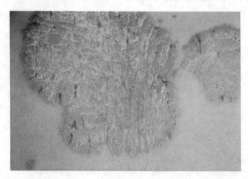

Fig. 2.11 Psoriasis

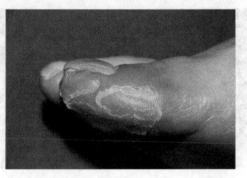

Fig. 2.12   Gouty tophus

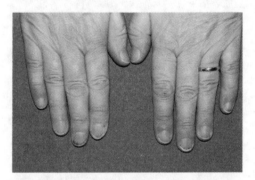

Fig. 2.13   Splinter haemorrhages

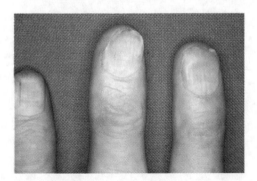

g. 2.14   Leuconychia and koilonychia

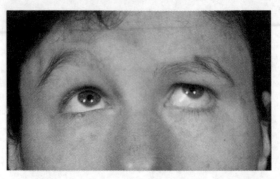

Fig. 2.15   Facial palsy (Courtesy of Dr Pierre-Marc Bouloux)

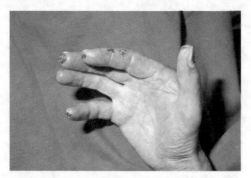

Fig. 2.16   Raynaud's phenomenon

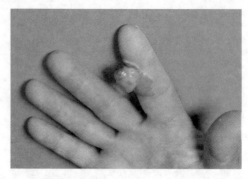

Fig. 2.17   Pyogenic granuloma

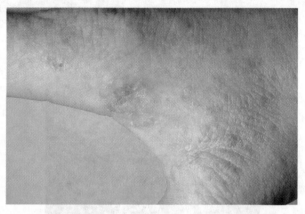

Fig. 2.18   Scabies

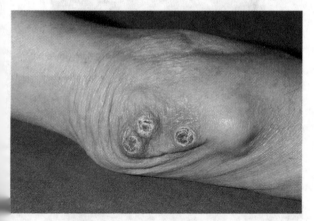

Fig. 2.19   Rheumatoid nodule

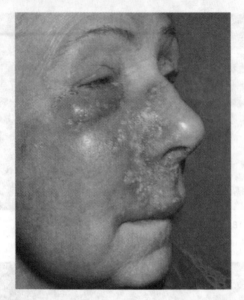

Fig. 2.20   Herpes zoster (Courtesy of Dr Pierre-Marc Bouloux)

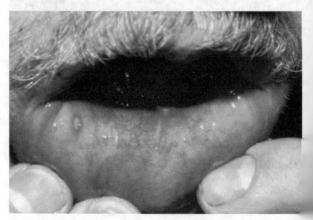

Fig. 2.21   Aphthous ulceration

Section 2:
Clinical specialties

3

Cardiovascular disease

38

INVESTIGATIONS

All patients suspected of cardiac disease should have a thorough history and physical examination which will often establish the diagnosis. Commonly required investigations include:

CXR This will identify cardiac enlargement, mediastinal abnormalities and in some instances the cardiac chamber involved and any associated pulmonary congestion or pulmonary oedema (→ Fig. 4.3, p 66).

ECG This can confirm ischaemic heart disease showing ischaemia at rest or myocardial infarction. However a normal ECG does not exclude IHD. The ECG is also essential in the diagnosis of cardiac arrhythmias and conduction abnormalities. Characteristic abnormalities may occur in LVH, mitral stenosis, pulmonary embolism, pericarditis, ventricular aneurysm and hypothermia.

Exercise ECG This test is performed under medical supervision and is useful in the assessment of the patient with suspected angina or following myocardial infarction. A standardized protocol (eg, Bruce) should be followed to allow objective assessment of performance.

Ambulatory ECG and BP monitoring These are useful in the assessment of suspected cardiac dysrhythmias and of suspected hypertension, respectively.

Echocardiography Useful in assessing ventricular function (systolic and diastolic), valvular abnormalities and investigation of possible pericardial effusions. 2-dimensional scans have now largely replaced the M-mode echo and allow, in expert hands, visualization of all four chambers, their wall thickness, valves in the heart and pericardium. Combined with Doppler studies the flow of blood across valves or septal defects can be determined and quantitated. Transoesophageal echocardiography is increasingly used for assessment of LA, interatrial septum, aorta and mitral valve functional abnormalities and imaging of the descending thoracic aorta.

Angiography This can be used to outline the coronary circulation and is essential in the assessment of coronary atheromatous disease in those who would be candidates for coronary surgery or angioplasty. Cardiac catheterization with contrast studies, pressure measurement and O_2 saturation allows accurate assessment of ventricular size and function, valvular heart disease or intracardiac shunts. Coronary revascularization can also be performed (PTCA and intracoronary stenting).

Isotope scans These can be used in the assessment of ventricular function, myocardial ischaemia and myocardial infarction.

Isotope-labelled perfusion tracers allow demonstration of areas of reduced myocardial perfusion. Cardiovascular stress can be provided by exercise or by drugs, eg dobutamine (an inotrope) or dipyridamole or adenosine (vasodilators), in patients who are unable to exercise. The isotope is administered at peak exercise and images are taken after exercise with a gamma camera. Pulmonary perfusion scans are commonly used in the diagnosis of pulmonary embolism.

ANGINA

Science basics Angina pectoris is the commonest and most important symptom of ischaemic heart disease and is due to an imbalance between the myocardial oxygen supply and demand. Ischaemia is usually produced if the coronary arterial luminal diameter is reduced by ≥70%. If reduction is ≥90% symptoms may occur at rest. Variants of classical angina include micro-vascular angina (Syndrome X) and Prinzmetal angina, due to coronary artery spasm, and unstable angina which increases in severity until occurring at rest and commonly is the forerunner of MI. Conditions other than ischaemic heart disease which may produce angina include cardiomyopathy, coronary artery spasm and aortic stenosis. The major risk factors for IHD are cigarette smoking, hypertension, male sex, age, family history, diabetes mellitus and hyperlipidaemia.

Clinical features

Symptoms: severe chest pain described variably as gripping, crushing or tight. The pain frequently radiates down the left arm and into the neck and jaw. It is typically induced by exercise and stress and relieved within 1–2 minutes by nitroglycerin.

Signs: often none. Risk factors such as hypertension or aggravating factors such as anaemia may be identified.

Investigations • ECG: although this may be entirely normal between attacks, particularly in those without a history of MI, it is usually abnormal during an attack. The classical abnormalities include ST segment depression and T-wave inversion. ST segment elevation occurs in coronary artery spasm (Prinzmetal angina) or myocardial infarction. In patients with a suggestive history but normal resting ECG an exercise test should be undertaken, using either a bicycle or treadmill, providing aortic stenosis and unstable angina have been excluded. This is performed until a required heart rate is reached or the patient becomes symptomatic, develops an arrhythmia or hypotension. Monitoring throughout is essential and should include blood pressure, heart rate, duration of exercise, quantitation and duration of any ECG abnormality. ECG and blood pressure are also monitored during the recovery period after exercise • Radio-isotope thallium scanning may provide additional information and helps to distinguish reversible from irreversible myocardial ischaemia. • Coronary angiography is the gold standard in the diagnosis of coronary artery disease and is required in those being considered for coronary artery surgery or angioplasty, ie those with refractory angina, those who develop hypotension, more than 2 mm ST depression or severe limitation in exercise tolerance during mild exercise which indicates high risk of triple or left main-stem coronary disease (in whom surgery prolongs life).

Management box

▶ Recognize and correct risk factors such as hypertension, smoking, obesity and hyperlipidaemia. Advise regarding exercise, occupation and stress-management. Adequate investigation to identify those likely to benefit from surgery. HRT should be offered to all post-menopausal women with angina (but be cautious it there is a strong family history of breast carcinoma).

▶ *Drug therapy*:
  – *Aspirin*: 75 mg/day is recommended for all angina patients, if tolerated.
  – *Nitrates*: sublingual or buccal for symptomatic relief; oral for prophylaxis, allowing an 8–10-hour interval without therapy to prevent tolerance (eg isosorbide mononitrate 20 mg bd). Their effectiveness depends on their ability to provide nitric oxide (NO). GTN tablets (not the spray) deteriorate once the container is exposed to air and a new supply may be needed monthly.
  – *β-blockers*: β_1-selective antagonists reduce adverse reactions (eg atenolol 50 mg/day). Titrate dose to achieve a resting heart rate of approximately 60/min. Particularly indicated post-MI. Should be avoided if direct contra-indictations are present (COPD, asthma, severe LV dysfunction).
  – *Calcium antagonists*: relax vascular smooth muscle, eg nifedipine 10 mg tid, diltiazem 60 mg tid (or sustained release preparations) or amlodipine 5–20 mg/day for both stable and unstable angina, particularly where coronary artery spasm exists. The latter is suggested by rest pain associated with transient ST segment elevation, which may be identified only by 24-hour ECG monitoring.
  – *ATP-sensitive potassium channel activators*: nicorandil 10–20 mg bd produces vasodilation but avoids haemo-dynamic tolerance.

→

▶ *Coronary angioplasty revascularization* (PTCA and stents): useful and successful in treating proximal arterial stenoses, particularly in those with localized disease. Its role shortly after acute myocardial infarction is still controversial.

▶ *Coronary artery bypass surgery*: indicated in those with severe coronary artery disease, ie triple vessel disease and left main stem stenosis, where surgery prolongs survival. The main indication remains symptomatic relief in those refractory to medical management where bypass is anatomically possible.

E ▶ **UNSTABLE ANGINA** → page 419

E ▶ **MYOCARDIAL INFARCTION** → page 419

E ▶ **ARRHYTHMIAS** → page 428

CARDIAC AXIS AND BUNDLE BRANCH BLOCK

Science basics The cardiac axis is determined using the standard limb leads. The normal axis is between −30° and +110°. The lead with equiphasic QRS complexes should be sought and the axis lies at right angles to this. A look at the QRS complexes in the other leads should clarify whether the right angle is clockwise or anticlockwise of the equiphasic lead, ie, a tall R wave in I indicating anticlockwise rotation (L axis deviation; LAD) while a tall R in III, clockwise rotation (R axis deviation; RAD). The cardiac axis is useful in identifying L or RVH and bifascicular block (see below).

Bundle branch block describes the ECG pattern which appears with major interruption of the normal electrical conduction through the Purkinje system. The QRS complex is always greater than 0.12 s. Right bundle branch block (RBBB) (→ Fig. 3.1): M-shaped QRS complex in VI and W-shaped in V6. This may be congenital but also develops with ischaemic heart disease. Left bundle branch block (LBBB) (→ Fig. 3.2): W-shaped QRS in V1 and M-shaped in V6. This is usually acquired and associated with ischaemic heart disease. Less commonly BBB may be found in conjunction with atrio-ventricular cushion defects and cardiomyopathy. BBB may be present intermittently in such disorders as paroxysmal atrial tachycardia, where incomplete recovery in a bundle occurs due to the rate resulting in aberrant conduction.

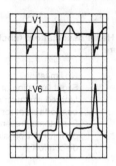

Fig. 3.2   Left bundle branch block.

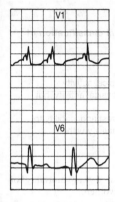

Fig. 3.1   Right bundle branch block.

Bifascicular block: combination of marked axis deviation and RBBB suggests a block in two bundles. Hence RBBB and LAD indicates block in the right and left anterior bundle; and LBBB blockage of both left bundles.

Trifascicular block: said to be present when first-degree heart block, RBBB and L anterior or posterior hemiblock coexist or first-degree HB and LBBB.

Bifascicular and trifascicular blocks may be found as complications of ischaemic heart disease but are also characteristic of ostium primum ASDs.

HEART FAILURE

Science basics   Heart failure exists when the heart is unable to pump sufficient blood to satisfy the body's metabolic requirement, while maintaining normal filling (preload) pressures. Although clinically failure is commonly divided into left or right-sided failure, it is rare for these to exist in isolation.

Aetiology   Heart failure is not a diagnosis but a clinical syndrome and the underlying cause must be sought. The commonest cause of heart failure is ischaemic heart disease (IHD) but it is important to identify the underlying cause in each patient in order to avoid missing correctable disorders. Other causes include: valvular heart disease, hypertension, arrhythmias, pulmonary embolism, anaemia, thyrotoxicosis, myocarditis, infective endocarditis, cardiomyopathy and thiamine deficiency (wet

Table 3.1
New York Heart Association: functional classification of heart failure

Class I	No limitation
Class II	Slight limitation of physical activity
Class III	Marked limitation of physical activity, but comfortable at rest
Class IV	Symptoms present at rest and inability to perform any physical activity without discomfort

beriberi). Systolic heart failure carries a 5-year mortality of approximately 60% for men and 50% for women.

Clinical features

Symptoms: in LVF dyspnoea on exertion, orthopnoea and paroxysmal nocturnal dyspnoea are common. In RVF ankle swelling and RUQ discomfort may occur. In both, fatigue and lethargy are usual.

Signs: ankle and sacral oedema, raised JVP, basal crepitations, hepatomegaly and gallop rhythm. Table 3.1 shows a classification of heart failure.

Investigations • CXR may show cardiomegaly, pulmonary venous distension, Kerley B lines, alveolar oedema, (often in a 'bat's-wing' distribution) and pleural effusions. It may also provide evidence of the underlying cause, eg L atrial enlargement in mitral stenosis • ECG may show LVH often due to chronic hypertension or aortic stenosis, P-mitrale of mitral stenosis or evidence of IHD • How well the LV is contracting, the chamber size and the state of the valves can be assessed by echocardiography. If no obvious cardiac disorder can be identified high cardiac output states such as thyrotoxicosis and thiamine deficiency should be excluded • Other causes of pulmonary or peripheral oedema should also be ruled out such as nephrotic syndrome, acute renal failure and liver disease.

Management box

▸ This should be directed to the cause in such correctable disorders as valvular heart disease and thyrotoxicosis. In most cases, however, usually due to IHD, treatment is purely symptomatic and includes:
  – Dietary salt reduction.

- Diuretics, usually a thiazide for mild CCF and loop diuretics in more severe cases. Combinations using loop thiazides and potassium-sparing agents (eg spironolactone) may be needed. Metolazone may be used with caution (monitor electrolytes).
- Digoxin in patients with associated AF. The role of digoxin in sinus rhythm remains controversial.
- Vasodilators can be used to reduce either pre load, such as the long-acting nitrates (avoiding tolerance by allowing an 8–10-hour treatment-free period daily), or after-load, such as ACE inhibitors, eg captopril or enalapril which have been shown to prolong life in heart failure. Other after-load reducers such as hydralazine and prazosin are used less commonly today.
- β-blockers (eg bisoprolol) may be given under specialist supervision.

In patients with refractory CCF, hospitalization and the administration of iv loop diuretics, vasodilators, eg isosorbide dinitrate infusion, and inotropes (dopamine, dobutamine) may be required. In young patients with severe, intractable cardiac failure, cardiac transplantation is now a viable therapeutic option.

⊟ LEFT VENTRICULAR FAILURE (ACUTE PULMONARY OEDEMA) → page 432

HYPERTENSION

Science basics It has been recognized for many years that high BP is associated with an increased risk of MI and strokes. However, the cut-off between normal pressure and hypertension remains controversial. It is generally agreed that individuals of less than 60 years with a BP consistently above 140/90 mmHg should be treated, as should those older patients with a BP above 160/100 mmHg. Clinical trials of treatment of such patients have shown a reduction in deaths from both IHD and strokes, although the benefit varies in different studies regarding such factors as sex and smoking. In Western societies up to 20% of the adult population may have hypertension with an increasing prevalence with age. It has been estimated that a reduction in diastolic BP of 6 mmHg maintained for 5 years could reduce the risk of stroke by 40% and CHD by 2.5%.

Screening The majority of individuals with hypertension are symptomatic and therefore detection depends in large part on screening. It is important that the BP should be checked on more than one occasion some weeks apart before a diagnosis of hypertension is made.

Aetiology In approximately 90% no obvious cause can be found and the patients are labelled as having essential hypertension. In the remaining minority the cause can be identified as due to: renal disease, such as renal artery stenosis due to fibromuscular dysplasia or atheroma, chronic glomerulonephritis or pyelonephritis, polycystic kidneys or renal vasculitis; endocrine causes including Conn's syndrome, Cushing's syndrome, acromegaly, diabetes mellitus and phaeochromocytoma; other causes including coarctation of the aorta, polycythaemia rubra vera, toxaemia of pregnancy and drugs (eg prednisolone).

Clinical features

Symptoms: usually none, occasionally headache, cardiac failure, MI and renal failure.

Signs: other than high BP, retinopathy, LVF and LV heave. Bruits may be heard in coarctation of the aorta and in renal artery stenosis. Four stages or grades of severity according to the retinal findings exist:

- Stage I: arteriolar narrowing
- Stage II: arteriolar irregularity
- Stage III: 'blot' and 'flame' haemorrhages and 'cotton wool' exudates
- Stage IV: papilloedema, associated with malignant hypertension

Investigations • In all patients CXR, ECG (→ Fig. 3.3), echocardiography, urinalysis, proteinuria, haematuria, U&E and creatinine, lipid and glucose levels. • In selected patients, especially if young or if biochemical or clinical results indicate, renal ultrasound IVU, urinary metadrenaline, urinary free cortisol and plasma aldosterone and renal angiography to exclude renal artery stenosis, phaeochromocytoma, Cushing's syndrome and Conn's syndrome respectively. 24-hour ambulatory BP measurement allows more accurate assessment if the diagnosis is in doubt (eg, 'white coat' hypertension) or in borderline or resistant cases.

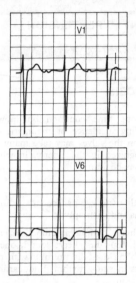

Fig. 3.3 Left ventricular hypertrophy.

Management box

This depends upon the cause. If a correctable lesion is found, such as renal artery stenosis or Conn's syndrome, treatment for this should be undertaken. For those in whom no cause is identified treatment is along the following lines:

▶ Reduction of excessive dietary salt intake.
▶ Reduction of stress, where possible.
▶ Weight and alcohol reduction, if appropriate.
▶ Thiazide (eg bendroflumethiazide (bendrofluazide) 2.5–5 mg) or β-blocker (eg atenolol 50 mg). Both have adverse reactions and treatment should be tailored to the individual. If hypertension remains:
▶ Add a vasodilator such as a calcium antagonist (eg nifedipine 10–20 mg tid), an ACE-inhibitor (eg captopril 25 mg tid) with a loop diuretic or hydralazine 25–50 mg bd. Again the treatment regimen, which often involves 3 or more drugs, should be tailored to the patient who may have to take such medications for many years. A close check should be kept on U&E and creatinine to ensure renal function is not compromised.

MALIGNANT HYPERTENSION → page 432

MITRAL VALVE DISEASE

MITRAL STENOSIS

Aetiology   At one time common but now relatively rare following the falling incidence of rheumatic fever. Since the scarring process on the valves may take many years, new cases may still be recognized in the elderly, in whom a history of rheumatic fever may be found.

Clinical features

Symptoms: breathlessness, particularly during pregnancy, cough, palpitations and haemoptysis.

Signs: malar flush, peripheral embolism, atrial fibrillation, tapping apex beat, loud first heart sound, opening snap and a low-pitched, rumbling diastolic murmur with presystolic accentuation in patients in sinus rhythm. Endocarditis is uncommon with pure mitral stenosis.

Investigations • CXR may show L atrial enlargement and pulmonary congestion • ECG P-mitrale or atrial fibrillation • Echocardiography is important in both diagnosis and assessing the severity of stenosis by chamber enlargement, valve motion and Doppler studies • Cardiac catheterization may be used to quantitate the gradient across the valve, the cardiac output and R heart pressures.

Management box

▸ Many patients, because of age or associated medical disorders, are treated with diuretics, digoxin for patients in AF and with warfarin because of the risk of peripheral embolism.

▸ Definitive treatment is either by mitral valvulotomy or balloon valvoplasty if the stenosis is not accompanied by regurgitation or by valve replacement if regurgitation or heavy calcification exists.

MITRAL REGURGITATION

Aetiology   Includes myxomatous degeneration, papillary muscle dysfunction, rheumatic heart disease, mitral valve prolapse secondary to LV dilatation due to cardiomyopathy or post-MI.

Clinical features

Symptoms: fatigue, palpitations and breathlessness.

Signs: large pulse pressure, LV heave, soft S_1, wide splitting of S_2, S_3, and an apical pansystolic murmur radiating towards the axilla.

Investigations • CXR may show cardiac enlargement and pulmonary oedema • ECG, LVH and AF • Echocardiography may reveal an enlarged LA, LV or abnormal mitral valve • Doppler studies can be useful in assessing severity • Cardiac catheterization may be used to quantitate the severity of regurgitation.

Management box

▶ In many patients treatment is of the associated cardiac failure and controlling associated arrhythmias.

▶ Valve replacement or repair should be considered in severe disease.

Mitral valve prolapse: often idiopathic and identified in otherwise entirely well young females. Some patients present with atypical chest pain or cardiac arrhythmias. Examination reveals a mid-systolic click and late systolic murmur. The diagnosis is confirmed by echocardiography and no treatment is required except prophylaxis against endocarditis ($\rightarrow$ p 52). In a small proportion progressive mitral regurgitation develops.

AORTIC VALVE DISEASE

AORTIC STENOSIS

Aetiology Congenital and rheumatic in younger age groups and calcification of congenital bicuspid valve and degenerative in the elderly. Subaortic stenosis may complicate hypertrophic cardiomyopathy and supravalvar stenosis may be associated with infantile hypercalcaemia (often with facial deformity).

Clinical features

Symptoms: dyspnoea, angina, syncope and sudden death (although often asymptomatic).

Signs: plateau pulse, small pulse pressure, heaving apex beat, basal thrill, ejection systolic murmur maximal in the right 2nd intercostal space radiating to the neck, with a quiet 2nd sound

Table 3.2
Heart murmur characteristics

Lesion	Murmur	Heart sounds	Radiation
MS	Mid-diastolic (patient on L side)	Loud S_1, opening snap	None
MR	Pansystolic	Soft S_1, split S_2, S_3 common	Axilla
AS	Ejection systolic	Soft delayed S_2, S_4 common	Neck
AR	Early diastolic (patient sitting forward)	Soft S_2, S_3 common	L sternal edge

and often a 4th sound (→ Table 3.2). An ejection click may be present and excludes supra- or subaortic stenosis.

Investigations • ECG: LV (+LA) hypertrophy • CXR: cardiomegaly and post-stenotic dilatation of the proximal aorta • Echocardiography: LV hypertrophy, valve orifice size, valve cusp appearance and opening abnormal • Doppler echocardiography: predicting gradient across valve • Cardiac catheterization: measuring valve gradient, LV function and coronary artery assessment.

Complications LVF, arrhythmias (including sudden death), infective endocarditis.

Management box
▶ Treat cardiac failure and angina avoiding after-load reduction.
▶ Avoid strenuous exercise.
▶ Valve replacement in symptomatic patients with gradient 50 mmHg.
▶ Balloon valvuloplasty in the elderly is controversial.
▶ Antibiotic prophylaxis for invasive procedures.

AORTIC REGURGITATION

Aetiology Congenital bicuspid valve, endocarditis, rheumatic. Uncommon: syphilis, connective tissue disease (SLE, ankylosing spondylitis, Reiter's and Behçet's syndrome), Marfan's syndrome, coarctation, aortic dissection and traumatic rupture.

Clinical features

Symptoms: often none, dyspnoea, palpitations, angina uncommon.

Signs: collapsing pulse, wide pulse pressure, cardiac apex displacement, early blowing diastolic murmur maximal at left sternal edge with patient sitting forward in full expiration. Systolic flow murmur common. Diastolic murmur at apex similar to mitral stenosis (Austin Flint). 2nd sound soft and 3rd sound common.

Investigations • ECG: LV hypertrophy • CXR: cardiomegaly • Echocardiography: dilated aortic root or valve cusp abnormality and mitral valve fluttering • Doppler studies: quantifying regurgitation • Cardiac catheterization with aortogram.

Complications Cardiac failure, endocarditis.

Management box
▶ Treat cardiac failure and underlying disease if possible.
▶ Valve replacement for severe regurgitation in symptomatic patients or those asymptomatic subjects with LV dysfunction or LV end systolic internal diameter 5.5 cm.
▶ Antibiotic prophylaxis for invasive procedures.

INFECTIVE ENDOCARDITIS

Science basics Infective endocarditis, the infection of cardiac valves usually by bacteria, is a serious but frequently preventable disorder. The valves involved are usually but not invariably abnormal before the infection. Clinically three types are recognized.

Subacute infective endocarditis: characterized by an insidious onset, pyrexia, night sweats and fatigue. Clinical features include haematuria, retinal infarcts, Osler's nodes, peripheral infarcts, changing murmur, joint pains and splenomegaly. The valve abnormalities at most risk are bicuspid aortic, rheumatic and prosthetic valves, particularly if regurgitant. Other sites of infection include VSD and PDA. The organism most often involved is *Strep. viridans;* others include staphylococci, *Strep. faecalis* and coliforms. Infection with *Strep. bovis* is associated with colonic cancer.

Acute or fulminant endocarditis: much less common and previously normal valves may be affected. For this reason the diagnosis may be delayed with dire consequences as the disorder is rapidly fatal. *Staph. aureus* is the usual organism. Features include pyrexia, retinal haemorrhages (Roth spots), petechiae and peripheral emboli.

Right-sided endocarditis: presents with pleuritic chest pain, pyrexia, breathlessness and fatigue. Risk factors are iv drug abuse and the presence of central iv lines. The tricuspid valve is most usually involved resulting in multiple pulmonary infarcts, abscesses and severe right-sided cardiac failure.

Investigations • The most important test is numerous sets of blood cultures (at least 4) over a 24–36-hour period • Antibiotics ideally should not be administered before these are taken • Supplementary investigations include transthoracic or transoesophageal echocardiography for vegetations (this may be negative in 30–40%), FBC showing a leukocytosis and a normochromic, normocytic anaemia and elevated ESR or CRP • Haematuria containing casts and a reduced serum C3 is common. Approximately 20% of cases are culture negative, either because antibiotics have been administered before blood cultures were taken or the infecting organism is difficult to identify, such as fungi or *Coxiella*.

Management box

▶ This should be tailored to the organism identified and bacteriological advice should be sought.

▶ Antibiotics should be administered parenterally for at least 2 weeks and for longer in many cases. For penicillin-sensitive streptococci benzylpenicillin 10–20 million units daily in divided doses along with gentamicin 1 mg/kg tid for 2 weeks followed by amoxicillin 500 mg tid for a further 2 weeks.

Prevention This is vitally important and all patients with abnormal or prosthetic valves and those with VSDs and hypertrophic obstructive cardiomyopathy should receive prophylaxis before procedures likely to produce bacteraemia.

Procedures: dental and oral surgery and bronchoscopy – 3 g oral amoxicillin 1 hour before (oral erythromycin should be used in penicillin-sensitive subjects or in those who have taken penicillin within 4 weeks, 1.5 g 1 hour before and 0.5 g 6 hours later); GI and GU surgery or endoscopy, bladder catheterization – ampicillin 1 g plus gentamicin 1 mg/kg before and ampicillin 500 mg 6 hours later. Prolonged or repeated courses of antibiotic encourage the emergence of antibiotic-resistant organisms.

CONGENITAL HEART DISEASE

Science basics Traditionally congenital heart disease is divided into cyanotic (R to L shunt) and acyanotic (L to R, or no shunt).

CYANOTIC

These are uncommon, particularly in adults since mortality without corrective surgery is high. The best known is Fallot's tetralogy which consists of pulmonary stenosis, VSD over which the aorta takes its origin and RVH. Eisenmenger's syndrome is said to exist when reversal of the L to R shunt in VSD occurs with pulmonary hypertension. The other form of cyanotic congenital heart disease is transposition of the great vessels. This is rapidly fatal without intervention by Rashkind's procedure or surgery.

ACYANOTIC

These include ASD, VSD, patent ductus arteriosus, aortic coarctation and pulmonary stenosis. In those disorders with L to R shunts the development of pulmonary hypertension may result in shunt reversal and cyanosis. Significant pulmonary hypertension is a contraindication to surgery and treatment must aim to prevent its development.

Atrial septal defect
This is often unsuspected until adult life when breathlessness and palpitations present.

Signs: prominent v-wave of JVP, L parasternal heave, fixed splitting of S_2 and parasternal systolic and tricuspid diastolic flow murmurs.

Investigations • CXR: prominent pulmonary vasculature and RV • ECG: partial RBBB and RAD (LAD with ostium primum defect, which is less common than secundum defects) • Echocardiography: enlargement of RA and RV • Doppler studies: transatrial and increased pulmonary flow.

Management box
▶ For those with a pulmonary flow 1.5 × greater than systemic flow, percutaneous or surgical repair is indicated unless pulmonary hypertension exists.

Ventricular septal defect
These are commonly asymptomatic and may close during childhood.

Clinical features In adults this is with fatigue and breathlessness.

Signs: systolic thrill, loud P_2, S_3, loud pansystolic murmur at lower L sternal border and a diastolic mitral flow murmur.

Investigations • CXR: prominence of pulmonary vasculature • ECG: may be normal, or show LV hypertrophy • Echocardiography: visualization of VSD in some, LA, RV and LV enlargement in those with large shunts • Doppler: demonstration of L to R flow.

> **Management box**
> ▶ As for ASD with same criteria for surgery. Prophylaxis against endocarditis.

Patent ductus arteriosus

The failure of closure of the ductus arteriosus, between the aorta and the pulmonary artery, which is commoner with maternal rubella, may be asymptomatic for years.

Clinical features

Symptoms: usually presents with fatigue and breathlessness on exertion.

Signs: thrusting apex beat, systolic-diastolic 'machinery' murmur at L upper sternal edge.

Investigations • CXR: prominent pulmonary vasculature, enlarged ascending aorta • ECG, LVH • Echocardiography: on 2-D echo the patent ductus may be visualized • Doppler may demonstrate turbulent flow in the PA • Cardiac catheterization.

> **Management box**
> ▶ Transcatheter intervention, using an umbrella or coil or surgical ligation, providing pulmonary hypertension has not developed. Prophylaxis against endocarditis.

Coarctation of the aorta

This disorder, a narrowing of the aorta just beyond the L subclavian artery, may be asymptomatic or present with hypertension, heart failure or poor perfusion in the lower limbs.

Signs: hypertension measured in the arm, radial-femoral pulse delay, visible collateral intercostal and periscapular vessels, systolic murmur posterosuperiorly.

Investigations • CXR: rib notching • ECG: LVH • Aortogram.

> **Management box**
> ▶ Surgery; prophylaxis against endocarditis.

Other congenital heart disorders

These include: bicuspid aortic valves which usually cause no symptoms until late in life when stenosis may develop, pulmonary stenosis when the patient may occasionally be cyanosed, and dextrocardia which usually causes more problems for the doctor than the patient!

PERICARDITIS

Science basics Pericarditis, inflammation of the pericardium, is common and causes include: MI, viral infection (particularly coxsackie), malignancy, renal failure, tuberculosis, Dressler's syndrome, connective tissue disorders and trauma.

Clinical features

Symptoms: usually sharp, localized chest pain characteristically relieved by leaning forward. It may occasionally have a pleuritic element, pleuropericarditis.

Signs: pericardial rub at L sternal edge, commonly present only transiently. Evidence of RVF, pulsus paradoxus and a rising JVP on inspiration (Kussmaul's sign) may accompany a pericardial effusion that is causing cardiac tamponade (→ Fig. 3.4).

Investigations • ECG: ST elevation without reciprocal ST depression • CXR may show globular cardiac enlargement suggestive of an effusion which should be confirmed by echocardiography.

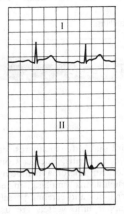
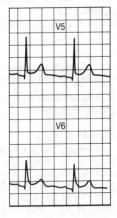

Fig. 3.4   Pericarditis.

Management box
▶ Treat the underlying disorder.
▶ Analgesia with NSAIDs.
▶ Large pericardial effusions, associated with pulsus para-doxus, RVF and hypotension require aspiration under ECG and echocardiographic monitoring and with cardiac surgical backup. This may also be necessary for diagnostic purposes. The aspirate should be examined biochemically, bacterio-logically and by cytology.

CONSTRICTIVE PERICARDITIS

A rigid pericardial sac which limits ventricular filling, may be caused by TB, malignancy, renal failure, viral infection and post-cardiac surgery.

Clinical features

Symptoms: include fatigue, ankle and abdominal swelling and breathlessness.

Signs: raised JVP which rises with inspiration (Kussmaul's sign), tachycardia with low volume pulse, ascites, ankle oedema and occasionally a pericardial knock after S_2.

Investigations • ECG may have low voltage • CXR: small cardiac shadow sometimes with peripheral calcification • Echo-cardiography shows a thickened pericardium and, unlike restrictive cardiomyopathy, a normally contracting ventricle.

Management box
▶ Surgical resection of the pericardium.

PERIPHERAL VASCULAR DISEASE

ARTERIAL DISEASE

Large vessel disease

In Western society this is almost invariably due to atherosclerosis. Other rare causes include giant cell arteritis, Buerger's disease and Takayasu's disease. Risk factors for atheroma include hyper-tension, diabetes mellitus, hyperlipidaemia, smoking, male sex, family history and age. The lower limbs and cerebral vessels are commonly involved while the upper limb vessels are usually spared. Cerebrovascular disease is discussed elsewhere (p 167).

Clinical features These depend upon whether the arterial insufficiency develops acutely, eg arterial emboli, or over a long period.

Symptoms: depend upon the vessel involved and the speed of onset but the commonest include hemiparesis and intermittent claudication.

Signs: vary with the vessel involved and include carotid bruit, hemiplegia, absent peripheral pulses, peripheral ulceration and gangrene, absent digits and cold, cyanosed peripheries.

Investigations • Angiography of the implicated vessels is the investigation of choice and will demonstrate the site and severity of the stenosis. Other less invasive tests include • Thermography • Doppler flow studies.

Management box
▸ All patients with atheromatous disease of medium and large arteries should be strongly advised to stop smoking which is the single most important risk factor.
▸ Treatment of hyperlipidaemia and hypertension.
▸ Increased perfusion to ischaemic tissues can be realized by reducing blood viscosity and venesection, if the patient is polycythaemic, and iv dextran may be useful.
▸ Aspirin (75–300 mg/day) reduces platelet aggregability and may produce benefit in reducing thrombi but is associated with increased risk of cerebral haemorrhage.
▸ Oral anticoagulation with warfarin is of value when cardiac emboli are the cause of ischaemia.
▸ Where localized arterial disease is identified surgery offers most benefit in the form of angioplasty and bypass.
▸ Endarterectomy, formerly popular for carotid stenosis, has been shown to be of limited value.

Small vessel disease

Disorders which result in disease or occlusion of small vessels include diabetes mellitus, arteritides such as polyarteritis nodosa, rheumatoid disease and SLE, hyperviscosity such as myeloma, Waldenström's macroglobulinaemia, polycythaemia and cryoglobulinaemia, and Raynaud's syndrome. Disease or occlusion of arterioles results in clinically apparent lesions in the peripheral circulation (fingers and toes) but also lesions in the circulation to internal organs such as the kidneys, heart, eyes and brain.

Clinical features

Symptoms: depend upon the site of disease but common symptoms include cold hands and feet, often with pain, and changes in colour.

Signs: small infarcts of extremities and ulceration, haematuria, retinal infarcts and haemorrhages and cold peripheries with good peripheral pulses.

Investigations • For diabetes: fasting blood glucose and HbA$_{1c}$ • Myeloma: immunoelectrophoresis, Bence-Jones proteinuria and serum calcium • Haematological disease: haemoglobin, haematocrit, platelet count • Connective tissue disease: ESR, ANF, C3 and renal angiography.

> **Management box**
> ▶ This depends upon the underlying disease.

VENOUS DISEASE

Two forms of venous thrombosis are recognized, thrombo-phlebitis, where the endothelium of the vein is inflamed and phlebothrombosis, a primary thrombosis in an otherwise normal vessel which carries a higher risk of pulmonary embolism. Risk factors include sluggish peripheral circulation, increased viscosity of the blood, damage to the vein, and malignancy (eg pancreatic cancer).

Clinical features Usually pain with accompanying signs of localized inflammation in thrombophlebitis and swelling, super-ficial venous distension, increased temperature, red dis-colouration and tenderness in deep venous thrombosis. The differential diagnosis includes musculoskeletal disorders, cellulitis, lymphangitis and a ruptured Baker's cyst.

Investigations • The diagnosis of thrombophlebitis is usually obvious but deep venous thrombosis is notoriously difficult; diagnosis on the basis of physical signs is erroneous in a large minority, while signs may be absent in those with venous thrombosis • The definitive test is venography and is essential for the diagnosis of thrombosis in the pelvic veins • Doppler ultrasound is useful in the diagnosis of proximal DVTs • Thermography and radio-labelled fibrinogen scans and venous plethysmography are useful in the diagnosis of more distal thrombosis.

> **Management box**
> ▶ Thrombophlebitis usually requires only symptomatic therapy and anticoagulation is not indicated unless the deep veins are also involved.
> ▶ Phlebothrombosis with its accompanying risk of pulmon-ary emboli and chronic venous insufficiency should be treated initially with subcutaneous low molecular weight heparin (→ p 380).

> ▶ Prophylactic measures, such as subcutaneous heparin, should be considered in bed-bound patients at risk of, or with a past history of, DVT.

CARDIOMYOPATHY AND MYOCARDITIS

Cardiomyopathy and myocarditis represent diseases of cardiac muscle excluding IHD. The term cardiomyopathy is used to denote an abnormality of the myocardium capable of producing heart failure, while myocarditis is applied to those where there is an inflammatory process, most often infective.

CARDIOMYOPATHIES

These can be divided into three main groups:

Dilated: characterized by dilatation of the R and L ventricles and impaired ejection fraction; clinically the apex beat is diffuse and displaced, S_1 is often quiet and a gallop rhythm and MR common ● Echocardiography is invaluable diagnostically although the clinical history, ECG and coronary angiography are important in excluding alcoholic and IHD ● Treatment is of the associated cardiac failure and the prognosis poor ● Warfarin should be considered because of the risk of systemic emboli.

Hypertrophic: this is commonly familial (autosomal dominant inheritance in 50% of cases, others are sporadic. A linkage to the β myosin heavy chain gene on chromosome 14 may be present, although other chromosomes (1, 7, 11 and 15) may be involved) and characterized by marked hypertrophy of the ventricle and/or interventricular septum; the latter commonly resulting in obstruction to LV outflow (HOCM) ● Clinical examination may reveal a 'jerky' pulse, double apical impulse and a systolic murmur ● Echocardiography usually confirms the diagnosis ● Treatment is with β-blockers or calcium antagonists to reduce the heart rate and contractility, and amiodarone to prevent ventricular arrythmias. Digoxin and vasodilators may increase outflow obstruction and should be avoided. Permanent pacing may be necessary ● The prognosis is variable and the condition is not infrequently identified at autopsy in young adults with sudden death.

Restrictive: characterized by reduced compliance (or increased stiffness) of the ventricles which reduces ventricular filling. It occurs in endocardial eosinophilia, cardiac amyloid and tropical endomyocardial fibrosis ● The diagnosis should be suspected in patients with cardiac failure and normal systolic function.

Cardiac biopsy will differentiate pericardial constriction from endocardial disease • Treatment is symptomatic, most usually with diuretics.

MYOCARDITIS

Aetiology Causes include • infective: viral (influenza and coxsackie B), bacterial (diphtheria) and protozoal (Chagas' disease) • metabolic: pregnancy, thyroid disease, haemochromatosis, thiamine deficiency and amyloidosis • connective tissue disease: SLE • infiltrative: leukaemia and sarcoidosis • neuromuscular: muscular dystrophy and Friedreich's ataxia • drugs: alcohol, phenothiazines and arsenic • radiation.

Clinical features May present like IHD of sudden onset with pain, sinus tachycardia with or without a third heart sound, cardiac failure and arrhythmias.

Investigations • ECG for arrhythmias and to exclude MI • CXR often reveals cardiomegaly and LVF • Echocardiography to exclude pericardial effusion, valvular disease and assess LV function • Serology to identify recent viral infection or connective tissue disease.

Management box
▶ This depends upon the underlying cause but in many is symptomatic.
▶ Steroids therapy (prednisolone initially 40 mg/day) is indicated in those with connective tissue disease.
▶ The prognosis in the majority of patients is good.

CARDIAC TRANSPLANTATION

First performed in 1967, cardiac transplantation is being increasingly used to treat debilitating heart disease. Selection of recipients is important. The basic criterion is that of severe cardiac disease (NYHA Grade IV → p 44), not amenable to other forms of therapy, and an estimated survival of less than 6 months. Cardiomyopathy and coronary artery disease are the commonest indications. Pulmonary vascular disease is a contraindication – donor hearts cannot pump against a high pulmonary vascular resistance, and unresolved pulmonary infarcts have a high probability of developing into abscesses. Age is a relative contraindication, but survival is little influenced up to 69 years. Body size and ABO blood group compatibility are the two most important matching criteria.

Rejection and infection are the main causes of death in the first year. However, after this time rapidly progressive graft coronary disease is the major cause of mortality and complications.

Current 1-year survival is 80%, 5-year 60% and 10-year 40%.

4

Respiratory disease

INVESTIGATIONS

Much can be learned of a patient's respiratory disorder from a thorough history and examination. Common investigations include:

CXR This is the single most important investigation in respiratory medicine and provides essential information concerning the underlying disease process in many patients, eg pneumonia, pulmonary fibrosis, tuberculosis, sarcoidosis and carcinoma. Some patients may have serious or advanced respiratory disease with a normal CXR eg asthma. Ideally both a PA and lateral view should be obtained. A PA CXR has an advantage over an AP (anteroposterior) film because the heart size is not exaggerated. It is always useful to compare the current CXR to any previous films.

Sputum microscopy and culture This is of considerable importance in order to select the appropriate antibiotic. Cytological examination of sputum, especially if repeated on three samples, is a reasonably sensitive test for bronchial carcinoma.

Peak expiratory flow rate This is a useful bedside and out-patient method for monitoring the severity of asthma and response to therapy. It reflects airway calibre but may underestimate the degree of airway obstruction present.

Arterial blood gas analysis Because clinical signs such as cyanosis may be unreliable, all patients with acute respiratory disease should have PaO_2, $PaCO_2$, $H+$ and HCO concentrations measured in arterial blood and related to inspired O_2 concentration.

Spirometry This again is a simple side-room test which allows measurement of the vital capacity and FEV_1 and allows separation of restrictive from obstructive airway disease ($\rightarrow$ Figs 4.1 & 4.2).

Pulmonary gas exchange The size and integrity of the lung surface available for gas exchange can be assessed by the carbon monoxide transfer factor (T_LCO) measured during 10 seconds of breath-holding after full inspiration from RV to TLC. Correction for lung volume can be made by calculating the transfer co-efficient (T_LCO/alveolar volume). The T_LCO falls in conditions producing interstitial fibrosis or emphysema and rises in lung haemorrhage.

Bronchoscopy This allows direct visualization of the proximal bronchial tree with the facility to take cytological specimens and biopsies from bronchi and lung parenchyma. Lavage fluid obtained is useful in the diagnosis of interstitial lung disease and infection (including TB and *Pneumocystis carinii* pneumonia).

Radio-isotopic ventilation and perfusion scans These are important in the diagnosis of pulmonary embolism if the CXR is normal.

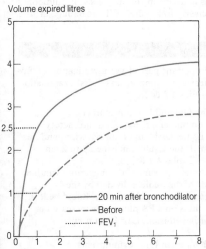

Volume expired litres

Fig. 4.1 Reversibility test. Forced expiratory manoeuvres before and 20 minutes after inhalation of a β_2-adrenoreceptor agonist. Note the increase in FEV_1 from 1.0–2.5 l. An improvement in FEV_1 of ≥15% and more than 300 ml, after the administration of 200 µg salbutamol (or equivalent) by inhalation is consistent with significant airway reversibility.

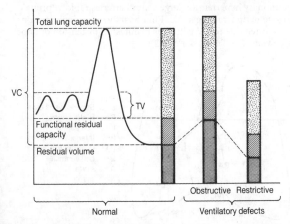

Fig. 4.2 Normal lung volumes and the changes which occur in obstructive and restrictive ventilatory defects.

Percutaneous pleural biopsy This is useful in the diagnosis of tuberculosis, carcinoma and mesothelioma.

CT scanning This has largely replaced tomography in the accurate localization and staging of pulmonary lesions. High-resolution CT scanning is useful in the diagnosis of pulmonary fibrosis and bronchiectasis and spiral CT scanning in the diagnosis of PE.

CHEST X-RAY

The chest X-ray is an important part of the investigation of any patient with either cardiac or lung disease. Its examination should be systematic (→ Figs 4.3 & 4.4):

- Check the name on the film and L and R markers.
- Check whole chest is on film and penetration satisfactory.
- Note trachea is central, mediastinum of normal width and hila position and size normal (the L hilum may be up to 2 cm higher than the R). (→ Tables 4.1 & 4.2).
- Assess cardiothoracic ratio (the sum of the maximum width of the heart on either side of the midline divided by the maximum internal diameter of the chest): this should be less than 50% in healthy adults on a PA film and is increased in cardiac failure, pericardial effusion, L or R ventricular hypertrophy.
- Pulmonary vessels: plethoric in L to R shunts and hyperdynamic states; oligaemic in recent pulmonary emboli, cardiac tamponade, RV failure and R to L shunts. In pulmonary hypertension large central arteries rapidly 'prune' to give peripheral oligaemia. Pulmonary venous hypertension, most often due to LV failure, is manifest as distension of upper lobe veins (→ Tables 4.1 & 4.2).

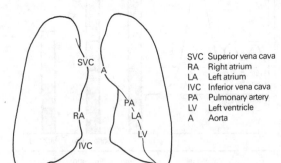

SVC	Superior vena cava
RA	Right atrium
LA	Left atrium
IVC	Inferior vena cava
PA	Pulmonary artery
LV	Left ventricle
A	Aorta

Fig. 4.3 A normal CXR.

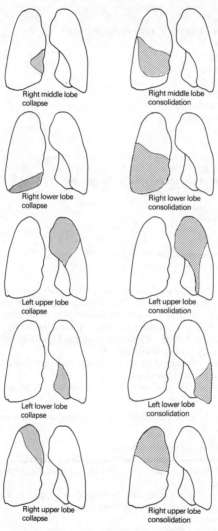

Fig. 4.4   Common CXR abnormalities.

Table 4.1
Causes of bilateral hilar enlargement

Sarcoidosis
Lymphoma
Tuberculosis
Pulmonary hypertension
Pulmonary embolism
Septal defects
Silicosis

Table 4.2
Causes of unilateral hilar enlargement

Bronchial carcinoma
Tuberculosis
Sarcoidosis
Lymphoma
Pulmonary embolism

- Lung fields: identify any obvious abnormality and then move on to comparing the two sides. Look particularly at the lung markings on the two sides and follow them to the lung edge. The apices and costophrenic angles should be closely scrutinized. Lobar collapse is a common finding in bronchial carcinoma ($\rightarrow$ Tables 4.3 & 4.4).
- Bones: these should be systematically studied looking for erosion, notching and fractures.
- Soft tissues: surgical emphysema, air in the soft tissues, may be missed if not looked for, as may a mastectomy.

If a CXR in an exam initially looks normal the following should be excluded:

- A small apical pneumothorax.
- A fluid level behind the heart due to hiatus hernia.
- R middle lobe collapse with loss of clarity of the R heart border.
- L lower lobe collapse with absence of the outline of the L diaphragm behind the heart (sail sign).
- A deviated trachea.
- Paratracheal lymphadenopathy.
- Air beneath the diaphragm.
- Rib notching.
- A mastectomy.
- Dextrocardia with the film reversed.

Table 4.3
Causes of pulmonary nodules

Bronchial carcinoma
Metastases
Pulmonary infarct
Adenoma/hamartoma
Tuberculoma
Abscesses
Arteriovenous malformation
Rheumatoid nodule
Wegener's granulomatosis
Sequestrated lobule
Fluid in oblique fissure ('vanishing tumour')
Granulomas (miliary TB, histoplasmosis, sarcoidosis)

Table 4.4
Causes of complete opacification of one lung field

Massive pleural effusion
Pneumonectomy
Complete lung collapse
Complete lung consolidation
Mesothelioma

UPPER RESPIRATORY TRACT INFECTION

Science basics The upper respiratory tract extends from the oropharynx to the trachea. This region is the entrance to the lungs and is the boundary between the mouth, which contains numerous commensal microorganisms, and the sterile pulmonary apparatus. Infections in this region are common but usually self-limiting.

Acute coryza (common cold)

This common disorder is due to infection with rhinoviruses, corona-, entero- and adenoviruses and respiratory syncytial virus.

Clinical features

Symptoms: usually start acutely with sneezing, dry sore throat, headache and rhinorrhoea. Although usually rapidly self-limiting, complications may occur and include sinusitis, otitis media and pneumonia. Symptoms of coryza which recur frequently during the summer are usually due to allergy rather than persistent viral infection.

Acute sinusitis

This disorder which frequently follows an acute viral upper respiratory tract infection is most often due to *H. influenzae*, *Strep. pneumoniae* or *Strep. pyogenes*.

Clinical features These include localized pain and tenderness over the involved sinus, pyrexia and headaches.

Investigations The diagnosis is usually clinical although X-rays usually demonstrate thickening of the sinus mucosa or a fluid level.

> **Management box**
> ▶ Antibiotics.
>   – amoxicillin 500 mg tid.
>   – erythromycin/clarithromycin.
> ▶ Nasal vasoconstrictors/steam inhalation.
> ▶ Delayed or unsuccessful treatment may lead to chronic sinusitis, meningitis, venous sinus thrombosis or osteomyelitis.

Acute pharyngitis

This is most often due to viral infection (eg EBV) or *Strep. pyogenes*.

Clinical features Usually there is only a sore throat but in more severe attacks dysphagia may occur. Examination reveals pharyngeal inflammation, lymphoid hypertrophy and, in some, an exudate.

> **Management box**
> ▶ Usually only symptomatic.
> ▶ If bacterial infection is suspected (pus present) take a throat swab before starting antibiotics.
> ▶ Antibiotics.
>   – amoxicillin 50 mg tid
>   – erythromycin/clarithromycin.
> ▶ Avoid ampicillin/amoxicillin with EBV as this may lead to a generalised rash.

Complications In cases of bacterial pharyngitis complications include peritonsillar and parapharyngeal abscess, both of which may require surgical intervention.

Acute laryngitis

This is usually a complication of coryza or an infectious disease such as measles. It is characterized by a sore throat with a hoarse voice accompanied by a non-productive cough and is usually rapidly self-limiting although repeated attacks may predispose to chronic laryngitis.

Acute epiglottitis

This potentially lethal disorder is usually due to *H. influenzae* infection in young children.

Clinical features These include cough, sore throat without hoarseness. In more severe cases stridor may progress to laryngeal obstruction. Where acute epiglottitis is suspected direct visualization of the epiglottis using tongue depressors should be avoided, as such instrumentation may precipitate obstruction of the airway.

> *Management box*
> ▸ Oxygen.
> ▸ Adequate hydration.
> ▸ iv antibiotics, ampicillin 500 mg qid.

Acute laryngotracheobronchitis (croup)

This disease of young children is caused by viral infection usually with the parainfluenza group. Superinfection with bacteria is not uncommon.

Clinical features These include bouts of coughing, breathlessness, fever, stridor and cyanosis.

> *Management box*
> ▸ Use humidified oxygen.
> ▸ Antibiotics if superinfection is suspected.
> ▸ Bronchoscopy/intubation may be necessary to clear secretion but should be done by an experienced operator as it may be technically hazardous.

Acute bronchitis

This disorder is usually a complication of viral upper respiratory tract infection and is due in most cases to pneumococcal, *H. influenzae* or *Staph. aureus* infection. Risk factors include cigarette smoking and damp or dusty conditions.

Clinical features

Symptoms: include cough, retrosternal pain and wheeze.

Signs: rhonchi and coarse crepitations and then productive sputum from which the infecting organism can be cultured.

Management box
▶ Antibiotics.
 – amoxicillin 250–500 mg tid.
 – erythromycin/clarithromycin.
▶ cough linctus.

Influenza

This deserves special mention as a cause of upper respiratory tract infection because of its potential severity. It is caused by a group of myxoviruses, influenza viruses A and B. Different strains of these viral types exist and cause epidemics or pandemics.

Clinical features

Symptoms: include headache, myalgia, anorexia and fever.

Signs: commonly absent other than pharyngitis, unless complications develop.

Management box
▶ Prevention is important – 'at-risk' individuals (patients with chronic lung/systemic disorders, eg COPD, severe asthma, diabetes) should receive yearly vaccination (in autumn).
▶ Symptomatic – fever, aches, pains.
▶ Regular paracetamol in adults.

Complications Secondary bacterial infection, eg *Staph. aureus*, of the upper and lower respiratory tract is common and should be treated with flucloxacillin in combination with amoxicillin. Viral encephalitis and demyelinating encephalopathy may occur as may cardiomyopathy. The mortality during epidemics, particularly in the elderly and infirm, may be high.

E **RESPIRATORY FAILURE** → page 433

CHRONIC OBSTRUCTIVE PULMONARY DISEASE (COPD)

This term supersedes previously used labels such as 'chronic bronchitis' and 'emphysema'. COPD is defined by the British Thoracic Society (BTS) as a chronic, slowly progressive disorder characterized by airflow obstruction (reduced forced expiratory volume in 1 second (FEV_1) and reduced FEV_1/FVC ratio) which does not change markedly over several months. Most of the lung function impairment is irreversible. This condition causes approximately 30 000 deaths per annum in the UK (M>F) and accounts for 25% of all medical admissions.

Science basics COPD encompasses various pathological changes in the large airways (chronic bronchitis), small airways (bronchiolitis) and lung parenchyma (emphysema). Chronic mucus hypersecretion, airway inflammation, scarring, loss of elastic recoil and lung parenchymal destruction lead to progressive airway narrowing. The role of oxidants/antioxidants in producing emphysema is important. With advanced lung destruction, persistent hypoxaemia develops leading to vasoconstriction in the pulmonary circulation and pulmonary hypertension. This can produce right ventricular hypertrophy (cor pulmonale) and eventually right ventricular dilatation and failure, with subsequent activation of the renin-angiotensin system secondary to a reduction in renal blood flow, leading to salt and water retention and peripheral oedema.

Classification 'Blue bloaters': patients with cor pulmonale, hypoxia, at risk of CO_2 retention; 'pink puffers': those with hyperinflation, low PaO_2 and frequently low $PaCO_2$ levels.

Aetiology The most important risk factor for COPD is cigarette smoking. Other causes include occupational exposure to irritants such as coal dust. α_1-antitrypsin deficiency predisposes to emphysema. In many patients with subclinical lung disease an acute respiratory infection may precipitate respiratory failure as well as worsen the underlying pulmonary problem. Low birth weight and poor socioeconomic status may predispose to COPD.

Clinical features In 'blue bloaters' productive cough and breathlessness are characteristic with signs such as cyanosis, peripheral oedema, coarse crepitations and L parasternal heave. Respiratory failure, cor pulmonale and polycythaemia can all develop. In 'pink puffers' breathlessness is the predominant problem associated with signs of tachypnoea and chest hyperinflation with reduced breath sounds.

Investigations • A thorough clinical history including risk factors • CXR • Reduced PEFR • Spirometry revealing an obstructive pattern with increased residual volume • ABG • Reduced transfer factor • Sputum microscopy and culture • ECG.

Management box
▶ The BTS have produced convenient guidelines based on the severity of the COPD:

Stable disease
▶ Stop smoking.

→

▶ Prn bronchodilators (β-agonists) and regular anticholinergics often in combinations.
▶ Long-acting β-agonist.
▶ Antibiotics for infections (amoxicillin, erythromycin or clarithromycin).
▶ Inhaled corticosteroids if airway reversibility can be demonstrated.
▶ Flu vaccination.
▶ Pulmonary rehabilitation.
▶ Domicillary oxygen.

Acute exacerbation
▶ Oxygen (use controlled 24–28%) if type II respiratory failure is present.
▶ Regular nebulized bronchodilators (β-agonists) and anticholinergics.
  – use an air compressor + 2 l oxygen per minute via nasal cannulae if type II respiratory failure is present.
  – use nebulized bronchodilators driven by oxygen in type I respiratory failure.
▶ Appropriate antibiotics (the commonest pathogen in the UK in exacerbation of COPD is *Pneumococcus* – use amoxicillin/macrolide).
▶ Oral/iv corticosteroids may be useful as a short course (7–10 days).
▶ Theophyllines may produce symptomatic benefit.
▶ Prophylactic sc heparin.
▶ Diuretics.
▶ Non-invasive ventilation (NIPPV) or doxapram are useful in type II respiratory failure.
▶ Mechanical ventilation may be appropriate if the patient has sufficient respiratory reserve present to allow weaning and if a reversible cause for the exacerbation is present (eg pneumonia).

ASTHMA

Science basics Asthma is characterized by bronchial inflammation with inflammatory cell infiltration (mainly eosinophils) leading to bronchial hyper-reactiveness. This results in cough, wheeze, breathlessness and chest tightness. The inflammatory process is usually reversible and involves a molecular and cellular cascade mechanism with inflammatory cell activation and recruitment. If this process is unchecked, irreversible airway damage and thickening of the bronchial basement membrane may occur over time.

Aetiology This is incompletely understood but immunological mechanisms are undoubtedly important. The increased sensitivity of the distal airways may be to readily recognized antigens such as the house-dust mite, animal danders or pollens, non-specific trigger factors such as cold or exercise, drugs such as β-blockers and aspirin or to factors which cannot be pinpointed. Patients can generally be divided into those with extrinsic asthma (atopic) and those with intrinsic asthma (non-atopic). In extrinsic asthma allergens can be identified either by skin or provocation tests and a family history of atopy can frequently be established. An occupational history should be sought. In intrinsic asthma such trigger factors cannot be established by such methods and a family history is usually absent.

Clinical features

Symptoms: usually typical consisting of expiratory wheeze and breathlessness frequently worse at night. The patient may be well aware of any trigger factors. In children cough is often the major symptom.

Signs: during an attack chest hyperinflation, tachypnoea, prolonged expiration and an audible expiratory wheeze are typical. In more severe attacks tachycardia, restlessness, pulsus paradoxus and cyanosis occur. A silent chest, especially in a patient too distressed to speak, indicates a severe attack and requires urgent treatment. Between attacks the patient may have no signs although nasal polyps, sinusitis and skin rashes should be sought.

Investigations • CXR • Regular PEFR at home looking for evidence of diurnal variation • FEV_1/FVC less than 75% and which improves ≥15% with bronchodilator administration. The FEV usually falls with exercise • FBC (eosinophilia) • Sputum examination may reveal an eosinophilia • Curschmann's spirals (casts of small airways) may be found in the sputum • ABG analysis establishes the severity. Hypoxia with a low $PaCO_2$ is common but hypoxia with hypercapnia indicates severe disease and requires aggressive therapy and/or ventilation • Hypersensitivity skin tests are useful in identifying atopic individuals.

Management box
▶ No smoking and avoid precipitating factors where possible.
▶ Hyposensitization injections are potentially dangerous and are rarely performed in the UK.
▶ Antihistamine drugs are of no value.
▶ The British Thoracic Society (BTS) published guidelines for the management of asthma in 1993 with subsequent revision and the principles of management are outlined in Tables 4.5 and 4.6.   →

▸ Maintenance control of day-to-day symptoms is with bronchodilators, eg salbutamol inhaler 2 puffs prn, along with regular inhaled corticosteroid, eg beclometasone 100 2 puffs bd. It is vital to ensure adequate inhaler technique and in those not capable of using inhalers administer the drugs via devices such as 'spacers' or using dry powder preparations, eg Ventodisks/Becodisks. Disodium cromoglicate (Intal) 20 mg 4–8 times/day is a prophylactic inhaled medication of value in children and those with exercise-induced asthma.

▸ Nocturnal symptoms may be improved by long-acting β-agonists (salmeterol or formoterol (eformoterol)) inhalers or with leukotriene antagonist use (montelukast or zafirlukast). Alternatively, substained release theophyllines, eg Uniphyllin 200–400 mg nocte or Phyllocontin 225–450 mg nocte can be used, although adverse reactions are common, eg nausea, dyspepsia, and occasionally life-threatening from cardiac arrythmias. Their use should be undertaken only when plasma levels are checked regularly. Sustained release oral bronchodilators, eg salbutamol 4–8 mg nocte are available but rarely used due to adverse reactions such as palpitations and tremor.

▸ The management of severe acute asthma is outlined in Fig. 17.12, p 435. This requires urgent assessment and aggressive management as it is life-threatening and approximately 2000 deaths still occur annually in the UK. (Indications for mechanical ventilation are indicated in Table 17.4, p 435).

Table 4.5
Asthma: aims and principles of management

Aims of management
- To recognize asthma
- To abolish symptoms
- To restore normal or best possible long-term airway function
- To reduce the risk of severe attacks
- To enable normal growth to occur in children
- To minimize absence from school or work

Principles of management
- Patient and family participation
- Avoidance of identified causes where possible
- Use of lower effective doses of convenient medications minimizing short- and long-term side-effects

Table 4.6
BTS Guidelines: management of chronic asthma in adults

Check that inhaler technique is adequate, prescribe PEFR meter, treatment may be stepped up or down as appropriate. Rescue course of prednisolone may be needed at any time and at any step.

Step 1: Occasional use of relief β-agonist (ie < once daily)

Step 2: Regular inhaled anti-inflammatory agents (eg beclometasone or budesonide 100–400 μg/24 hrs) or fluticasone 50–200 μg/24 hrs. Alternatively, use cromoglicate or nedocromil sodium.

Step 3: Move to high-dose inhaled steroid (800 μg–2000 μg/24 hrs) via large volume spacer (and mouth rinse). Add long-acting β-agonist (salmeterol or formoterol (eformoterol)) or leukotriene antagonist (montelukast or zafirlukast).

Step 4: High-dose inhaled steroids and regular bronchodilators (eg ipratropium, oxitropium, sustained release theophylline β-agonist tablets).

Step 5: Addition of regular steroid tablets in a single daily dose (rarely needed).

Step 6: Step down treatment once control is achieved. Review treatment regularly and try to step down slowly.

E▶ ACUTE ASTHMA → page 434

PNEUMONIA

Science basics Infection of the parenchyma of the lung can be divided into primary (specific) pneumonia, due to microorganisms with special pathogenicity for lung, or secondary (aspiration) pneumonia, where organisms affect already damaged lung tissue or where predisposing factors for aspiration exist. Upper respiratory tract viral infections may alter host defences and allow secondary bacterial infection to occur.

Primary pneumonia

The microorganisms commonly responsible for this are listed in Table 4.7. In immunosuppressed patients the number of potential organisms is greatly increased.

Clinical features

Symptoms: productive cough, rigors, chest pain and breathlessness. Systemic upset, confusion, haemoptysis.

Table 4.7
Microorganisms which cause primary pneumonia and treatment

Organism	Treatment
Streptococcus pneumonia	Benzylpenicillin 1.2 g qid or Amoxicillin 500 mg tid
Streptococcus pyogenes	Amoxicillin 500 mg tid
Staphylococcus aureus	Flucloxacillin 500 mg qid
Klebsiella pneumonia	Mezlocillin or gentamicin
Mycoplasma pneumonia	Tetracycline 500 mg qid or Erythromycin 500 mg qid or Clarithromycin 500 mg qid
Chlamydia psittaci	Tetracycline 500 mg qid
Coxiella burnetii	Tetracycline 500 mg qid
Legionella pneumophilia	Erythromycin or rifampicin
Pneumocystis carinii	Cotrimoxazole 1920 mg qid
Influenza viruses A and B	No antibiotic effective

Signs: pyrexia, herpes labialis, reduced chest expansion, dull to percussion, bronchial breathing, crepitations, tachypnoea.

Investigations • Leukocytosis • Sputum microscopy and culture • Blood cultures • CXR showing segmental or lobar consolidation • Serological tests are important in confirming aetiology • Less often bronchoscopy may be indicated when the patient fails to respond to therapy. • Pneumococcal antigen identification in sputum, blood or urine. • CRP (C-reactive protein) is useful in following the course of infection.

Management box
▶ Liaise closely with microbiologist.
▶ Refer to the BTS community-acquired pneumonia guidelines.
▶ Antibiotics after blood and sputum taken for culture, initially on a best-guess basis and subsequently modified according to the results of culture.
▶ General measures:
  – oxygen
  – rehydration
  – treat arrhythmias
  – prophylactic sc heparin
▶ Specific antibiotics (→ Table 4.7).
▶ Physiotherapy may be useful if copious secretions/mucus are present (but avoid in exhausted patients).
▶ NIPPV may be useful in type I respiratory failure.

- ITU care may be necessary.
- Inadequate or delayed treatment predisposes to the formation of lung abscess, which invariably results in permanent lung damage, empyema, respiratory failure or septicaemia.
- Pneumococcal infections may be prevented in immuno-suppressed patients (eg AIDS, chemotherapy, splenectomy) by pneumococcal vaccination (one dose of 0.5 ml sc/iv repeated after 5–10 years).

Secondary pneumonia

Many of the organisms which can cause pneumonia in healthy lungs are commonly responsible for the infection in those with underlying pulmonary disease. *H. influenzae* and other Gram-negative and anaerobic organisms may also be responsible. Access to the lungs is usually by aspiration of upper respiratory tract commensals. Predisposing factors include chronic illness, anaesthesia, vomiting, bronchial carcinoma, drugs which suppress cough or respiration, gastro-oesophageal reflux and immuno-compromised patients.

Clinical features

Symptoms: worsening of underlying pulmonary disease such as chronic bronchitis, with cough, increased sputum and rigors.

Signs: pyrexia, cyanosis, basal dullness to percussion, bilateral basal crepitations. Signs of consolidation often absent.

Investigations • Leukocytosis • Sputum and blood cultures • CXR looking for patchy, often bilateral, areas of consolidation.

Management box
- Recognition is important as late diagnosis results in lung damage.
- Liaise closely with microbiologist.
- Physiotherapy/oxygen/NIPPV support antibiotic therapy.
- Specific antibiotics:
  - Broad spectrum penicillins or cephalosporins (azlocillin or cefotaxine) combined with an aminoglycoside (gentamicin or tobramycin)
  - Monitor drug levels
  - Add metronidazole if anaerobic infection is suspected.
- Prevention of bacterial infection in those with chronic lung disease is better than treatment.
- Vaccination against influenza is important.

Reasons for failure of treatment
- Incorrect diagnosis
  - pulmonary embolism
  - bacterial carcinoma
  - pulmonary oedema
  - pulmonary fibrosis/alveolitis
  - pulmonary eosinophilia
- Incorrect antibiotic – resistant pathogen
- Immunocompromised patient
- Complication:
  - empyema
  - lung abscess
  - pulmonary embolism

Atypical pneumonia

Describes a pneumonic illness without purulent sputum, or absence of a bacterial pathogen in Gram-stain of sputum. Includes infection by *Mycoplasma pneumoniae*, *Legionella pneumophilia*, *Coxiella burnetii* (Q fever), viral infection, PCP and *Chlamydia psittaci*. Mycoplasma infection can occur in winter epidemics every 4–5 years.

Clinical features   Often have mild respiratory symptoms with marked systemic effects. The CXR is often much worse than the symptoms.

Symptoms: non-productive cough, low-grade fever, headache, myalgia, arthralgia, confusion, meningism, abdominal pain.

Signs: often few chest signs, occasional basal crackles, erythema multiforme.

Investigations   • CXR • Paired serology • ABG • U&E (often hyponatraemia) • LFTs • Cold agglutinins suggest mycoplasma • FBC (lymphopenia may be present).

Management box
▶ As for primary pneumonia (see Table 4.7 p 78 for antibiotic guidance).

PULMONARY ABSCESS

Science basics   Pulmonary consolidation with damage to the lung parenchyma may result in abscess formation. Predisposing factors include infection with *Staph. aureus* and *Klebsiella pneumoniae*, inhaled foreign bodies, pulmonary infarction, malignancy, TB, fungal infection, aspiration and immunosuppression, inadequately treated primary pneumonia.

Clinical features

Symptoms: usually very ill with large volumes of purulent sputum, haemoptysis, rigors and sweating.

Signs: include pyrexia, finger clubbing (which may develop rapidly), signs of consolidation or pleural effusion, pleural rub and metastatic abscesses (eg cerebral).

Investigations • CXR usually confirms the diagnosis with consolidation with cavitation and a fluid level • Chest US is useful in identifying fluid collection and allows diagnostic aspiration • Bronchoscopy is indicated in all patients with evidence of bronchial obstruction to exclude foreign-body aspiration and bronchial carcinoma.

Management box

▶ Surgery is rarely necessary provided appropriate and adequate antibiotic therapy, eg 6 weeks treatment with ampicillin 500 mg qid, flucloxacillin 500 mg qid and metronidazole 400 mg tid, is instituted. Erythromycin 500 mg qid should be substituted for penicillin in hypersensitive patients.

▶ Regional pulmonary fibrosis is an invariable sequela.

BRONCHIECTASIS

Science basics Respiratory airways that are permanently damaged and dilated are common sites for recurrent infection due to pooling of mucus. Such infections result in further damage resulting in a spiral of deterioration. The pathogenesis of bronchiectasis involves inflammation leading to airway damage and repair. The inflammation may be triggered by host defence defects (immunological), localized bronchial obstruction or following infection. Three pathological variants of bronchiectasis can occur: follicular (commonest), saccular or atelectatic.

Aetiology Otherwise normal respiratory airways may be damaged by infections such as measles, pertussis or tuberculosis. The airways of patients with cystic fibrosis, bronchopulmonary aspergillosis, Kartagener's syndrome, α_1-antitrypsin deficiency and immunosuppression are susceptible to infection because of impaired airway defence or clearance mechanisms.

Clinical features

Symptoms: frequent respiratory infections, chronic cough productive of large volumes of purulent sputum, weight-loss and haemoptysis. Respiratory failure, pleurisy, empyema and distant abscesses, eg cerebral, are all recognized complications.

Signs: finger clubbing, rhonchi and coarse crepitations.

Investigations • Sputum culture • CXR showing fibrosis, cysts and tramlines due to bronchial oedema • Spirometry revealing reduced vital capacity • Bronchography showing bronchial irregularity • High resolution CT scanning may be useful in certain cases • Proteinuria may develop due to amyloidosis.

Management box

▶ Physiotherapy with postural drainage is important.

▶ Appropriate antibiotics (eg amoxicillin 500 mg qid or clarithromycin 500 mg bd) for episodes of respiratory infection. In patients with cystic fibrosis *Pseudomonas aeruginosa* infection is common and requires specific therapy (eg iv ceftazidime, ciprofloxacin or azlocillin).

▶ Bronchodilator therapy and humidifier therapy are useful in those with bronchospasm and thick, tenacious secretions.

▶ Prophylactic antibiotics may be useful in reducing the number of infections, eg cyclical courses of amoxicillin, clarithromycin or quinolones.

▶ If the disease is localized surgical resection may be an option.

BRONCHIAL CARCINOMA

This is the commonest tumour in males in Western society and the mortality has continued to increase over the last 30 years. Its prevalence to a large part is due to cigarette smoking. Four main types can be identified: • squamous • adenocarcinoma (including alveolar cell) • large cell and • small cell. Identification of type is important since treatment regimens vary with pathology.

Science basics Lung cancer arises in the bronchial mucosa (or rarely in the lung parenchyma). 80% arise in the main lobar or segmental bronchi. Carcinogens in tobacco smoke produce recurrent, cumulative genetic abnormalities during cell growth and division, secondary activation of oncogenes, deletion of tumour suppressor genes and decreased levels of apoptosis.

Clinical features

Symptoms: cough, sputum, haemoptysis, breathlessness, chest pain, dysphonia, dysphagia, stridor and persistent chest infection or slowly resolving pneumonia.

Signs: include finger clubbing, cachexia, consolidation, cavitation or pleural effusion, Horner's syndrome, SVC obstruction.

Investigations • CXR, including a lateral, reveals the majority of tumours, although those centrally situated may be obscured by the heart or great vessels • Sputum cytology especially if repeated on at least three samples has a sensitivity of approximately 80%

• Fibreoptic bronchoscopy is the investigation of choice, particularly because it allows direct visual confirmation as well as histological confirmation in central tumours • FBC, LFT, abdominal and cranial CT mediastinoscopy and abdominal US may indicate disseminated disease, while thoracic CT scans are helpful in determining local invasion and staging the disease • Small cell tumours (APUDomas) may secrete substances such as ACTH, resulting in Cushing's syndrome, or ADH-producing hyponatraemia • Squamous carcinoma may present with hypercalcaemia due to secretion of a PTH-like substance • Before treatment can be considered the extent of the disease must be determined (staging).

Management box

▶ This depends upon the histological type of tumour.

▶ Peripheral small cell tumours may be amenable to resection while larger lesions may respond well initially to chemotherapy and/or radiotherapy.

▶ Non-small cell tumours if small and localized may be resected while larger lesions may respond to radiotherapy.

▶ Radiotherapy should be considered for symptomatic metastatic lesions in bone and the CNS, SVC obstruction, haemoptysis or large airway obstruction.

▶ Palliation of obstructive lesions by endoscopic laser therapy or radiotherapy should be considered where appropriate.

▶ It is vital that the diagnosis is disclosed in a professional and caring manner.

▶ Support services (MacMillan nurses, OT, physiotherapy, social worker, district nurse) are vital in the ongoing management process.

▶ The GP should be informed immediately once the diagnosis is confirmed.

Prognosis At the time of diagnosis three-quarters of patients have unresectable disease and of the quarter of patients with localized disease only one-third of these will be alive at five years.

SARCOIDOSIS

Science basics This is a disease of unknown aetiology characterized by non-caseating granulomas which may affect many organs in the body, particularly the respiratory tree. The granulomata cause fibrosis and damage to the parenchyma of involved organs. The highest incidence occurs in young adults, especially females. Two main clinical types of sarcoidosis are recognized: subacute which is self-limiting and chronic.

Clinical features These depend upon the organ system involved, although weight-loss, tiredness and fever are common.

Skin: lupus pernio, subcutaneous nodules, erythema nodosum, maculopapular rashes.

Lungs: most commonly affected organ but is frequently asymptomatic until extensive pulmonary fibrosis exists. In many only hilar lymphadenopathy is found incidentally on CXR (stage 1). Transient pulmonary infiltrates may be recognized in addition to hilar lymphadenopathy (stage 2). Interstitial fibrosis may occur in chronic sarcoidosis (stage 3) and be accompanied by pulmonary hypertension.

Liver: granulomata common (70%) but usually asymptomatic.

Kidneys: nephrocalcinosis related to hypercalcaemia and hypercalciuria, renal calculi.

Eyes: uveitis and corneal calcification.

Nervous system: both the CNS and peripheral nerves may be involved.

Haematological: anaemia and thrombocytopenia.

Heart: arrhythmias, conduction defects and impaired contractility.

Salivary glands: parotid swelling.

Joints: phalangeal cysts and arthritis.

Investigations • CXR for hilar lymphadenopathy and pulmonary infiltration • FBC • U&E • serum calcium • urinary calcium • Bronchoscopy allows bronchial/transbronchial biopsies and bronchoalveolar lavage which contains increased numbers of lymphocytes • serum ACE, derived from the pulmonary capillaries, is often increased and correlates with disease severity but is not specific for sarcoidosis • Mantoux to exclude TB • Intradermal Kveim test using antigen from human sarcoid spleen, although it takes 6 weeks for a positive result • Isotope gallium scanning reveals lung tissue actively involved • Reduced vital capacity, lung volumes and CO transfer factor • Biopsies from skin lesions or the liver may also identify granulomata.

Management box

▶ Subacute sarcoidosis is self-limiting and treatment usually unnecessary, although short courses of steroids may be required to treat skin lesion, uveitis or systemic disturbance such as pyrexia or fatigue.

▶ Chronic sarcoidosis commonly requires long-term steroid therapy to control pulmonary and/or eye disease. The initial dose should be prednisolone 40–60 mg/day for 1–2 months followed by a reducing dose to a maintenance level of 10 mg/day. Disease progression should be monitored by serial lung function tests, CXR and ACE levels. The prognosis is good unless extensive pulmonary fibrosis is present.

PULMONARY FIBROSIS

Science basics Three types of fibrosis occur within the lung:
• replacement fibrosis secondary to damage caused by disorders like infarction, TB and pneumonia • focal fibrosis in response to irritants such as coal-dust and silica • diffuse parenchymal lung disease (DPLD) which occurs in cryptogenic fibrosing alveolitis and extrinsic allergic alveolitis.

FOCAL FIBROSIS

The most common cause for this is occupational lung disease, the commoner of which are listed in Table 4.8.

Science basics The fibrogenic dusts involved are inhaled and carried by macrophages to nearby lymphoid tissue where fibrosis starts. The three most important diseases are coal-miner's pneumoconiosis, asbestosis and silicosis.

Coal-miner's pneumoconiosis
This is caused by the inhalation of coal-dust particles most of which are less than 5 μm in diameter and is often made worse by cigarette smoking. The disease can be subdivided into the simple type and progressive massive fibrosis. The former is categorized according to the severity of radiological changes and is non-progressive if dust exposure is halted. Progressive massive fibrosis, which is associated with dusts containing high proportions of quartz, is characterized by large often confluent masses predominantly in the upper zones and progresses even if exposure is

Table 4.8
Forms of occupational lung disease

Dust	Disease	Tissue reaction
Coal-dust	Coal miner's pneumoconiosis	Marked
Asbestos (chrysotile, amosite and crocidolite)	Asbestosis, mesothelioma	Marked
Silica	Silicosis	Marked
Beryllium	Berylliosis	Moderate
Iron oxide	Siderosis	Mild
Tin dioxide	Stannosis	Mild
Aluminium	Aluminosis	Moderate
Barium sulphate	Baritosis	Mild

stopped. The clinical features of coal-miner's pneumoconiosis are essentially the same as chronic bronchitis. In certain patients ANF and rheumatoid factor may be found in the serum. In Caplan's syndrome rheumatoid arthritis coexists and fibrotic nodules can be seen within the lung. The diagnosis of coal-miner's pneumoconiosis is important since industrial compensation may be available.

Asbestosis

Exposure may occur in such occupations as mining, the building trade, pipe-fitting and demolition. The two main types of asbestos involved are chrysotile and crocidolite (blue asbestos). The major medical problems are pulmonary fibrosis and malignancy of the respiratory tract, pleura and peritoneum. The fibrosis is related to the severity and duration of exposure, while malignancy has a less-clear correlation and a longer latency period (15–20 years). Cigarette smoking substantially increases the risk of bronchial carcinoma but has little influence on the development of mesothelioma. Bilateral pleural plaques indicate past exposure to asbestos and have little significance otherwise. Fibrosis tends to be more severe in the lower lung fields and develops in those with heavy exposure.

Silicosis

Exposure to crystalline quartz (silica) occurs in such industries as mining, sand-blasting and stone-cutting. Two types of silicosis are recognized: acute due to high intensity exposure over a short period (months) and chronic in those with protracted (>10 years) but limited exposure. The former results in rapidly increasing, severe and frequently fatal pulmonary fibrosis. Chronic silicosis results in fibrosis mainly in the upper zones associated with an increased risk of pulmonary tuberculosis. The CXR shows pulmonary fibrosis and often 'egg-shell' calcification of enlarged hilar lymph nodes.

DIFFUSE PARENCHYMAL-LUNG DISEASE (DPLD)

Fibrosis of the alveolar walls and production of exudates or transudates in the alveolar air result in reduced pulmonary compliance and maldistribution of ventilation. The commonest causes include fibrosing alveolitis, either idiopathic or related to connective tissue disorders, and extrinsic allergic alveolitis.

Fibrosing alveolitis

This results in generalized pulmonary alveolar fibrosis for no identifiable reason (idiopathic) or associated with underlying connective-tissue disease, eg RA, scleroderma, SLE.

Clinical features

Symptoms: include progressive exertional breathlessness and a dry cough.

Signs: finger clubbing, tachypnoea, reduced chest expansion and end-inspiratory crepitations. Pulmonary hypertension and cor pulmonale may develop.

Investigations • CXR: widespread lung opacities and elevated diaphragm • High-resolution CT scan (HRCT) is more sensitive and specific than CXR and allows distinction between active inflammation producing 'ground glass' appearance and chronic 'burnt out' honeycomb lung • Increased FEV_1/FVC, reduced vital capacity, total lung capacity and CO transfer factor • ABG reveal hypoxia and hypocapnia • Bronchoscopy, with lavage containing increased neutrophils and eosinophils • Transbronchial or open-lung biopsy allows histological analysis • Rheumatoid factor and ANF positive in some even without evidence of connective tissue disease • Differential diagnosis includes idiopathic pulmonary haemosiderosis, sarcoidosis, extrinsic allergic alveolitis, Langerhans cell hystiocytosis (histiocytosis X) and tuberous sclerosis.

> *Management box*
> ▶ Steroids (combined with azathioprine 2–3 mg/day) effective in 20–30% but requires high doses, eg prednisolone 60 mg/day at least initially and response should be monitored by serial pulmonary function tests.
> ▶ Cyclophosphamide 50–100 mg/day may be used as an alternative to azathioprine if the latter cannot be tolerated.
> ▶ Diuretics, oxygen, NIPPV may be necessary
> ▶ Single lung transplantation for patients under 65 years in whom drug treatment has failed and T_LCO and or VC < 50% predicted, pulmonary hypertension and resting hypoxaemia is present.

Extrinsic allergic alveolitis

This is caused by the inhalation of organic dusts which provoke a diffuse immunological reaction within the respiratory tree. Some of the agents responsible are listed in Table 4.9. Prolonged exposure results in permanent pulmonary damage with fibrosis, leading to pulmonary hypertension, cor pulmonale and eventually death.

Science basics In acute EAA there is an intense mononuclear inflammatory infiltrate of the alveolar and small airway walls, with the formation of non-caseating granulomata. If the disease is untreated, chronic interstitial fibrosis occurs.

Table 4.9
Causes of extrinsic allergic alveolitis

Disease	Antigen	Source of antigen
Farmer's lung	*Micropolyspora faeni* *Aspergillus fumigatus* *Thermoactinomyces vulgaris*	Mouldy hay
Maltworker's lung	*Aspergillus clavatus*	Malt, mouldy hay
Bird fancier's lung	Pigeon droppings and feathers	Pigeons, parrots budgerigars
Mushroom worker's lung	*Micropolyspora faeni*	Mushroom compost
Bagassosis	*Thermoactinomyces sacchari*	Mouldy bagasse
Humidifier fever	*Thermophilic actinomycetes, Amoeba*	Air humidifiers

Clinical features

Symptoms: 4–12 hours after exposure breathlessness without wheeze, tiredness, fever, sweating and non-productive cough.

Signs: after exposure pyrexia, cyanosis, crepitations.

Investigations • CXR: diffuse reticular fibrosis • FBC: neutrophilia or eosinophilia • Spirometry: reduced vital capacity and a restrictive defect • ABG: hypoxia with normal or reduced $PaCO_2$ • Reduced carbon monoxide transfer factor • Serology: positive precipitin test • Provocation test to the suspected antigen • Transbronchial/open lung biopsy.

Management box
▶ Oxygen.
▶ Oral steroids.
▶ Avoid exposure to triggering antigenic stimulus.

E **PNEUMOTHORAX** → page 435

PLEURAL DISEASES

PLEURAL EFFUSION

Fluid within the pleural space may be due to pleural or systemic

Table 4.10
Causes of pleural effusions

Transudate	Exudate
Cardiac failure	Empyema
Nephrotic syndrome	Pneumonia
Liver failure	Malignancy including mesothelioma
Fluid overload	Pulmonary infarction
	Connective tissue disease
	Subphrenic abscess
	Pancreatitis (L sided with high amylase content)
	Haemothorax
	Tuberculosis

disease. Traditionally, pleural effusions are divided into transudates, with a protein concentration below 30 g/l, and exudates, in which the protein concentration is higher than 30 g/l, but account must be taken of the plasma albumin level. All pleural effusions should be investigated by diagnostic aspiration and the fluid examined for protein content, bacteria and cell-type. A pleural biopsy is useful in the investigation of pleural exudates. Large effusions that are interfering with respiration may need to be aspirated for symptom relief but no more than 1000 ml should be removed at one sitting.

Aetiology The causes are shown in Table 4.10.

PLEURISY

Inflammation of the pleura, pleurisy, may be due to underlying pneumonia, viral infection, pulmonary infarction, malignancy or TB. The condition is characterized by pain which is localized, sharp and exacerbated by deep inspiration or coughing. Such pain in the absence of radiological lung disease may occur in pulmonary infarction (haemoptysis common), viral intercostal myalgia (pleurodynia or Bornholm's disease) or rib fractures.

ADULT RESPIRATORY DISTRESS SYNDROME

Science basics Adult respiratory distress syndrome (ARDS), is a common and serious disorder characterized by acute respiratory failure due to pulmonary injury and accompanied by hypoxia and respiratory distress. ARDS represents the severe end of the spectrum of 'acute lung injury' (ALI). The precise pathogenesis

Table 4.11
Causes of ARDS

Infections	Bacteria, fungi, pneumocystis, TB, septicaemia
Embolism	Fat, air, amniotic fluid
Hypovolaemia	
Aspiration	Vomit, water
DIC	
Drugs	Opiates, barbiturates, aspirin
Pancreatitis	
High altitude	
Intracerebral haemorrhage	
Smoke inhalation	
High inhaled oxygen concentration	

is unclear but a leaky alveolar epithelial/endothelial membrane develops and is followed by fibrous-tissue deposition. Precipitating factors are shown in Table 4.11. Lung injury scoring systems can be used to quantify the severity of the ALI and are based on CXR appearance, lung compliance measurements, degree of hypoxaemia and the level of positive end-expiratory pressure (PEEP) required when ventilated.

Clinical features The usual presentation is a few days after the recognition of a serious underlying disease and not uncommonly during convalescence.

Symptoms: include breathlessness and deterioration in clinical condition.

Signs: tachypnoea, cyanosis, intercostal indrawing and hypotension.

Investigations • CXR shows a 'white-out' with sparing of the costophrenic angles in the early stages. This helps in the differentiation from LVF in which a more central infiltration occurs associated with cardiomegaly • ABG: hypoxia with hypocapnia and respiratory alkalosis, the hypoxia is relatively resistant to oxygen administration and progressive • Swan Ganz catheterization shows a PCWP <18 mm/kg (with normal plasma oncotic pressure).

> **Management box**
>
> This can be divided into two parts; treatment of the underlying disorder and treatment of the lung problem.
>
> ▶ The underlying disease may not be obvious.
> - Shock, if present, should be corrected aggressively but once an adequate circulation has been restored fluid administration, particularly crystalloids, must be administered with care as pulmonary oedema develops readily.
> - Inotropic support (eg dobutamine) is commonly required.
> - The use of high-dose steroid therapy is controversial particularly in septic shock but is recommended in fat embolism and following aspiration.
> - Sepsis when present should be treated aggressively with intravenous antibiotics and surgical drainage or resection of septic foci.
> - Where large volumes of blood require to be transfused, filters to remove particulate material reduce the risk of ARDS.
>
> ▶ The pulmonary problem in ARDS
> - Requires mechanical ventilation with sufficient oxygen to maintain an adequate but not increased PaO_2. High concentrations of oxygen may lead to further lung damage.
> - Control of respiration with increased tidal and minute volumes and PEEP are usually required with careful monitoring of the cardiac output and blood pressure.
> - Prevention of pulmonary oedema by careful fluid balance, loop diuretics and salt-poor colloid administration is important.
>
> ▶ Early recognition and adequate treatment of ARDS greatly improves survival. The mortality remains around 70% due most often to multi-organ failure and many patients are left with permanent restrictive lung damage.

CYSTIC FIBROSIS

This autosomal recessive condition is the commonest serious inherited disorder, occurring in 1:2000 live births and being carried as heterozygotes in 5% of the population.

Science basics Cystic fibrosis is characterized by a generalized abnormality of all exocrine glands resulting in the production of unusually viscous secretions, probably because of an abnormality in the glycoprotein component of cell membranes rendering them relatively impermeable to chloride. This leads to changes in the composition of the airway surface liquid and predisposes the lung to chronic infections and bronchiectasis. The pathogenesis is unclear at present but the gene responsible has recently been identified on the long arm of chromosome 7.

The gene encodes the cystic fibrosis-transmembrane conductance regulator (CFTR).

Clinical features Presentation usually in infancy with meconium ileus, intussusception and failure to thrive. In older children repeated chest infections leading to bronchiectasis and steatorrhoea is usual. In adolescents and adults repeated chest infections, often due to *Pseudomonas*, pneumothorax, haemoptysis, malabsorption, RVF and cirrhosis with portal hypertension and pancreatic insufficiency are common features. Eventually pulmonary fibrosis leads to death from ventilatory failure or cor pulmonale. Males but not females are infertile. Intestinal obstruction (meconium ileus equivalent) may occur in adults.

Investigations • In children sweat test reveals a high concentration of sodium in sweat >70 mmol/l • In adolescents sweat test is unreliable and the diagnosis remains clinical with repeated chest infections and pancreatic insufficiency • Diagnosis may be confirmed by DNA analysis for mutations of CFTR gene on chromosome 79 • CXR shows hyperinflation and signs suggestive of bronchiectasis (thickened bronchial walls, 'tramlines', nodular and ring shadows) • PFTs • Flow-volume loops suggestive of airways obstruction • ABG • Sputum (and *Aspergillus*) culture • GTT • Pancreatic function tests.

Management box

▶ Chest
 – Prompt and adequate treatment of all respiratory tract infections is essential. *H. influenzae* should be treated with ampicillin 500 mg qid or erythromycin 500 mg qid and *Staph. aureas* with flucloxacillin 500 mg qid.
 – *Pseudomonas* colonization is much more troublesome and eradication is seldom possible. Treatment is with aminoglycosides, eg gentamicin, tobramycin or netilmicin (the dose depending upon the patient's height, weight and renal function and should be monitored by peak and trough blood levels) in combination with a broad-spectrum penicillin, eg azlocillin or carbenicillin or with ceftazidime or ciprofloxacin. Intravenous treatment should be for at least 2 weeks. Nebulized Colomycin may be useful in children colonized with *Pseudomonas*.
 – Physiotherapy with breathing exercises and postural drainage of secretions is important.
 – Bronchodilators and/or inhaled saline administered before physiotherapy may be helpful to clear bronchial secretions.

▶ Pancreas
 – Replacement of pancreatic enzymes with such preparations as Pancrex V and Creon reduce malabsorption and improve nutrition including vitamin supplements.

Prevention Genetic counselling should be given to parents and older cystic fibrosis patients.

PULMONARY VASCULAR DISEASE

The main disorder of the pulmonary vasculature is pulmonary arterial hypertension. This may be acute, as in pulmonary embolism, or chronic.

PULMONARY EMBOLISM/INFARCTION

($\rightarrow$ Ch. 16, p 355 and **E** Ch. 17, p 437)

Thrombi, most often from DVT in the large veins of the upper leg and pelvis, may break off and arrive in the pulmonary artery via the right ventricle. Risk factors for this are the same as for DVTs and include bed-rest, low cardiac output, polycythaemia and thrombocythaemia. Pulmonary embolism not uncommonly occurs without signs of DVT and it should never be excluded on this basis.

Clinical features In the case of a small or medium-sized embolism the pain is well localized, often severe and knife-like and accompanied by shortness of breath and considerable distress. There may be haemoptysis. When the embolism is large the pain is often central and accompanied by faintness, collapse and hypotension, ($\rightarrow$ also Ch. 17, p 437). In many the signs and symptoms are few and once the diagnosis has been considered it must be excluded urgently since subsequent emboli may be rapidly fatal.

An important pointer to the diagnosis of pulmonary embolism is the presence of one or more predisposing factors (Table 16.5).

Symptoms: acute breathlessness, pleuritic chest pain, haemoptysis and collapse.

Signs: hypotension, tachycardia, dyspnoea, raised JVP, pleural rub, cyanosis.

Examination you should look especially for: • pallor or cyanosis • raised jugular venous pressure (JVP) without peripheral oedema • tachycardia • hypotension • area of dullness in the chest with crackles, bronchial breathing or a pleural friction rub • gallop rhythm • do not forget to check the legs for evidence of a DVT.

Investigations • CXR may be normal or show atelectasis • ECG: the $S_1 Q_3 T_3$ pattern may be found with or without R heart strain (but remember that a normal CXR and ECG do not exclude the diagnosis) • The commonest ECG finding is a sinus tachycardia • If the CXR is normal a paired isotope ventilation and perfusion scan may help to identify mismatched defects which suggest pulmonary embolism. The results of such isotopic scans are often reported as showing low, intermediate or high probability of embolism • If the CXR is abnormal a CT pulmonary angiogram (CTPA) is useful in the identification of thrombi in the central pulmonary vessels, as far distally as segmental vessels • Where doubt remains, pulmonary angiography is requried • ABG shows hypoxaemia and hypocapnia • Doppler ultrasound/ascending lower limb venography looking for evidence of DVT • D-dimers in the blood; a positive D-dimer is of no diagnostic value but a negative result makes a PE unlikely.

Management box

▶ Prevention is the best cure for both DVT and pulmonary embolism and many methods have been advocated including elastic stockings and iv dextran. The most commonly used prophylaxis is subcutaneous heparin (5000 units tid) during the period of increased risk, eg during bed-rest post-MI.

▶ Once the diagnosis has been made treatment depends upon the degree of haemodynamic disturbance. If minimal, treat with sc low molecular weight heparin or iv heparin. For larger emboli (→ page 437). For larger emboli associated with haemo-dynamic compromise treatment with thrombolytic agents such as tPA is indicated.

▶ Following treatment with such intravenous agents oral anti-coagulants, most often warfarin, should be introduced and continued for 3–6 months, the dose being adjusted to maintain the INR 2–4 × normal.

▶ Surgery and thrombectomy is indicated only for those with massive pulmonary emboli with circulatory collapse. Patients in whom medical management is contraindicated or unsuccessful, particularly if the risk of further emboli is high, may be treated by the insertion of filters in the inferior vena cava. A thrombophilia screen may be checked (before starting anticoagulation) in young patients with no obvious risk factors for PTE.

CHRONIC PULMONARY HYPERTENSION

This may be due to repeated pulmonary emboli, cardiac disease, cor pulmonale or primary pulmonary hypertension. The first three are discussed elsewhere.

Primary pulmonary hypertension

This uncommon and serious disease of unknown aetiology usually affects young females. Fenfluramine, used as an appetite suppressant, may cause pulmonary hypertension.

Clinical features

Symptoms: fatigue, chest pain, breathlessness and ankle swelling.

Signs: these vary from prominent 'a' waves, R ventricular heave and loud P_2 in the early stages to frank RVF later.

Investigations • CXR: prominent central pulmonary vasculature with peripheral pruning • ECG: R axis deviation and R-sided strain • Echocardiography: R atrial and ventricular enlargement • Cardiac catheterization is required to measure pulmonary arterial pressure • Other investigations may be required to exclude other causes of pulmonary hypertension such as chronic pulmonary emboli, valvular disease and chronic lung disease.

> **Management box**
> ▶ Once established the disease is incurable and treatment is palliative.
> ▶ Oral anticoagulant therapy if started early may prolong life.
> ▶ Other drugs such as β-blockers and pre-load and after-load reducers (eg diltiazem) may help control symptoms.
> ▶ Cardiopulmonary transplantation currently is the only curative procedure in selected patients.

MEDIASTINAL MASSES

Science basics Many structures and tumours can give rise to mediastinal masses and it is easiest to divide masses according to their position.

Anterosuperior: retrosternal thyroid, aneurysm, thymoma (malignant in 25% and frequently associated with myasthenia gravis), metastatic carcinoma.

Anteroinferior: dermoid cyst, metastatic carcinoma, teratoma, pericardial cyst, Morgagni hernia.

Middle: lymphoma, bronchial cyst, metastatic carcinoma.

Posterior: ganglioneuroma, lymphoma, enterogenous cyst, Bochdalek hernia, achalasia, aortic aneurysm, paravertebral abscess, hiatus hernia.

Skin or subcutaneous lesions may appear on a single CXR as a thoracic mass but different views and clinical examination reveal their true position. Presentation of mediastinal masses is variable but commonly with vague chest pain, cough, superior vena caval obstruction or incidentally on routine CXR.

SLEEP APNOEA/HYPOPNOEA SYNDROME (SAHS)

Science basics SAHS is a disorder characterized by repetitive episodes of pharyngeal collapse/obstruction during sleep, leading to arousal from deep sleep and sleep fragmentation. The consequences of this are unrefreshing, restless sleep, nocturnal choking episodes, snoring and uncontrollable excessive daytime sleepiness with loss of normal concentration and reduced cognitive function. There is also increasing evidence of a link with hypertension which may lead to an increased risk of MIs and strokes in later life. SAHS may occur in 2–4% of middle-aged men and 1–2% of women and forms the mid part of the spectrum of sleep-disordered breathing problems with simple snoring at the mild end and profound nocturnal hypoventilation with significant hypoxaemia and hypercapnia at the other end.

Definitions *Apnoea*: complete cessation of airflow for at least 10 seconds; *Hypopnoea*: 50% reduction in thoracic/abdominal movement; *Obtructive apnoea*: cessation of airflow despite persistent respiratory efforts of the chest wall/abdomen; *Central apnoea*: cessation of both oronasal airflow and chest wall/abdominal respiratory efforts; *Apnoea/hypopnoea index (AHI)*: the number of apnoeas and hypopnoeas per hour slept (> 15/hour is consistent with significant SAHS).

Aetiology The main factor producing obstructive SAHS is narrowing or collapse of the pharyngeal airway during sleep and this may be caused by a variety of factors:

- A genetic tendency towards a small cross-sectional airway.
- Retrognathia.
- Loss of pharyngeal/tongue muscular tone during sleep.
- The degree of peri-pharyngeal fat deposition.

The net result is a narrowed pharyngeal space exacerbated by the negative pressure present during inspiration in the pharyx, leading to snoring and recurrent obstructive apnoeic episodes. This may in turn produce oxygen desaturations (>4% dips × 15/hour). These apnoeic episodes are sensed by the brain leading to an increase in EEG activity (arousal) which produces activation of the pharyngeal dilating muscles leading to a transient awakening and sleep disruption. Many of these awakenings are too short-lived to be remembered but occur repeatedly throughout the night resulting in poor-quality, restless sleep.

Clinical features

Symptoms: excessive daytime sleepiness, snoring, witnessed apnoeic episodes, nocturnal choking, unrefreshing/restless sleep, nocturia, reduced libido, mood changes (irritability/temper/depression).

Signs: central obesity, collar size > 17 inches, retrognathia, uvula swelling, tonsillar hypertrophy, exclude hypothyroidism/acromegaly/nasal obstruction.

Investigations • Subjective assessment of sleepiness (patient and partner), the Epworth sleepiness scale assesses the likelihood of falling asleep in a variety of situations. Score > 10/24 is consistent with excessive sleepiness: 0 = would never doze; 1 = slight chance of dozing; 2 = moderate chance of dozing; 3 = high chance of dozing. Each *situation* is scored: *Chance of dozing* sitting and reading, watching TV, sitting inactive in a public place (eg theatre or meeting), as a passenger in a car for an hour without a break, lying down to rest in the afternoon when circumstances permit, sitting and talking to someone, sitting quietly after a lunch without alcohol, in a car while stopped for a few minutes in traffic; giving a possible total score of 24: with a final question: are you experiencing any difficulty with driving due to sleepiness? • Assessment of apnoeic episodes: pulse oximetry may show characteristic desaturations but these are not always evident even with significant SAHS; portable home-based equipment (pulse oximetry, airflow, chest wall movement, pulse rate) do not assess quality/amount of time asleep; polysomnography 'gold standard', allows confirmation and characterization of sleep and accurately assesses the severity of SAHS.

> **Management box**
> ▸ Treat any underlying conditions (acromegaly, hypothyroidism).
> ▸ Weight-loss (if appropriate) – rarely successful.
> ▸ Mandibular advancement device – intraoral devices which move the lower jaw and tongue forward thereby increasing the upper pharyngeal cross-sectional area.
> ▸ CPAP (continuous positive airway pressure) applied via a closely-fitting nasal/full-face mask. Acts as a pneumatic 'splint' to maintain upper airway patency (usually 5–10 cm H_2O).
> ▸ Complex maxillofacial surgery to correct deformity/retrognathia – rarely undertaken.
> ▸ Uvulopalatopharyngoplasty (UP3) – not successful and should not be performed.
> ▸ Tracheostomy – effective but has significant morbidity.

5

Gastroenterology

100

INVESTIGATIONS

There are probably more investigations available in the diagnosis of gastrointestinal disease than for any other system. The most important are:

Endoscopy Direct visualization of parts of the GI tract and the taking of biopsies can be achieved by endoscopy. Flexible fibreoptic instruments have largely replaced rigid scopes except for sigmoidoscopy. Disorders in the oesophagus, stomach and proximal duodenum can be investigated with the gastroscope under light sedation. 'Push' enteroscopy allows visualization of the jejunum. Full endoscopic assessment of the small bowel is possible with an enteroscope and the help of a laparoscopic surgeon. The pancreas and biliary tree can be visualized following the injection of contrast medium into their ducts, using endoscopic retrograde cholangio-pancreatography (ERCP) which uses a longer endoscope and where the view is from the side of the instrument rather than end-on. The large bowel and terminal ileum can be investigated using the colonoscope, although an examination of the whole large bowel is only possible in approximately 85–90% of subjects. Diseases of the rectum can be investigated with the sigmoidoscope. The flexible instrument allows visualization of the sigmoid colon and descending colon. Endoscopy allows, as well as visualization of the bowel, biopsies to be taken, polyps removed, strictures dilated, vessels injected or ligated and laser therapy to be administered.

Laparoscopy This is a method of inspecting the abdominal organs directly, through one or more small incisions, and a fibreoptic system is usually employed. Laparoscopy may be performed under local or general anaesthesia and is particularly useful in the investigation of abdominal pain of unknown cause and in the investigation of liver disease.

Radiology The whole of the GI tract can be investigated radiologically once contrast medium, usually barium, is applied to the appropriate region. The commonest investigations are the barium swallow, meal and enema. The small intestine can be investigated with the barium meal and follow-through and the small bowel enema, in which barium is introduced into the proximal small intestine through an oro-duodenal tube.

Crosby capsule This is used to obtain jejunal biopsies usually in the investigation of coeliac disease.

Faecal fat collection The collection of faeces for 3 or 5 days to quantitate the fat content is important in the diagnosis and investigation of malabsorption.

Faecal occult blood   The detection of small quantities of blood in faeces can be made by simple bed-side methods which detect haemoglobin.

Breath tests

Urea breath test: based on the production of urease by *H. pylori* which splits ^{14}C-labelled urea to labelled $^{14}CO_2$ and ammonium ions. This test is useful in documenting the presence or absence of *H. pylori* in dyspeptic patients, before and after treatment.

^{14}C-labelled glycocholic breath test: is based on the fact that many bacteria deconjugate bile acids. If this happens in the small intestine due to bacterial overgrowth ^{14}C-labelled glycine is released, absorbed and metabolized producing $^{14}CO_2$, which is exhaled. Appearance of $^{14}CO_2$ at 2–3 hours is suggestive of bacterial colonization of the small intestine, although rapid transit through the intestine to the colon gives false-positive results. Similar results may be obtained with the glucose hydrogen breath test.

Lactose hydrogen breath test: used to detect disaccharidase deficiency. After an oral 50 g lactose load patients with lactase deficiency exhale more than 20 ppm compared with values of less than 5 ppm in normal subjects.

Pancreatic function tests   No ideal test to assay pancreatic exocrine function exists. Traditionally a standard fatty meal (Lundh meal) is given after a tube has been positioned in the 2nd part of the duodenum. Pancreatic secretions are aspirated and enzymes assayed. Tubeless tests have been devised which include urinary excretion of PABA which results from hydrolysis of administered N-benzoyl-L tyrosyl-PABA and radiolabelled fatty meals with subsequent analysis of serum radioactivity.

Intestinal motility   This can be assessed crudely by observing the speed of transit of radio-opaque markers along the GI tract.

Oesophageal manometry   The measurement of intra-oesophageal pressures during swallowing helps in the diagnosis of oesophageal dysmotility. Similarly, ano-rectal manometry helps in the diagnosis of incontinence.

pH monitoring   The investigation of gastro-oesophageal reflux has been greatly advanced by the introduction of portable pH probes which are positioned above the gastro-oesophageal junction and connected to a 24-hour recording system.

OESOPHAGITIS

Science basics   Inflammation of the oesophagus is usually due to reflux of acid from the stomach. The prevalence of such gastro-oesophageal reflux disease appears to be increasing. The squamous epithelium is not resistant to low pH and inflammation develops. The severity can be graded into four categories from mild (grade 1) to ulcerative (grade 4). Other factors which can result in oesophagitis include alcohol, bile and drugs, particularly if their passage is slowed by a stricture. Infection may affect the oesophagus, the commonest being due to herpes simplex and candida. This latter is commoner in immunosuppressed patients due to drug therapy such as steroids, or AIDS. Reflux of acid, the commonest cause of inflammation, occurs in all of us but the frequency and duration of reflux episodes is greater in those with reflux oesophagitis. Predisposing factors include pregnancy, hiatus hernia, obesity and smoking.

Clinical features

Symptoms: heartburn, a dull retrosternal ache, is the commonest symptom and is often triggered by food, sometimes particular factors such as coffee or alcohol. It may be aggravated by bending or lying flat. This symptom may be indistinguishable from angina pectoris. Less common symptoms include dysphagia or lethargy due to anaemia.

Signs: Commonly there are none; however, pallor due to anaemia caused by occult bleeding or haematemesis may complicate ulcerative oesophagitis. Severe reflux may be associated with aspiration accompanied by coarse crepitations at the lung bases. Barrett's oesophagus.

Investigations • Upper GI endoscopy is the most sensitive means of diagnosing and grading oesophagitis and may reveal the underlying cause such as hiatus hernia • Barium swallow may show mucosal changes of inflammation and/or ulceration and may demonstrate reflux and/or aspiration • 24-hour pH and motility studies may be useful in identifying gastro-oesophageal reflux • Symptomatic gastro-oesophageal reflux may be present despite an apparently normal endoscopy.

Management box

▶ Mild symptomatic reflux causing occasional heartburn is commonly treated only with antacids. In many, acid-suppressing agents such as cimetidine or ranitidine are required. Protein pump inhibitors (omeprazole 20 mg, lansoprazole 30 mg) are useful for those with ulcerative oesophagitis or in those with symptoms refractory to H_2 antagonists.

▶ For those resistant to such therapy the addition of mucosal protecting agents such as alginates or sucralfate are useful. Agents to increase the lower oesophageal sphincter pressure such as metoclopramide and prokinetic agents such as domperidone are useful in some.

→

▶ In all patients advice regarding loss of weight (where appropriate), smaller meals, avoiding late-evening snacks, stopping smoking and sleeping with the head of the bed elevated should be given.

OESOPHAGEAL CARCINOMA

Science basics Carcinoma of the oesophagus occurs most frequently in the distal third of the oesophagus either as adenocarcinoma, from gastric-type epithelium, or squamous carcinoma. More proximal tumours are usually squamous. Risk factors include alcohol abuse, smoking, achalasia, symptomatic gastro-oesophageal reflux disease, Barrett's oesophagus, Plummer– Vinson syndrome, tylosis and radiation exposure. It is commoner in males in whom it is the fifth-commonest tumour. It is especially common in certain regions such as China and Iran.

Clinical features

Symptoms: dysphagia, initially for solids; weight-loss; chest pain, cough and hoarseness.

Signs: include cough, anaemia and pulmonary signs due to aspiration.

Investigations • Upper GI endoscopy will identify the stricture and enable biopsies and brushings to be taken • Barium swallow reveals an irregular stricture.

Management box
▶ Cure is only possible for those with localized disease. If localized, oesophagogastrectomy is indicated, and offers the best chance of cure.
▶ In extensive malignancies, where cure is not possible, palliation of dysphagia should be sought by either surgical or endoscopic means. The insertion of prosthetic tubes allows the patient to swallow semisolid foods. Laser therapy and endoscopic ethanol injection also improves swallowing. Radiotherapy or surgery may offer the best palliation in certain cases.

Prognosis The 5-year survival is less than 10% and palliation, particularly to avoid the distressing inability to swallow saliva, is the goal in many patients.

DYSPHAGIA

Science basics   Difficulty in swallowing is a relatively common complaint and should always be treated seriously and investigated, usually with a barium swallow and/or endoscopy where appropriate. The most frequent causes follow.

Reflux oesophagitis → p 102

Benign stricture

This is usually a complication of peptic ulcerative oesophagitis. Patients may, however, have complained little of heartburn until the dysphagia develops, which is usually for solids initially. Endoscopy is necessary to confirm the diagnosis histologically and in many cases to allow endoscopic dilatation. This latter may have to be repeated regularly.

Oesophageal carcinoma → p 104

Achalasia

This is due to a failure of the lower oesophageal sphincter to relax. The cause is probably due to abnormal innervation of the lower oesophagus and closely resembles Chagas' disease. Dysphagia is invariable and is present for liquids as well as solids. Chest pain and pulmonary aspiration are common complications. The barium swallow gives a highly characteristic appearance with proximal dilatation and distal smooth tapering. Endoscopy is necessary to exclude carcinoma and to allow hydrostatic or pneumatic dilatation. Alternative treatment is a surgical cardiomyotomy (Heller's operation). Both methods of treatment may be followed by gastro-oesophageal reflux. Local injection of *Botulinum* toxin into the lower oesophageal sphincter gives temporary improvement for those patients unfit for dilatation or surgery.

Oesophageal spasm

This is relatively uncommon. It usually affects the elderly and is associated with muscular hypertrophy of the lower oesophagus. It is accompanied by chest pain which may mimic angina pectoris. Barium swallow shows abnormal peristalsis with uncoordinated contractions, which can be confirmed by manometry. Treatment is with muscle relaxants such as isosorbide mononitrate 10–20mg bd and nifedipine 10–20 mg tid and advice regarding avoiding factors which may provoke spasm, such as hot or cold liquids. Oesophageal dilatation may be required

Miscellaneous

Other causes of dysphagia include stomatitis, tonsillitis, head, neck and mediastinal tumours, pharyngeal pouch, scleroderma,

Plummer–Vinson syndrome and bulbar or pseudobulbar palsy, neuromuscular incoordination and globus hystericus. In those in whom swallowing cannot be improved, particularly after stroke, insertion of a percutaneous endoscopic gastrostomy (PEG) is becoming increasingly popular.

PEPTIC ULCERATION

Science basics   Peptic ulcers are divided into two main categories, gastric and duodenal ulcers. Ulcers form when there is an imbalance between damaging (acid) and protecting factors. In both types, acid secretion is important and when acid is neutralized or secretion inhibited, ulcers heal. Over-secretion of acid is associated with duodenal ulcer disease, while for gastric ulcers impaired mucosal protection is important. *Helicobacter pylori* infection is recognized as the cause of 90% of duodenal ulcers and 70% of gastric ulcers. Cytotoxin-associated gene A (CagA) strains of *H. pylori* are associated with a higher incidence of duodenal ulceration. Other causes include NSAIDs, Crohn's disease and Zollinger-Ellison syndrome (hypergastraemia).

Clinical features   Ulcers may be truly asymptomatic or cause mild discomfort or severe abdominal pain. Most common is localized epigastric pain and the patient may be able to point to the site of maximum pain. Some association with eating is recognized, DUs tending to give rise to pain between meals and during the night while GUs often give rise to pain while eating.

Symptoms: tend to wax and wane over a period of weeks or months. Exacerbations may occur at times of stress or be triggered by such factors as drugs or alcohol.

Signs: localized epigastric tenderness is common but not invariable. Anaemia may be obvious in those who have had a recent bleed. A succussion splash may be elicited in those with gastric outlet obstruction due to prepyloric oedema or scarring.

Investigations   • GUs may be malignant and should always be biopsied. If identified on a barium meal, an endoscopy with biopsies must follow with a further endoscopy after treatment to ensure healing • DUs on the other hand are almost never the site of malignancy and biopsies are not usually necessary • Diagnosis can therefore be made by either barium meal or endoscopy and a follow-up endoscopy to ensure healing after treatment if the patient has become asymptomatic is usually unnecessary • *H. pylori* status should be determined in all patients. This can be assessed in a number of ways. Gastric biopsies taken at the time of endoscopy can be tested for urease activity (CLO test) or histologically for the presence of *Helicobacter*. Serology can confirm *Helicobacter* infection but it is less effective in assessing response to treatment. Urea breath tests are a useful non-invasive assessment of *H. pylori* status. • In certain patients with numerous or difficult to treat ulcers, serum gastrin levels should be checked to exclude Zollinger–Ellison syndrome • Acid-output studies are not commonly required except to assess the success or otherwise of surgical procedures to reduce acid production.

Management box

▸ Mainstay of medical management is *H. pylori* eradication. This can be obtained in approx. 90% of patients with a combination of a proton pump inhibitor (omeprazole 20 mg bd, lansoprazole 30 mg bd) and two antibiotics (amoxicillin 500 mg tds, metronidazole 400 mg tds, clarithromycin 500 mg bd) for 1 week. Eradication may be confirmed by endoscopy or urea breath test if necessary.

▸ Some advocate the empirical treatment of new-onset dyspepsia with *H. pylori* eradication, however, new dyspepsia in patients older than 45 years should be investigated.

▸ *H. pylori*-negative ulcers may be treated with either maintenance quantities of proton pump inhibitors or H_2-receptor antagonists (cimetidine 400 mg bd or ranitidine 150 mg bd) and avoidance of cause (eg NSAIDs).

▸ Mucosal-protecting agents such as sucralfate 1 g qid, coloidal bismuth (De-Nol) 240 mg bd and misoprostol are helpful in some cases, and misoprostol particularly reduces the ulcerogenic potential of NSAIDs.

▸ As well as drug treatment patients should be given advice regarding stopping smoking and avoiding NSAIDs. There is no place for special ulcer diets although foods that exacerbate symptoms should be avoided.

▸ Operations are indicated only in those patients resistant to medical treatment and those who have suffered complications such as perforation or haemorrhage. Cutting the vagal nerves at the level of the lower oesophagus effectively reduces acid secretion but is frequently followed by adverse reactions such as post-prandial hypoglycaemia (late dumping) or dizziness and lethargy soon after eating, due to the osmotic effect of large volumes of food in the proximal small intestine (early dumping). These adverse reactions can be largely overcome by a highly selective vagotomy, where the nerve supply to the pylorus is left intact removing the need for a drainage procedure such as pyloroplasty or gastroenterostomy. Ulcer relapse after highly selective vagotomy is, however, higher than after truncal vagotomy. The numbers of gastric operations for peptic ulceration have reduced drastically in recent years.

GASTRIC CARCINOMA

Science basics The frequency of distal gastric cancer is decreasing, although it still remains a relatively common and lethal tumour. 60% involve the prepyloric region and antrum but spread into the duodenum is very rare. The cause is unknown but dietary factors and N-nitroso compound ingestion are believed important. It is particularly common in certain countries such as Japan and Chile and is more frequent in individuals with blood group A. Other predisposing factors include atrophic gastritis, pernicious anaemia and previous gastric surgery. The role of *H. pylori* is now established. It is now not believed that benign gastric ulcers can become malignant and believed that malignant ulcers are malignant from the outset even though they may initially appear to heal with drug therapy.

Clinical features

Symptoms: develop late and include epigastric pain, weight-loss, dysphagia (tumours in the cardia) and vomiting (tumours in the antrum).

Signs: epigastric mass, haematemesis, melaena, pallor, acanthosis nigricans, succussion splash, ascites, supraclavicular lymph-adenopathy (Virchow's node, Troisier's sign) and hepatomegaly (due to metastatic spread).

Investigations • Barium meal commonly shows an irregular ulcer or filling defect. Occasionally a thick-walled contracted stomach without peristalsis is identified (linitus plastica); this latter may be missed both at endoscopy and with endoscopic biopsies as the tumour infiltrates deep to the mucosa • Gastroscopy is the investigation of choice allowing visualization, biopsies and cytology • US is useful to exclude hepatic spread and may identify thickening of the gastric wall • CT scanning may be needed for staging.

Management box
▸ Surgery offers the only hope of cure but unfortunately only for small localized tumours. The vast majority of gastric cancers diagnosed in Western society do not fall within this category having already spread. This is not true for Japan where screening programmes exist and early diagnosis and treatment is common.
▸ Even for patients where curative resection is not possible, surgery offers the best form of palliation, particularly for antral tumours where gastric outlet obstruction is a complication and for cardial lesions which may result in complete dysphagia. The patient's clinical condition should be ▸

optimized prior to surgery by blood transfusion, correction of biochemical derangements and parenteral nutrition, if indicated.
▸ Radiotherapy is of no value, while chemotherapy may produce remission in a minority.

Prognosis This depends upon the tumour stage. The 5-year survival for early gastric cancer is over 75% but less than 10% for the later and commoner lesion. Screening programmes for high-risk groups such as post-gastric surgery and pernicious anaemia are advocated by some. Early endoscopy should be considered in all patients over 45 years with new-onset dyspepsia.

E UPPER GASTROINTESTINAL HAEMORRHAGE
→ page 438

COELIAC DISEASE

Science basics Coeliac disease is characterized by mucosal villous atrophy, which improves after gluten withdrawal from the diet. Gluten has two main compontents, glutenin and α-gliaden. It is components of the latter which are believed to be antigenic, leading to immunologically mediated injury. Genetic association exists with a high prevalence of HLA B8 and DR3, although environmental influences are also important. Anti-endomysial antibodies are highly sensitive and specific for coeliac disease. This condition is increasingly diagnosed.

Clinical features Usually children of 1–5 years, but can occur as a first presentation in adulthood.

Symptoms: diarrhoea, steatorrhoea, weight-loss and failure to thrive. Abdominal pain, irritability and delayed puberty are recognized. Presentation in adulthood occurs usually with diarrhoea or consequences of malabsorption such as anaemia.

Signs mouth ulcers, peripheral oedema, muscle wasting, skin pigmentation and dermatitis herpetiformis (see below).

Investigations ● FBC showing anaemia and Howell–Jolly bodies (hyposplenism) ● LFTs may reveal hypoalbuminaemia ● The xylose tolerance test is usually abnormal ● Jejunal or distal duodenal biopsy is essential and demonstrates subtotal or total villous atrophy along with a chronic inflammatory cell infiltrate and increased intra-epithelial lymphocytes.

Management box
▶ Gluten withdrawal and dietary education. All barley, wheat, oats and rye-containing foods are potentially harmful.
▶ A useful booklet containing diets and recipes can be obtained from the Coeliac Society (PO Box 220, High Wycombe, Bucks, UK).

Complications An increased incidence of intestinal lymphoma and adenocarcinoma as well as oesophageal and pharyngeal tumours exists. Intestinal ulceration and stricture formation are recognized.

Dermatitis herpetiformis
This condition with an itchy, blistering skin eruption is also associated with jejunal villous atrophy which responds to a gluten-free diet. Dapsone is effective in treating the skin rash.

CROHN'S DISEASE

Science basics This is a chronic inflammatory disease of any part of the GI tract, the cause of which is unknown. An interplay between an infective agent and an abnormal immune response is currently believed important. The inflammation, unlike UC, affects the entire thickness of the bowel wall. The terminal ileum and proximal colon are the most commonly affected sites.

Epidemiology The annual incidence in the UK is approximately 5/100 000 with an equal sex distribution occurring most commonly between 15–35 years. Familial clustering occurs and involves UC as well as Crohn's disease.

Clinical features It is a chronic, relapsing and remitting disease with symptomatology depending upon the site of involvement in the GI tract.

Symptoms: include malaise, anorexia, nausea, weight-loss, fever, abdominal pain, diarrhoea, arthralgia and rectal bleeding.

Signs: pallor, malnutrition, oral ulcers, abdominal mass, perianal abscesses and fistulae, finger clubbing, erythema nodosum, pyoderma gangrenosum and uveitis.

Investigations • FBC: anaemia due to blood loss and/or folate or vitamin B_{12} deficiency, leukocytosis, increased platelet count which correlates with disease activity • ESR: elevated • Biochemistry: hyponatraemia, hypokalaemia, acidosis, hypoalbuminaemia, abnormal LFTs if associated autoimmune hepatitis or pericholangitis • Elevated levels of C-reactive protein correlate with disease activity • Radiology: plain abdominal film may show obstruction, toxic dilatation or perforation. Barium meal, follow-through and enema are useful both in making the diagnosis and in assessing its extent and severity ● US is useful in detecting abscesses ● Endoscopy: both upper and lower GI endoscopy allow direct visualization and biopsies to be taken. Strictures within reach of the endoscope may be treated by balloon dilatation in selected cases ● Radionuclide scanning: technetium and indium-labelled WBC scans may be useful in detecting areas of disease activity ● Histology: the diagnosis of Crohn's disease should, where possible, have histological confirmation; features of Crohn's disease include full-thickness inflammation, non-caseating granulomata, fissuring, ulceration and erosions.

Complications Malnutrition, stricture formation, perianal disease, severe haemorrhage, toxic dilatation, abscess formation, fistulae, renal calculi, gallstones and psychological problems. The risk of developing small or large bowel cancer is increased slightly.

Management box

▶ Symptoms due to inflammation usually respond to medical measures while those due to strictures require surgical intervention.

▶ General medical measures include replacement of fluid and electrolytes, haematinics if required, nutritional supplements and advice and psychological support.

▶ Corticosteroids, usually prednisolone 40 mg/day, are effective in controlling acute exacerbations in the majority. Large doses should be reduced when possible to minimize adverse reactions and maintenance steroid therapy should be avoided, as it does not reduce the frequency of relapse. 5-ASA preparations may be useful in active disease, and may reduce frequency of relapse. Other immunosuppressive drugs such as azathioprine and 6-mercaptopurine may be useful as steroid-sparing agents in selected cases.

▶ Antibiotics should be used where there is sepsis and when bacterial overgrowth is suspected. Metronidazole is particularly useful for perianal disease.

▶ Monoclonal antibody against TNFa may be used for severe, refractory, or fistulating disease.

▶ Dietary therapy is important for maintaining adequate nutrition; elemental diets have been shown to induce remission in many cases. Their use is particularly indicated in children to reduce the adverse effects of steroids on growth.

▶ Surgical indications include:
  – Intractable disease with persistent ill-health despite drug therapy →

- Intestinal obstruction not settling medically
- Perforation and abscess or external fistula formation
- Toxic dilatation of the colon
- Ureteric obstruction due to periureteric inflammation.

Prognosis   Acute ileitis is atypical in that it does not recur unlike all other forms of Crohn's disease. Patients with colonic Crohn's disease usually respond well to medical treatment, although 50% will require surgery at some time. 70% of those with both large and small bowel disease require surgery at some time. Conservative surgery such as stricturoplasty should be undertaken whenever possible. The overall mortality in patients with Crohn's disease is approximately twice that of the general population due to complications of active disease.

ULCERATIVE COLITIS

Science basics   This is a chronic inflammatory disease of either part or the whole of the colon. The inflammation is confined to the mucosa, almost invariably affecting the rectum and extending proximally to varying degrees in a continuous fashion. The cause is unknown but immunological, dietary, genetic and psychological factors have all been implicated.

Epidemiology   The sex distribution is approximately equal, the majority presenting between 25–35 years with an annual incidence of 4–7/100 000. As for Crohn's disease familial clustering is recognized.

Clinical features   The clinical course may be acute fulminating, relapsing-remitting or chronic continuous.

Symptoms: include diarrhoea, rectal bleeding, mild abdominal pains, fever and weight-loss.

Signs: pallor, mouth ulcers, dehydration, abdominal tenderness, erythema nodosum, pyoderma gangrenosum, arthritis and uveitis. Severe colitis should be recognized when there is bloody diarrhoea > 6x/day, tachycardia, fever and anaemia.

Investigations   • FBC: anaemia due to blood loss, leukocytosis • ESR: increased correlating with disease severity • Biochemistry: hyponatraemia, hypokalaemia, acidosis, hypocalcaemia and hypomagnesaemia, abnormal LFTs due to associated auto-immune hepatitis ($\uparrow$ ALT) or sclerosing cholangitis ($\uparrow$ alk phos) • Radiology: the plain abdominal film is essential in severe acute attacks to exclude toxic dilatation (> 5.5 cm in diameter); the double-contrast barium enema is useful in the diagnosis and determining the extent and severity of disease; it is contra-indicated in those at risk of toxic dilatation • Colonoscopy: this allows direct visualization and biopsies to be taken which is essential both for the diagnosis and for surveillance of colonic cancer in patients with chronic disease; again contraindicated in those at risk of toxic dilatation • Histology: the diagnosis of UC should be supported by histological evidence although the appearances are not usually pathognomonic.

Complications (→ Table 5.1)

Table 5.1
Complications of ulcerative colitis

Local	Extra-colonic
Haemorrhage	Seronegative arthritis
Rupture	Uveitis, rashes
Carcinoma	Chronic liver disease, eg autoimmune hepatitis, sclerosing cholangitis

Management box

▸ Acute severe colitis should be managed with iv fluids, blood transfusion and parenteral nutrition where indicated and high-dose parenteral steroids (hydrocortisone 100 mg qid).

▸ The commoner relapsing-remitting course should be treated with high-dose steroids (40 mg prednisolone daily) to control symptoms, followed by their withdrawal once remission occurs. 5-amino salicylic acid preparations, eg mesalazine (Asacol) 1.5–3 g/day or olsalazine 1 g/day in divided doses, should be used to reduce the frequency of relapse.

▸ Distal colitis and proctitis may be adequately controlled without systemic steroids but with steroid enemata for relapses and 5-ASA preparations for maintenance.

▸ Indications for surgery are:
  – Acute UC not responding to medical management
  – Relapsing-remitting disease responding poorly to drug therapy
  – Long-standing disease where severe dysplasia or carcinoma has been identified.

▸ The commonest operation is pancolectomy with ileostomy. Ileorectal anastomosis is preferred by some, although continued disease activity may occur in the retained rectum and long-term surveillance of the rectum for malignancy is required. Ileoanal pouch operations are popular but are not without their problems.

Cancer surveillance   The risk of developing colorectal cancer in UC is well recognized. This depends upon the extent of the disease and its duration. In pancolitis the risk is increased after 10 years to 1%, after 20 years to 13% and after 30 years to 34%. Left-sided colitis is associated with a lower but still significant increased risk after 20 years. It is believed that neoplasms in patients with UC are preceded by initially mild and later severe dysplasia of the colonic epithelium and the aim of surveillance is to identify such premalignant changes. Colonoscopy with multiple biopsies should be performed every 18–24 months and more frequently once early dysplasia is recognized.

IRRITABLE BOWEL SYNDROME

Science basics   Irritable bowel syndrome (IBS) is the commonest GI disorder, affecting females more often than males and commonest in the 3–4th decades. The principal symptoms of change in bowel habit associated with abdominal pain and bloating may closely resemble other GI pathology and a diagnosis by exclusion is common.

Pathogenesis   Abnormalities in muscular tone of the GI tract are present and are responsible for the symptoms. A family history is common. Emotional and psychological factors are often important.

Clinical features

Symptoms: poorly localized abdominal pain most commonly in the L iliac fossa or epigastrium. The pain may be exacerbated by eating, stress and premenstrually and relieved by defaecation. Abdominal bloating is common. Alternating diarrhoea, often on rising in the morning, and constipation is characteristic although one usually predominates. The passage of mucus is common but rectal bleeding is not a feature and should never be attributed to IBS.

Signs   usually few but include abdominal distension, tenderness over the colon and mucus on PR examination.

Investigations   • No diagnostic tests are available although in the young the diagnosis can be confidently made in those with a characteristic history • Sigmoidoscopy, barium enema, and upper GI endoscopy are required in many subjects to exclude such disorders as peptic ulceration and colorectal cancer • In many subjects with IBS such common disorders as gallstones or diverticular disease may be identified and symptoms should not necessarily be attributed to these.

Management box
- An adequate explanation of the disorder is essential and some patients benefit greatly from psychotherapy.
- Dietary manipulation to gradually increase the fibre content to approximately 7 g may be useful, particularly in those with constipation, and foods which exacerbate symptoms should be identified and omitted.
- Drug therapy is not necessary in many patients and where used is directed at symptoms – antispasmodics such as anticholinergics and Colpermin for pain, drugs such as loperamide for diarrhoea and bulking agents such as hydrophilic colloids for constipation.
- In a small number of patients low-dose antidepressants (eg amitriptyline 25 mg/day) are of value whereas sedatives such as benzodiazepines should not be used.

INFECTIVE BOWEL DISEASE

These can be divided into those which produce acute diarrhoea and specific GI infections and infestations.

ACUTE INFECTIOUS DIARRHOEA

Three clinical syndromes are recognized: ($\rightarrow$ also p 279).

Acute food poisoning
This is characterized by vomiting and diarrhoea within 24 hours of ingesting contaminated food and is due to a bacterial toxin within the food. The commonest organisms are toxin-producing strains of *Staph. aureus*, *Cl. perfringens* and *Bacillus cereus*. A rare and atypical cause is *Cl. botulinum*, the toxin of which causes progressive paralysis.

Acute watery diarrhoea
Due to enterotoxin-producing or invasive organisms transmitted via contaminated water or food or occasionally from person to person. Pathogens include enterotoxin-producing *E. coli* and *V. cholerae*: invasive organisms include Rotavirus, *Salmonella*, *E. coli*, Norwalk virus and *Giardia lamblia*.

Bloody diarrhoea
The organisms causing this form of diarrhoea, in which blood is obvious within the faeces, include both invasive and enterotoxin-producing forms such as *Salmonella*, *Shigella*, *Campylobacter jejuni*, *Y. enterocolitica*, *E. coli* and *E. histolytica*. *Cl. difficile* may cause pseudomembranous colitis after antibiotic therapy due to

toxin production. Antibiotics most frequently implicated are ampicillin, clindamycin and lincomycin. In those where the organism is commensal the cytotoxin is not present.

Investigations • Faecal culture and parasite screen will identify many organisms although jejunal aspiration or small-bowel biopsy may be necessary to identify *Giardia* • Numerous WBC in the faeces identified by methylene blue staining is suggestive of colonic inflammation of either infective or inflammatory origin • Sigmoidoscopy and biopsy is useful in the diagnosis of amoebiasis and excluding inflammatory bowel disease and pseudomembranous colitis • Serological tests are available for *Salmonella*, *Campylobacter* and *Yersinia* infections as well as *E. histolytica Cl. difficile* toxin testing.

Management box

▶ Rehydration, where indicated by such features as tachycardia, postural hypotension, reduced skin turgor and ocular pressure and oliguria, can usually be oral using fluids containing sodium, potassium, bicarbonate, chloride and glucose.

▶ Intravenous fluids are indicated in those with persistent vomiting.

▶ No restriction on food intake is generally indicated although temporary milk intolerance may occur due to secondary lactase deficiency.

▶ Anti-diarrhoeal drugs such as codeine phosphate, diphenoxylate or loperamide may be useful in controlling symptoms but should be avoided in moderate to severe cases as they prolong infection.

▶ Antibiotics are listed in Table 5.2.

**Table 5.2
Antibiotics for infective bowel disease**

Pathogen	Antibiotic	Indication
Salmonella	Ampicillin, Ciprofloxacin, Cotrimoxazole	Only if bacteraemia
Shigella	Cotrimoxazole, Cyrofloxacin	Symptomatic cases
Yersinia	Tetracycline	Symptomatic cases
Campylobacter	Erythromycin, Tetracycline	Severe or persistent cases
Clostridium difficile	Vancomycin, Metronidazole	Only when cytotoxin present
Giardia lamblia	Metronidazole, Mepacrine	Repeated courses may be necessary

SPECIFIC INFECTIONS

Intestinal tuberculosis

This is an uncommon disorder in the UK but still prevalent worldwide. Infection of the GI tract with *Mycobacterium tuberculosis* most often affects the ileocaecal region and is usually identified in patients under investigation for suspected malignancy or inflammatory bowel disease.

Clinical features

Symptoms: abdominal pain, fever, weight-loss and diarrhoea.

Signs: RIF mass, splenomegaly and signs of associated pulmonary TB.

Investigations • CXR to identify current or previous TB • Positive Mantoux test and examination of sputum, urine, faeces and gastric aspirates • Barium studies of large and small bowel to identify wall thickening, ulceration and stricture formation similar to Crohn's disease • Colonoscopy and biopsy where appropriate • Laparotomy may be required to confirm the diagnosis.

> #### Management box
> ▶ 6 months' therapy with isoniazid and rifampicin. Ethambutol and pyrazinamide should be included for the first 2 months (→ p 269–270).
> ▶ Surgery is indicated for perforation, abscess formation, major haemorrhage and intestinal obstruction.

Traveller's diarrhoea

This is common in travellers to developing countries due to ingestion of contaminated food or water. The most frequent pathogens are: enterotoxigenic *E. coli*, *Shigella*, *Salmonella* and *Campylobacter*. Prophylactic treatment with cotrimoxazole or ciprofloxacin reduces the incidence of infective traveller's diarrhoea. Less severe episodes of diarrhoea in travellers may just be due to a change in the bacterial flora and not truly infective.

Sexually transmitted intestinal infection

This is becoming more common and principally affects homosexuals and women practising receptive anal intercourse (Table 5.3).

In patients with AIDS other GI problems include enterocolitis due to *Giardia*, *Strongyloides* and *Cryptosporidia*; oesophagitis due to *Candida*, cytomegalovirus and herpes simplex; cytomegalovirus vasculitis of the colon and Kaposi's sarcoma (p 289).

Table 5.3
Sexually transmitted intestinal infections

Problem	Cause
Anal lesions	Herpes simplex, secondary syphilis
Proctitis	*Neisseria gonorrhoeae*, *Chlamydia trachomatis*, herpes simplex, syphilis
Proctocolitis	*Chlamydia trachomatis*, *Shigella*, *Salmonella*, *Campylobacter*

HELMINTH INFESTATIONS

Although relatively uncommon in the UK they represent a major health problem in many areas of the world.

Nematodes (roundworms)

Ascariasis   Usually due to *Ascaris lumbricoides*, this is the commonest worm infestation in man. The adult worm resides in the upper small intestine and releases eggs which pass in the faeces. Infection is via the faeco-oral route. Ingested eggs release larvae which penetrate the intestinal wall and migrate to the lungs where they are coughed up and swallowed. Complications include anaemia, biliary obstruction, pancreatitis and appendicitis.

Treatment: mebendazole 100 mg bd for 3 days.

Enterobiasis (threadworm)   Infestation with *Enterobius vermicularis* is the commonest infestation in the UK. The adult worm resides in the caecum although the female worm migrates to the anus to lay eggs. Transmission is via the faeco-oral route with children often reinfecting themselves as a consequence of pruritus ani.

Treatment: mebendazole.

Hookworms   Most often *Ancylostoma duodenale* and *Necator americanus*. The adult worm resides in the upper small intestine and eggs are released and pass out in the faeces. These hatch outside the body and the larvae infect man by penetrating the skin (eg soles of feet). They pass then to the lungs, are coughed up and swallowed.

Clinical features   include local or generalized allergic reactions, anaemia and abdominal pain.

Treatment: mebendazole.

Trichuriasis (whip worm)   The adult *Trichuris trichuira* worm resides in the lower intestine and releases eggs which pass in the faeces. These are ingested and the eggs hatch within the GI tract. No visceral stage exists.

Clinical features   include abdominal pain, diarrhoea, eosinophilia and appendicitis.

Treatment: mebendazole.

Strongyloides stercoralis   The larvae of this worm may invade the host tissues especially in the immunosuppressed.

Clinical features   include colitis, malabsorption, pulmonary disease and neurological symptoms.

Treatment: tiabendazole 25 mg/kg bd for 2–3 days.

Cestodes (tapeworms)

The commonest in man are *Taenia saginata* (beef tapeworm), *T. solium* (pork tapeworm), *Hymenolepis nana* (dwarf tapeworm) and *Diphyllobothrium latum* (fish tapeworm). The adult worm attaches to the intestinal wall by its head (scolex) and the fertilized eggs are passed in the faeces. The intermediate host ingests these and the larvae invade their viscera. Human infestation follows ingestion of poorly cooked or raw tissue from the intermediate host.

Clinical features   include nutritional deficiency, abdominal pain, pruritus ani, intestinal obstruction or perforation.

Treatment: praziquantel.

Hydatid disease   This is due to *Echinococcus granulosis* (or less often *E. multilocularis* or *E. oligarthus*) infection. Man is an intermediate host with the dog being the definitive host. Ova from dog faeces are ingested and pass to the liver via the portal vein and there develop into hydatid cysts.

Clinical features   include abdominal pain, hepatomegaly, cholangitis, cough and allergic reaction including anaphylaxis.

Investigations   • Abdominal X-ray may reveal the calcified rim of the cyst although US is more sensitive • Serological tests and the Casoni skin test are available but may be negative in those where cyst leakage has not occurred.

Treatment: surgical resection where possible, otherwise mebendazole.

Trematodes (flukes)

These are responsible for Schistosomiasis (bilharziasis), liver flukes (*Clonorchis*) and *Fasciola hepatica* infestation.

MALABSORPTION

Science basics   Malabsorption is the term used to describe the presence of nutrients, usually absorbed, in the faeces. In clinical practice it is usually only the fat content of the faeces that is measured. As well as abnormalities of absorption, disorders of digestion and intestinal transit are usually included.

Aetiology

Mucosal: coeliac disease, tropical sprue, Whipple's disease, abetalipoproteinaemia.

Structural: intestinal resection, Crohn's disease, amyloidosis, intestinal ischaemia, lymphangiectasia, lymphoma.

Infective: acute enteritis, parasites, eg *Giardia*, bacterial overgrowth, TB.

Maldigestion: pancreatic insufficiency, biliary obstruction.

Systemic disease: hyper/hypothyroidism, diabetes mellitus, Addison's disease, dermatitis herpetiformis, connective tissue disease.

Investigations These can be divided into tests of • nutrient malabsorption • mucosal disease and • structural abnormality.

Fat malabsorption: the commonest test of malabsorption is the 3-day faecal fat collection during which the patient must be taking a normal-fat diet of approximately 100 g/day. The ^{14}C triolein breath test is based on the release of $^{14}CO_2$ after metabolism of absorbed ^{14}C-labelled oleic acid. Gross steatorrhoea is suggestive of pancreatic disease.

Carbohydrate malabsorption: impairment of absorption of monosaccharides can be tested by the glucose and xylose tolerance tests. Disaccharide malabsorption: lactose tolerance test, with normal giving a rise in blood glucose of >1 mmol/l, sucrose tolerance test abnormal in isomaltase deficiency. Radiological studies mixing the appropriate sugar with barium demonstrates intestinal hurry and dilatation.

Protein malabsorption: true malabsorption very rare. Excessive dietary protein catabolism occurs in bacterial overgrowth identified by the ^{14}C glycocholate breath test. Protein-losing enteropathy can be identified by faecal loss of ^{51}Cr-labelled albumin or of α_i anti-trypsin.

Bile salt malabsorption: detected by ^{14}C glycocholate breath test which is abnormal with terminal ileal disease and bacterial overgrowth. The ^{75}SeHAT test is also abnormal with terminal ileal disease but normal with bacterial overgrowth.

Vitamin B_{12} malabsorption: the Schilling test using dual isotopes can differentiate between pernicious anaemia and ileal disease.

Pancreatic functions (→ page 123)

Radiology: Malabsorption may give abnormal appearances on the small bowel meal which include: barium flocculation, rapid transit, strictures or ulceration, oedematous mucosal folds and evidence of previous surgery.

Intestinal histology: • Biopsies of the small intestine can be obtained at endoscopy or with a Crosby capsule • Total villous atrophy – coeliac disease, tropical sprue, severe malnutrition, idiopathic mucosal enteropathy and cows' milk or soya sensitivity • Subtotal villous atrophy – partially treated coeliac disease, bacterial overgrowth, dermatitis herpetiformis, intestinal ischaemia and Zollinger–Ellison syndrome • Non-villous abnormality – Whipple's disease (PAS-positive macrophages), giardiasis, Crohn's disease, lymphoma, radiation enteritis, lymphangiectasia and abetalipoproteinaemia • Intestinal biopsies may be processed to assay brush border enzymes in some laboratories to aid diagnosis of malabsorption due to enzyme deficiency • Duodenal aspirates allow quantitative bacteriological studies to be performed in cases where bacterial overgrowth is suspected.

PANCREATIC CARCINOMA

Science basics This is the second commonest tumour of the GI tract causing 5% of all cancer deaths. Two main types of pancreatic tumour occur, exocrine, principally adenocarcinoma, and the less common endocrine tumours, such as insulinomas and glucagonomas. The cause of pancreatic cancer is unknown but cigarette smoking, chronic pancreatitis and diabetes mellitus have all been incriminated.

Clinical features

Symptoms: epigastric pain which radiates posteriorly is present in the majority, weight-loss, jaundice in tumours involving the head of the pancreas, anorexia, nausea and vomiting. In the rare insulinoma, confusion due to hypoglycamia is characteristic.

Signs: include steatorrhoea, palpable gallbladder (Courvoisier's law) and occasionally thrombophlebitis migrans. In glucagonomas a necrolytic migratory erythematous rash may develop.

Investigations • An increased alkaline phosphatase and bilirubin occur with tumours obstructing the CBD • Impaired glucose tolerance or frank diabetes may be found • CEA levels may be increased in those with hepatic metastases • US and CT scanning are the two most useful tests which identify a pancreatic mass and/or dilatation of the CBD • ERCP may identify a stricture of the CBD or pancreatic duct • A tissue diagnosis should be obtained by US- or CT-guided fine needle biopsy.

Management box

▸ Cure can only be achieved by surgery but this is only applicable for those with small, localized tumours. Radical pancreatoduodenectomy (Whipple's operation) should be considered for such lesions. In the majority of patients, who are usually elderly, curative resection is not possible due to early localized spread.

▸ Palliation of jaundice and associated itch can be achieved by endoscopic stenting through the CBD stricture or surgery to create biliary diversion such as cholecystojejunostomy.

▸ Enteric bypass may be necessary for vomiting due to duodenal involvement.

▸ Pain relief is usually required using opiates and/or coeliac plexus block.

▸ The use of chemotherapy remains controversial.

▸ Endocrine tumours should be resected if localized.

▸ Streptozotocin is useful in the treatment of insulinomas.

Prognosis This is very poor with a one-year survival of less than 10%.

PANCREATITIS

Science basics Inflammation of the pancreas can be divided into acute pancreatitis including relapsing acute pancreatitis, and chronic pancreatitis including relapsing chronic pancreatitis. Differentiation into these categories, particularly the relapsing type may not be obvious and depends upon the permanency of abnormalities on pancreatic function testing.

Aetiology The causes of acute and chronic pancreatitis overlap (Table 5.4). The pathogenesis of pancreatitis is incompletely understood but interruption of the flow of pancreatic juice and/or reflux of bile into the pancreatic duct may be important. The severity of damage to the pancreas varies from mild inflammation with oedema to haemorrhagic necrosis. In chronic pancreatitis the ongoing inflammation results in fibrosis initially around ducts and acini but later within the acini.

Ⓔ ACUTE PANCREATITIS → page 441

CHRONIC PANCREATITIS

This is a relatively common disease, the commonest cause of which is chronic alcohol abuse. The pathophysiology is ill-understood but may be related to alcohol-induced change in the

Table 5.4
Pancreatitis

Acute	Chronic
Gallstones	Alcohol
Alcohol	Obstruction of pancreatic duct
Drugs, eg thiazides, azathioprine, oestrogen, furosemide (frusemide)	Hyperparathyroidism
	Hyperlipidaemia
Trauma	Haemochromatosis
Post-operative, post ERCP	Idiopathic
Pancreatic carcinoma	Hereditary
Hyperparathyroidism	Tropical calcific pancreatitis
Viral infection, eg mumps, coxsackie, E-B virus	

composition of pancreatic juice, resulting in precipitation and obstructive plug formation. Damage to acini results with fibrosis which often appears to involve nerve fibres. Less common causes include hypercalcaemia, hyperlipidaemia and heredity.

Clinical features

Symptoms: commonest is epigastric pain which may radiate posteriorly. Weight-loss, steatorrhoea, nausea and vomiting are common. Diabetes mellitus, with polydipsia and polyuria is common particularly in calcific pancreatitis.

Signs: are few other than abdominal tenderness. Jaundice may occur if the CBD is obstructed. Splenic vein thrombosis may result in splenomegaly and portal hypertension.

Investigations ● Faecal fat: gross steatorrhoea is highly suggestive of pancreatic disease ● Blood glucose may confirm diabetes ● Pancreatic function tests are necessary to confirm exocrine pancreatic insufficiency; the tubeless tests such as the PABA and the Pancreolauryl test are replacing older tests, eg Lundh test meal ● Plain abdominal X-ray may reveal pancreatic calcification ● US in experienced hands is fairly sensitive and both it and CT scanning are useful in excluding pancreatic cancer ● ERCP usually shows abnormalities both in the main pancreatic duct and side branches but a normal pancreatogram does not exclude chronic pancreatitis.

Management box

▶ Revolves around adequate pain relief and treating mal-absorption, with dietary manipulation to maintain calorie intake while reducing fat, and pancreatic enzymes, eg Pancrex Forte or Creon 1–5 tablets with food, and controlling diabetes mellitus.

▶ Achieving adequate pain relief is often difficult; commonly patients become dependent on opiates and suicide is well recognized. Absolute abstinence from alcohol is essential.

▶ Surgical procedures advocated to relieve pain where medical means fail include distal pancreatectomy, pancreato-duodenectomy, pancreaticojejunostomy and sphincteroplasty (for sphincter of Oddi disease).

Prognosis This is dependent upon age and continued alcohol intake and overall approximately 25–30% die within 10 years.

APPENDICITIS

Science basics Inflammation of the vermiform appendix is usually due to normal bowel flora and is commonly preceded by obstruction of the appendiceal lumen by lymphoid tissue or faecoliths. Inflammation results in oedema and ischaemia of the wall which may lead to gangrene and perforation. It is commonest in children and young adults and is the most frequent cause for acute surgery in this age group.

Clinical features

Symptoms: pain which characteristically starts periumbilically and moves to the RIF as visceral and parietal peritoneum respectively are involved. Nausea, vomiting and anorexia are common as is recent constipation.

Signs: fever, tenderness over McBurney's point (1/3 along a line from the anterior superior iliac spine to the umbilicus). Guarding and rebound tenderness suggest parietal peritoneal inflammation. Pain on passive hyperextension of the thigh (psoas sign) may be present, as may tenderness on rectal examination. Ureteric colic may be simulated by an appendix lying beside the R ureter. A mass in the RIF suggests abscess formation.

Investigations • A leukocytosis is usually present • US may be useful • Diagnosis is essentially a clinical one and a large differential diagnosis exists (Table 5.5).

Table 5.5
Differential diagnosis in appendicitis

Diagnosis	Useful features
Mesenteric adenitis	Less guarding and pain
Acute regional ileitis	Diarrhoea or constipation
Pancreatitis	Hyperamylasaemia
Renal colic	Radio-opaque stone and haematuria
Volvulus/intussusception	Characteristic radiograph
Cholecystitis	HIDA-scanning
Pyelonephritis	Urine microscopy

Management box
▶ Early surgery is standard treatment. In mild cases or when surgery is contraindicated iv fluids and antibiotics may produce resolution but careful surveillance for deterioration or signs of perforation is essential.
▶ A fixed mass indicates abscess formation due to a sealed perforation and conservative treatment with delayed surgery is appropriate.
▶ Perforation carries a significant mortality and resolution of an appendix abscess may take several weeks.

COLORECTAL CARCINOMA

Science basics This is the second commonest malignancy in the UK and is increasing, particularly those of the right side of the colon.

Aetiology Factors implicated include dietary mutagens, deficiency of dietary anti-mutagens, lack of dietary fibre, low dietary calcium and bile acids. Patients at increased risk include those with IBD (especially UC), previous colonic polyps or tumours, a history of ovarian or breast cancer and a family history of colonic cancer or familial adenomatous polyposis syndromes such as familial polyposis, Gardner's and Turcot's syndromes.

Clinical features

Symptoms: abdominal discomfort, rectal bleeding, weight-loss and change in bowel habit.

Signs: include pallor, abdominal mass, rectal mass or ulcer on rectal examination and jaundice. Occasionally presentation may be acute with intestinal obstruction or perforation.

Investigations • Rectal examination reveals a palpable mass in less than 50% of cases but when combined with rigid sigmoidoscopy the percentage is significantly increased • These investigations in combination with barium enema will detect the majority of lesions • The sensitivity of colonoscopy by an experienced operator is high and allows histological confirmation • In 20% more than one tumour is identified.

Management box
▶ Depends upon the size and extent of the tumour. Staging is usually according to Duke's classification (→ Table 5.6). Small tumours confined to polyps may be removed endoscopically. Surgery is indicated for all other lesions and even in Duke's class D surgical palliation prevents intestinal obstruction.
▶ Adjuvant chemotherapy with 5-fluorouracil and folic acid is of benefit for Dukes' C patients.
▶ Radiotherapy may be of use in rectal carcinoma.

Table 5.6
Staging in colorectal carcinoma

Duke's class	Extent	5-year survival (%)
A	Limited to muscularis propria	95
B	Through wall but not involving regional lymph nodes	70
C_1	Regional lymph nodes involved, resection complete	35
C_2	Nodes proximal to resection line involved	15
D	Distant metastases present	5

DIVERTICULAR DISEASE

Science basics This is the commonest structural disorder of the large bowel, and affects approximately 50% of the population over the age of 70 years. It is generally asymptomatic unless diverticulitis develops. This latter is a complication caused by obstruction of the diverticular neck by faecal material.

Aetiology It is commonly believed that deficiency of dietary fibre results in hypertrophy of both the longitudinal and circular muscle of the colon, leading to hypersegmentation and increased intraluminal pressure with the development of pulsion diverticulae. The evidence for this theory is however scanty and normal aging of the bowel is probably important.

Clinical features

Symptoms: largely if not entirely due to complicating diverticulitis, with abdominal pain, fever, nausea and vomiting.

Signs: include LIF tenderness and rectal bleeding. Fistula formation may occur between the colon and bladder, vagina and small bowel presenting with pneumaturia, vaginal discharge and malabsorption respectively. Colonic stricture formation may develop with constipation, colic and later vomiting.

Investigations • The diagnosis of diverticular disease is made on barium enema • Diverticulitis can be presumed in those with diverticular disease associated with fever, leukocytosis and pain • The barium enema may reveal signs of active inflammation • The presence of rectal bleeding or stricture formation requires the exclusion of colorectal cancer • Colonoscopy with biopsy is useful but may be difficult in those with large diverticulae • Other diseases which may require exclusion include ischaemic colitis, UC and Crohn's disease.

> #### Management box
> ▶ In those with diverticular disease the risk of developing diverticulitis is reduced by a high-fibre diet.
> ▶ Treatment of diverticulitis includes bed-rest, iv fluids and antibiotics, analgesics and antispasmodics.
> ▶ Surgical intervention is required in only a minority and is indicated for peritonitis, fistula formation, pericolic abscess formation, persistent haemorrhage, bowel obstruction and repeated attacks of diverticulitis despite medical therapy.

RECTAL BLEEDING

Science basics Rectal bleeding is common and may indicate serious disease and must not just be attributed to haemorrhoids without proper investigation.

Clinical features The freshness of the blood and whether it is mingled within the faeces should be noted and may be of use in determining the site of bleeding (Table 5.7). Fresh blood streaking the faeces is typical of bleeding from haemorrhoids unlike the mixture of blood and diarrhoea in UC.

Table 5.7
Clinical features of rectal bleeding

Profuse bleeding	Minor bleeding
Ulcerative colitis	All causes of profuse bleeding
Haemorrhoids	Colorectal cancer
Diverticulitis	Infective colitis
Arteriovenous malformation	Crohn's disease
	Polyps
	Ischaemic colitis
	Idiopathic colonic ulcers

Investigations • All patients should undergo sigmoidoscopy which allows identification of active bleeding from haemorrhoids, rectal tumours and UC • Colonoscopy is the investigation of choice although may be difficult in the face of active bleeding. It allows histological confirmation of lesions such as colonic tumours and allows treatment of such lesions as polyps by polypectomy and a-v malformations by laser • Double-contrast barium enema also identifies many causes of colonic bleeding but is not useful during active bleeding • Arteriography may be invaluable in identifying bleeding lesions, particularly when active bleeding at a rate of 1–2 ml/minute exists • Radionuclide studies using radio-labelled erythrocytes may be useful in identifying the site of occult bleeding providing significant bleeding takes place at the time of investigation.

Management box
▶ This depends upon the cause although investigation should not be undertaken until the patient has been adequately resuscitated.

GALLSTONE DISEASE

Science basics By the sixth decade 20% of women and 10% of men have gallstones and with advancing age the prevalence increases, although always higher in females. In Western society cholesterol or mixed cholesterol-calcium-bilirubin stones account for the majority of stones. The pathogensis is incompletely understood but factors which may produce lithogenic bile include increased cholesterol content, reduced bile acids and biliary stasis. In the majority of cases gallstones are asymptomatic and only 10% develop symptoms after 5 years. Gallstones are responsible for three main disorders: cholecystitis, biliary colic and choledocholithiasis.

CHOLECYSTITIS

Gallstone impaction in the cystic duct is the commonest cause of cholecystitis. Less common causes include primary infection (eg *Salmonella typhi* or *Ascaris lumbricoides*), trauma, surgery, chemotherapy and TPN.

Clinical features

Symptoms: RUQ pain often with radiation to the R shoulder, nausea, vomiting and fever.

Signs: RUQ tenderness, gallbladder tenderness demonstrable on inspiration (Murphy's sign), gallbladder usually impalpable and jaundice in a minority of patients.

Investigations ● FBC usually demonstrates a leukocytosis ● Abdominal X-ray reveals radio-opaque stones in a minority and occasionally a sentinel loop or air in the biliary tree ● US demonstrates gallbladder stones and thickening of the mucosa ● Radio-isotopic scanning (HIDA; PIPIDA) is useful in identifying obstruction of the cystic duct.

Complications Empyema, gangrene and gallbladder perforation, pancreatitis, perihepatic abscesses, portal pyaemia and septicaemia.

> #### Management box
> ▸ Initially supportive with iv fluids, analgesics and antibiotics, eg amoxicillin and tobramycin.
> ▸ Cholecystectomy (now usually laparoscopic) once the patient is stable is the treatment of choice, although the timing of surgery (ie early or delayed (interval) cholecystectomy) is controversial and depends upon the patient's condition and age.
> ▸ Percutaneous cholecystotomy may be indicated in seriously ill patients.

BILIARY COLIC

This is usually due to stone impaction in the cystic duct.

Clinical features

Symptoms: a constant epigastric or RUQ pain which usually increases over 2–3 hours before settling. Pain for more than

6 hours should suggest cholecystitis. Nausea and vomiting are common.

Investigations • The diagnosis is largely clinical particularly since gallstones are so prevalent. Many patients with gallstones and dyspepsia are not helped by cholecystectomy and in many the abdominal discomfort is due to IBS (hepatic flexure syndrome) • Transient increases in bilirubin and alkaline phosphatase support the diagnosis of biliary colic • Biliary scintigraphy may demonstrate cystic duct obstruction if performed during an attack.

Management box
▸ Analgesia until the attack has passed. Morphine increases the sphincter of Oddi pressure and should be avoided.
▸ Cholecystectomy is indicated for those fit for surgery.
▸ In those unfit or who refuse surgery gallstone dissolution therapy with ursodeoxycholic acid is appropriate for those with radiolucent stones less than 1.5 cm in diameter and with a functioning gallbladder on oral cholecystography. Complete dissolution occurs in approximately 30% at 12 months.

CHOLEDOCHOLITHIASIS

Common bile-duct stones most commonly arise from gallbladder stones but may form in the bile ducts due to biliary strictures, primary or secondary sclerosing cholangitis or in Caroli's disease.

Clinical features May be asymptomatic.

Symptoms: include biliary colic, intermittent or constant RUQ pain, nausea and vomiting.

Signs: fluctuating jaundice, RUQ tenderness and palpable gallbladder in 15%. Fever and rigors indicate cholangitis.

Investigations • FBC reveals a leukocytosis and LFTs an increased bilirubin, alkaline phosphatase and gamma GT; a mild elevation of transaminases is not uncommon • A prolonged PT is common • Abdominal X-rays may reveal radio-opaque stones or rarely air within the biliary tree • US may reveal dilatation of the biliary tree but is not sensitive in identifying the stones within the CBD, which usually requires ERCP or PTC.

Complications Pancreatitis, cholangitis, septicaemia, hepatic abscess and secondary sclerosing cholangitis or biliary cirrhosis.

Management box

▶ Initially analgesia, iv fluids and antibiotics (eg amoxicillin or tobramycin).

▶ Stone removal is best achieved by ERCP, sphincterotomy and extraction with a Dormia basket or balloon.

▶ Large stones may be dissolved or reduced in size chemically with methyl-tert-butyl-ether or mono-octanion administered via a vaso-biliary tube.

▶ Mechanical fragmentation of stones by lithotripsy may prove to be a useful alternative.

6

Hepatology

INVESTIGATIONS

FBC A macrocytosis is common in chronic liver disease particularly of alcoholic origin. A reduced platelet count is also common due partly to hypersplenism.

LFTs These reflect hepatic dysfunction rather than function and are discussed in more depth on pp 350–352.

Serology
- AntiHBsAg – previous HBV infection or vaccination
- IgM antiHBcAg – recent HBV infection
- HBeAg and HBV-DNA – ongoing active infection
- IgM antiHAV – recent hepatitis A infection
- AntiHDV – previous Delta virus infection
- AntiHCV – usually chronic hepatitis C infection
- HCV-RNA – active HCV infection
- Antimitochondrial Ab – positive in the vast majority of patients with primary biliary cirrhosis
- ANF and anti-smooth muscle Ab – positive in many patients with autoimmune CAH
- Anti-LKM antibody – positive in some patients with chronic HCV and some children with autoimmune CAH.

Other blood tests • α-fetoprotein increased in hepatomas • low levels of α_1-antitrypsin in patients homozygous for PiZ or PiS • Caeruloplasmin low in Wilson's disease • cholesterol high in Zieve's syndrome (along with haemolysis and leukocytosis) and chronic cholestasis • Hypoglycaemia in fulminant hepatic failure and some patients with hepatoma • Ferritin very high in haemochromatosis.

Radiology • The plain abdominal X-ray may reveal air within the biliary tree after sphincterotomy or in patients with gallstone ileus • US is an important investigation looking both at the liver parenchyma and the diameter of the biliary tree • ERCP is invaluable in investigating the biliary tree • PTC is useful in investigating those with dilated intrahepatic ducts • CT scanning is important in identifying lesions within the hepatic parenchyma • MRI is increasingly used for disorders of the liver, biliary tree and the pancreas • Angiography of the hepatic artery and, during the venous phase, the portal system, may be essential in investigating those with hepatic tumours or portal hypertension • A measure of the portal pressure can be obtained by hepatic venous catheterization using a balloon catheter (wedged hepatic venous pressure).

Endoscopy Valuable in identifying gastro-oesophageal varices and portal gastropathy.

Liver biopsy   Obtained either percutaneously or at laparoscopy, is usually required in either the diagnosis or staging of most hepatic disorders. In those with coagulopathy or ascites a transjugular route for biopsy may be used, reducing the risk of haemorrhage.

ACUTE VIRAL HEPATITIS

Science basics   Acute viral hepatitis is common and may be caused by a large variety of viruses, the best known of which are hepatitis A, B, C, D and E viruses, non-A non-B agents, and Epstein-Barr virus. Damage to the liver may be directly due to the virus or the immune response. Histologically the various viral causes generally cannot be separated, all causing hepatocyte death, inflammation and regeneration. The clinical picture in each may vary from mild anicteric disease to fulminant hepatic failure. Patients may present with acute hepatitis due to other causes which require to be excluded, especially where viral serology is negative. Other causes include drugs (eg paracetamol poisoning, isoniazid, allopurinol, halothane, methyldopa, sulphonamides), Wilson's disease, poisons (eg *Amanita phalloides*), Reye's syndrome (in children), lymphoma and Budd-Chiari syndrome.

> **Management box**
> ▸ No specific treatment exists. Supportive measures include bed-rest, alcohol abstinence and a low fat, high carbohydrate diet.
> ▸ Steroid therapy improves the LFTs in many but does not influence the natural history favourably and should be avoided.
> ▸ Lamivudine may be effective in acute HBV infection.
> ▸ Prevention is best and includes the use of immune globulin and vaccines and reducing the risk of transmission by screening blood donors for HBsAg, anti-HBc and anti-HCV antibodies and those with elevated serum transaminase levels.

HEPATITIS A VIRUS

A 27–30 nm, single-stranded RNA virus. Infection never becomes chronic and immunity measured by anti-hepatitis A titres is usually life-long. Active or recent infection is diagnosed by IgM anti-HAV.

HEPATITIS B VIRUS

Consists of a central structure, the Dane particle, made up of the core antigen HBcAg (the e antigen, HBeAg, is part of the core

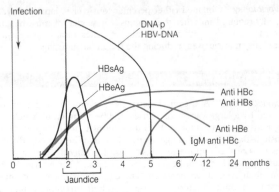

Fig. 6.1   Acute hepatitis B infection.

antigen) within which is contained DNA-polymerase and double-stranded DNA. Surrounding the central particle is the surface antigen, HBsAg. The activity of the various antigens and antibodies during acute HBV infection is illustrated in Figure 6.1. Anti-pre-S antibodies appear early in the infection. Infection with HBV in the UK is most commonly venereal or via shared needles in iv drug abusers. Classically infection is followed by the onset of jaundice 2–3 months later accompanied by a serum-sickness-like illness with fever and arthralgia. Acute infection is confirmed by IgM anti-HBc. 10% of patients develop chronic carriage and this is more frequent in males. The population carriage rate in the UK is approximately 0.1%. Prophylaxis can be obtained in the short term by hepatitis B immune globulin and long-term with HBV vaccines.

HEPATITIS C VIRUS

Is an RNA virus, 30–60 nm in diameter, which resembles members of the flavirus family. It has a lipid envelope, nucleocapsule proteins and a single large open reading frame RNA, coding for structural and non-structural proteins including RNA polymerase. Transmission is parenteral, generally via blood or blood products or iv drug misuse, although sporadic infection does occur. Acute infection, classically post-transfusion hepatitis, occurs and is often anicteric. Diagnosis is by detection of anti HCV antibodies, which may take 4–6 months to appear after infection, or by detection of HCV RNA. Approximately 50–75% of patients progress to develop chronic hepatitis. The population carriage rate in the UK is around 0.5–1%. No vaccine is currently available.

HEPATITIS D VIRUS

This is a defective virus which requires co-infection with HBV to be pathogenic in man. It is rare in the UK and common in southern Europe. Co-infection with HBV and HDV results in a more severe illness with a higher rate of fulminant hepatic failure. HDV infection in carriers of HBV may result in relapse. Acute infection is diagnosed by IgM anti-Delta antibodies.

HEPATITIS E VIRUS

This is a DNA virus which is enterally transmitted (like hepatitis A) with a prevalence in the UK of perhaps as high as 1–2%. It presents as either a subclinical infection, typical acute hepatitis or rarely as fulminant hepatic failure (especially in pregnancy). Diagnosis is by anti-HEV antibodies or less often detection of HEV in faeces.

NON-A, NON-B HEPATITIS VIRUSES

Viruses, as yet unidentified, believed to cause viral-like hepatitis which may have a fulminant course. Approximately 50% are now believed to be probably due to hepatitis E virus.

EPSTEIN–BARR VIRUS INFECTION

Infection results in jaundice in 10–15% and is accompanied by pharyngitis, lymphadenopathy and splenomegaly. The diagnosis is confirmed by atypical lymphocytes in the blood and a positive monospot, although this latter test may be false-positive in hepatitis A. Chronic liver disease does not occur.

CHRONIC HEPATITIS

Science basics This is defined as inflammatory disease of the liver for longer than 6 months. Causes include:

- Chronic HBV or HCV infection
- Autoimmune CAH
- Alcohol abuse
- Drugs, eg isoniazid, methyldopa, nitrofurantoin
- Metabolic, eg Wilson's disease.

Histologically, varying degrees of inflammation are seen. If hepatocyte death is present (chronic active hepatitis) progression to cirrhosis is likely without treatment.

CHRONIC HEPATITIS DUE TO HBV CARRIAGE

Approximately 10% of patients, particularly males, with acute HBV infection do not clear the virus by 6 months.

Clinical features   Many are asymptomatic and may present only with complications of cirrhosis later. Others may show weight-loss, lethargy and hepatomegaly.

Investigations   • Serology divides patients into those in the replicative (HBsAg +ve, HBeAg +ve, DNA-polymerase +ve and IgM antiHBc +ve) and non-replicative phases (HBsAg +ve, HBeAg −ve, DNA-polymerase −ve, anti-HBe +ve and IgM anti-HBc −ve) • Those in the replicative phase are more often symptomatic and have more active liver disease, ie chronic active hepatitis (CAH) rather than chronic persistent hepatitis • In a few patients viruses persist which do not synthesize the eAg (precore mutation) and are therefore anti HBeAb +ve and HBV DNA +ve • Coexistent HDV infection should be excluded.

> **Management box**
> ▸ Steroids are not effective and although LFTs may improve viral replication is encouraged.
> ▸ Anti-viral drugs such as α-interferon 3–5 million units sc 3 × per week and lamivudine 100 mg daily may well be useful particularly in those in the replicative phase of HBV infection without cirrhosis.

CHRONIC HEPATITIS DUE TO HCV CARRIAGE

Approximately 70% of cases of acute HCV hepatitis, often subclinical, become chronic. This leads in most cases to a chronic low-grade hepatitis with mildly and variably abnormal LFTs. Approximately 20% develop cirrhosis over 20 years (50% by 30 years) which may progress to hepato-cellular carcinoma. Alcohol abuse and old age may accelerate liver damage.

Clinical features   Most are asymptomatic although features of cirrhosis and portal hypertension may be present. Associated with porphyria cutanea tarda.

Investigations   • Serology for anti HCV antibodies by RIA and ELISA (non-specific), with confirmatory recombinant immunoblot (RIBA) tests • HCV-RNA can be detected by PCR • Genotyping necessary for treatment planning • Liver histology (often characteristic) helps in staging the disease.

Management box
▶ The best treatment for chronic HCV hepatitis is combination therapy with α-interferon 3 million units, 3 times weekly for 6 months with ribavirin 1–1.2 g daily, with a response rate of 50% and sustained response in 30–40%.
▶ 12 months of therapy is indicated for genotype I infection and those with cirrhosis.

AUTOIMMUNE CAH

This is typically a disease of young and middle-aged women.

Aetiology Associated with HLA A1, B8, DRW3 and reduced numbers of suppressor T-cells. In most it presents insidiously but may mimic acute viral hepatitis.

Clinical features Spider naevi, amenorrhoea, hepatosplenomegaly. Associated disorders include diabetes mellitus, hypothyroidism, arthropathy, Coomb's positive haemolytic anaemia, fibrosing alveolitis and ulcerative colitis.

Investigations • HBV and HCV –ve • LFTs with 5–10 × increase in transaminases and 2–5 × increase in bilirubin • Anti-smooth muscle and ANF positive in 70% and antimitochondrial antibodies in 25% • Liver histology reveals large numbers of lymphocytes in the portal tract infiltrating into the hepatocyte lobules with little fatty change • Cirrhosis develops rapidly without treatment.

Management box
▶ Prednisolone 30–40 mg daily for 1 week reducing over next month to maintenance dose of 10 mg/day. If LFTs and liver histology do not normalize add azathioprine (50 mg/day). Continue steroids (and/or azathioprine) for 2 years before slowly withdrawing.
▶ Approximately 50% will remain in remission and for those who relapse steroids should be reintroduced and then changed to azathioprine for long term therapy.

Prognosis Steroid therapy has greatly improved survival although many patients still develop cirrhosis with its complications of variceal haemorrhage and ascites. Patients who develop liver failure should be considered for liver transplantation.

ALCOHOLIC LIVER DISEASE

Science basics Alcohol abuse is increasing in the UK and the incidence of alcoholic cirrhosis, which currently is approximately

10–15 per 100 000 per year, is also increasing. The threshold beyond which alcoholic liver disease may occur is 21 units (a unit being 10 g of alcohol or a $\frac{1}{2}$ pint of beer or one measure of spirits) per week for men and 14 units for women.

Aetiology Ethanol is metabolized in the liver mainly by alcohol dehydrogenase to acetaldehyde and hydrogen ions. The latter affects the NADH:NAD ratio in the cell, which affects the cell membrane and in conjunction with the toxic effect of acetaldehyde results in cell damage. Other enzyme systems such as the microsomal ethanol oxidizing system (MEOS) are also involved, particularly in heavy drinkers. Other factors implicated include female sex, associated malnutrition, HLA B8 and DW2 genotype and immunological responses against alcohol-induced antigens.

Classification

Fatty liver: this is the mildest form of hepatic injury and is reversible.

Alcoholic hepatitis: with perivenular (zone 3) hepatocellular damage, Mallory's hyaline and an inflammatory cell infiltrate; jaundice, fever and ascites are common.

Perivenular sclerosis with perisinusoidal fibrosis and collagenation of the space of Disse: leads to cirrhosis. It may accompany fatty change resulting in cirrhosis without alcoholic hepatitis.

Cirrhosis: characterized by fibrosis and nodule formation and is irreversible and usually accompanied by portal hypertension.

Clinical features

Symptoms: include nausea, vomiting, anorexia and fever.

Signs: include spider naevi, bruising, old rib fractures, hepatomegaly, splenomegaly, ascites, parotitis and macrocytic anaemia.

Investigations • An accurate history of alcohol intake is essential • FBC often reveals a macrocytosis • LFTs: an increased GGT reflects ethanol abuse and an abnormal ALT hepatocellular damage • An AST:ALT ratio of >2 is suggestive of alcoholic damage • An elevated serum IgA is common • In alcoholic hepatitis the ALT may not be particularly raised, although cholestatic jaundice is often pronounced, along with fever and leukocytosis.

Management box

▶ Total abstinence from alcohol is the only effective treatment and psychiatric referral may help compliance.

▶ In alcoholic hepatitis corticosteroids, eg prednisolone 40 mg/day, may be beneficial in those with marked cholestasis and/or encephalopathy but improvement in survival is debatable.

Prognosis   This depends upon the stage of the disease and the continued alcohol intake. Alcoholic hepatitis carries a mortality of 25–60%. In those with cirrhosis who abstain from alcohol the 5-year survival is approximately 70% compared with 35% for those who continue to drink. Adverse prognostic features include variceal haemorrhage, ascites and jaundice.

CIRRHOSIS

Science basics   This is defined as diffuse fibrosis and nodule formation. Classification into macronodular, frequently viral, and micronodular, often alcoholic, depends upon the size of the nodules. The main complications are: portal hypertension due to increased resistance to portal venous drainage and increased portal inflow secondary to splanchnic vasodilatation; hepatic decompensation due to a progressive reduction in liver cell mass; and hepatocellular carcinoma.

Aetiology

Infection: HBV and HCV infection.

Metabolic: alcohol, haemochromatosis, Wilson's disease, α_1-antitrypsin deficiency, galactosaemia.

Immunological: PBC, chronic active hepatitis (CAH), PSC.

Drugs: methotrexate, methyldopa, isoniazid.

Vascular: Budd-Chiari syndrome, veno-occlusive disease, constrictive pericarditis.

Miscellaneous: sarcoidosis, prolonged cholestasis, intestinal bypass, cryptogenic.

Clinical features

Symptoms: include lethargy, itch (especially PBC), ankle and abdominal swelling.

Signs: hepatomegaly, splenomegaly, bruising, spider naevi, finger clubbing, palmar erythema, parotitis, jaundice, testicular atrophy, ascites, gynaecomastia, reduced body hair and leukonychia.

Investigations   These can be divided into those to identify the aetiology, ie history of alcohol abuse, high MCV and GGTP, serum ferritin, α_1-antitrypsin, caeruloplasmin, viral serology, auto-antibodies • and those to determine severity, ie clotting studies, albumin, platelets, bilirubin, US (for spleen and liver size and ascites), endoscopy for varices, portal pressure measurements, EEG for encephalopathy • Liver histology is usually required to confirm the diagnosis and disease activity.

> **Management box**
> ▶ Cirrhosis is irreversible and no treatment reverses the pathological process.
> ▶ Treatment for certain causes, such as steroids for CAH, venesection for haemochromatosis and absolute alcohol abstinence for alcoholic cirrhosis, retard disease advancement.
> ▶ The complications of cirrhosis such as ascites, encephalopathy and variceal haemorrhage should be treated appropriately. Propranolol 160 mg LA/day may reduce the risk of variceal haemorrhage and is indicated in those with large varices where no contraindications exist.
> ▶ Endoscopic band ligation may also be indicated to prevent haemorrhage.
> ▶ Hepatic transplantation should be considered for patients with end-stage cirrhosis.

Prognosis This depends upon the cause and severity. For alcoholic cirrhosis the mortality for persistent drinkers is 65% at 5 years compared with 30% for those who stop. Assessment of severity can be assessed from the Child's-Pugh classification (Table 6.1).

PRIMARY BILIARY CIRRHOSIS

Science basics This is an autoimmune disease which causes destruction of intrahepatic bile ducts. It affects females predominantly (90%) in their fifth and sixth decades and is the commonest indication for liver transplant in the UK. Anti-

Table 6.1
Child's-Pugh classification of cirrhosis severity

Score	1	2	3
Encephalopathy	None	Mild	Marked
Bilirubin (µmol/l)	<34	34–50	>50
Albumin (g/l)	>35	28–35	<28
PT (s prolonged)	<4	4–6	>6
Ascites	None	Mild	Marked
Bilirubin (in PBC and sclerosing cholangitis)	<68	68–170	>170

Add the individual scores <7 = Child's A, 7–9 = Child's B and >9 = Child's C. The survival for Child's C, the poorest prognostic group, is less than 12 months.

mitochondrial antibodies (mainly directed towards the E2 component particularly of the pyruvate dehydrogenase complex) are usually present.

Clinical features May be asymptomatic and only diagnosed on screening of liver function tests. Generalized pruritus and lethargy are the earliest symptoms and usually precede jaundice. Hepatosplenomegaly is often present and xanthelasma may be found. It may be associated with kerato conjunctivitis sicca and other connective tissue diseases.

Investigations • Raised alkaline phosphatase and IgM • Mitochondrial antibodies in 95% (other antibodies such as ANA and smooth muscle may be present) • Liver biopsy shows a plasma cell and lymphocyte infiltrate in the portal tracts with granulomata.

Management box

▶ Ursodeoxycholic acid may improve pruritus and liver function tests. Pruritus can also be controlled by colestyramine.
▶ Supplementation of fat-soluble vitamins and treatment of hyperlipidaemia may be required.
▶ There is no effective medical therapy and patients should be considered for liver transplantation once the bilirubin has exceeded 100 μmol/l. Ursodeoxycholic acid may slow disease progression.

PRIMARY HAEMOCHROMATOSIS

Science basics Primary (or genetic) haemochromatosis is an autosomal recessive disorder which results in iron overload in various organs, particularly the liver, pancreas and heart. It is caused by mutations resulting in malfunction of the HFE gene product. The commonest genotype in genetic haemochromatosis is C282Y homozygotes with the H63D variant less common. The underlying genetic abnormality appears to be an inability to reduce iron absorption in situations where the body's iron content is normal (in secondary haemochromatosis regulation of intestinal absorption is normal and excess administration, usually parenterally, overloads the system).

Clinical features Phenotypic expression of the condition is less common in women because of menstruation. Presentation is usually with lethargy, abdominal pain, arthralgia and reduced libido. Signs include hepatomegaly, skin pigmentation, reduced body hair, splenomegaly, gynaecomastia, testicular atrophy, ascites and jaundice. Type I diabetes is common, particularly in those with cirrhosis. Cardiac failure and cardiac arrhythmias are also common.

Investigations • Serum ferritin > 700 µg/l, serum iron > 35 µg/l, hepatic iron content > 400 µ/100 mg dry weight • HLA typing has largely been replaced by HFE genotyping for the C282Y and H63D mutations.

Management box
▸ Regular venesection, initially 500 ml weekly then monthly, until the serum ferritin falls to <12 µg/l or mild iron deficiency anaemia develops.

Prognosis Without treatment once the condition is clinically apparent death within 5 years is common, chiefly due to cardiac failure, liver failure, variceal haemorrhage or hepatocellular carcinoma. The risk of the latter is not affected by venesection in patients with cirrhosis.

WILSON'S DISEASE

Science basics An inborn error of copper metabolism characterized by gross copper loading in the liver, low plasma caeruloplasmin levels, and a high urinary copper excretion. The gene for Wilson's disease has now been discovered (ATPTB) and the commonest mutation (H1069Q) causes functional failure of the protein involved in copper transport. This leads to hepatic cirrhosis which may present like acute liver failure or with the complications of cirrhosis often with associated extra pyramidal symptoms of rigidity and haemolysis. Kayser-Fleischer rings, brown copper deposits around the edge of the cornea, may be present. Treatment is with penicillamine or, if advanced, liver transplantation.

LIVER TUMOURS

Science basics The commonest tumour in the liver is metastatic disease. Two major primary liver tumours exist, hepatocellular carcinoma and cholangiocarcinoma.

HEPATOCELLULAR CARCINOMA

This is a tumour of hepatocytes and is one of the commonest tumours in the world due to the endemic infection of HBV and HCV in the Far East.

Aetiology Chronic HBV or HCV carriage, cirrhosis of any cause but especially haemochromatosis and α_1-antitrypsin deficiency, toxins such as aflatoxin and drugs such as the contraceptive pill and anabolic steroids.

Clinical features   Males $3 \times$ commoner than women, abdominal pain, weight-loss, ascites, jaundice, fever, hepatomegaly with a bruit. Paraneoplastic syndromes include hypoglycaemia, erythrocytosis, hypercalcaemia and ectopic gonadotrophin production.

Investigations   • Increased α-fetoprotein in 85% of cases complicating cirrhosis, much lower frequency in those with non-cirrhotic livers • US and CT scanning • Liver biopsy, often under laparoscopic or US guidance • Biopsy should be avoided in those in whom surgery is planned because of possible tumour seeding • Patients with cirrhosis should have HCC surveillance with 3–6-monthly α-fetoprotein and US.

Management box
▶ Resection or liver transplantation currently offers the only hope of cure. Unfortunately early spread and the presence of cirrhosis precludes this in the majority.
▶ Chemotherapy with adriamycin or combinations of 5-fluorouracil, methotrexate, vincristine and cyclophosphamide may be better but are toxic. Chemoembolization may reduce tumour mass and be valuable before surgery. Perfusion of chemotherapy drugs directly into the hepatic artery or hepatic artery ligation may be appropriate in certain cases.
▶ Pain control often requires opiates and/or coeliac plexus block.

CHOLANGIOCARCINOMA

A tumour of the biliary tree, which is much less common although is probably increasing in frequency.

Aetiology   Factors include PSC, Thorotrast (an obsolete contrast medium), gallstones and infestation with *Clonorchis sinensis*.

Clinical features   Similar to hepatocellular carcinoma although central tumours present with jaundice early.

Investigations   (as for hepatocellular carcinoma) α-fetoprotein is negative.

Management box
▶ Because early spread via the lymphatics occurs, resection or liver transplantation is rarely possible.
▶ Palliation of jaundice and pruritus may be achieved by surgical bypass or by endoscopic and percutaneous stent insertion.

E **ACUTE OR FULMINANT HEPATIC FAILURE** → page 443

E **OESOPHAGEAL VARICES** → page 440

ENCEPHALOPATHY

Science basics This is a neuropsychiatric syndrome in which changes in intellect and behaviour occur along with reduced conscious level in patients with acute or chronic liver disease. It occurs in the setting of fulminant hepatic failure where progression to coma, cerebral oedema and death is common and in those with portosystemic shunts usually as a consequence of chronic liver disease.

Aetiology It is believed that some substance derived from protein breakdown in the intestine is absorbed and reaches the brain, either because of shunting around the liver or when the liver is incapable of removing it. The exact nature of this substance is unclear but false neurotransmitters derived from aromatic aminoacids or gamma aminobutyric acid (GABA) are currently believed the most likely.

Clinical features In acute liver failure progression from drowsiness (grade I), through confusion (grades II and III) to coma (grade IV) occurs. Raised intracranial pressure and cerebral oedema may develop. Foetor hepaticus, a flapping tremor (asterixis) and hyperreflexia are characteristic. The condition behaves in parallel with the underlying liver function. In chronic liver disease encephalopathy usually develops along with some complication such as upper GI bleeding, infection, hypokalaemia, high protein intake, constipation or sedative drugs. In mild cases abnormalities can be detected by poor performance at joining sequences of scattered numbers (number connection tests) and constructional apraxia, eg drawing a five-pointed star. Progression to coma is unusual.

Investigations Diagnosis is largely clinical but can be confirmed by EEG which shows a reduced α-rhythm, increased Q activity and large-voltage slow waves.

> *Management box*
> ▸ In acute liver failure treatment is directed to supporting the patient while liver recovery takes place.
> ▸ Hypoglycaemia may mimic encephalopathy in these patients and should be avoided by careful monitoring of the blood glucose concentration.

▸ In those with chronic liver disease identification and correction of the underlying complication such as sepsis, variceal haemorrhage or electrolyte imbalance is essential.

▸ Additional measures include reducing protein intake, reducing faecal content by lactulose (20 ml tid) and enemas.

▸ The use of branch-chain aminoacids, vegetable protein diets and bromocriptine are still controversial and are not advocated in general clinical practice.

ASCITES

Science basics The presence of excess free fluid within the peritoneal cavity can occur in a large number of situations including cirrhosis, intra-abdominal malignancy, nephrotic syndrome, Meig's syndrome, constrictive pericarditis, Budd-Chiari syndrome and tuberculous peritonitis. Abdominal swelling due to fluid should be differentiated from fat, flatus, faeces and fetus.

Ascites in cirrhosis

Aetiology The current most popular theory for the pathogenesis of ascites is the peripheral vasodilatation hypothesis, which proposes that the first change is peripheral vasodilatation, leading to renal hypoperfusion. This in turn leads to salt and water retention, made worse by secondary hyperaldosteronism. The extravascular fluid tends to collect in the abdomen because of portal hypertension. Hypoalbuminaemia exacerbates extravascular fluid retention.

Clinical features

Symptoms: include abdominal swelling, rapid weight-gain and often ankle swelling.

Signs: bilateral shifting flank dullness and a fluid thrill. Other stigmata of chronic liver disease may be present.

Investigations • US is especially useful in confirming the diagnosis and identifying other features such as splenomegaly • A diagnostic paracentesis of 20 ml should be carried out in all patients to identify the protein content, exclude malignant cells and bacteria and determine the WBC concentration • WBC count >250/mm (predominantly polymorphs) is diagnostic of spontaneous bacterial peritonitis, commonly due to coliforms • Presence of more than one type of organism should raise the possibility of bowel perforation.

Management box

▶ Step-wise approach starting with bed-rest, reduced salt intake (no added salt) and spironolactone 50–100 mg daily. Aim for a weight-loss of 0.5 kg per day. If no response increase spironolactone gradually to 400 mg before adding 20–40 mg furosemide (frusemide).

▶ Care should be taken when introducing loop diuretics not to precipitate hepatorenal syndrome with rising creatinine, oliguria and hyponatraemia.

▶ Once the ascites has resolved maintenance doses of spironolactone of 50–200 mg are required along with dietary salt restriction (patients with malignant ascites may require large doses of furosemide (frusemide) 80–120 mg to control ascites).

▶ This approach fails in 10%, in whom one should perform a therapeutic total paracentesis accompanied by iv albumin (80 g for every 3 l of ascites removed). A low-salt diet of 40–60 mmol/day should be started.

▶ In refractory cases a Le Veen (peritoneo-venous) shunt or TIPSS may be the only way to control ascites.

▶ In those in whom spontaneous bacterial peritonitis is suspected by a high WBC count in the ascitic fluid, cefuroxime 500 mg qid with metronidazole 500 mg tid should be started and modified once the bacteriology is known. Norfloxacin has been shown to be effective in the prophylaxis of spontaneous bacterial peritonitis.

LIVER TRANSPLANTATION

This was first undertaken in 1963, and has been part of clinical practice since 1983. Two major types are recognized: auxillary homotransplantation where a liver is transplanted in an ectopic place leaving the existing liver in place; and orthotopic transplantation where a new liver is inserted in place of the old. The latter is by far the most popular. Successful liver transplantation is a joint medical and surgical effort.

Indications

Children: biliary atresia, if corrective surgery is delayed beyond 2–3 months, inborn errors of metabolism, eg α_1-antitrypsin deficiency, Wilson's disease, tyrosinaemia, glycogen storage disease and primary hepatic malignancy.

Adults: subacute or fulminant hepatic failure, eg due to paracetamol poisoning, and end-stage cirrhosis, eg due to PBC, CAH and cryptogenic and primary hepatic malignancy.

Selection • Less than 70 years, patent portal vein and hepatic artery, satisfactory renal and cardiopulmonary function and receptive psychological attitude • Correct timing: before the patient becomes too ill is important • Previous upper abdominal surgery makes the surgery more difficult • HLA typing is not necessary • Contraindications: metastatic disease, sepsis, recent variceal haemorrhage and active alcoholism.

Management box

▶ Triple therapy immunosuppression with prednisolone, azathioprine and ciclosporin or tacrolimus is the most popular regimen. The former two drugs can often be withdrawn over time. Over-immunosuppression should be avoided because of the risk of sepsis.

Complications

Early: acute rejection, vascular thrombosis, haemorrhage and sepsis.

Late: biliary infection, opportunistic infection, chronic rejection (vanishing bile-duct syndrome) and disease recurrence, eg malignancy.

Prognosis 1-year survival is 60–70% for adults and 80% for children. Transplantation for malignancy has a poorer outlook than for benign disease because of disease recurrence. Transplantation for acute liver failure in those predicted unlikely to survive, eg fulminant hepatic failure due to non-A, non-B hepatitis, halothane hepatitis or paracetamol poisoning accompanied by features of gross hepatic failure (such as acidosis, gross coagulopathy and renal failure), if performed before the development of cerebral oedema, has a good prognosis.

7

Nephrology

INVESTIGATIONS

A thorough history and examination are fundamental to the investigation of patients with suspected renal disease and will identify those with a history of analgesic abuse or associated diseases such as hypertension, diabetes mellitus and connective tissue disorders.

Biochemistry Urea, creatinine, calcium, urate and glucose. Creatinine, especially in the elderly is insensitive and severe impairment of renal function may exist with only minimal increases in serum creatinine. Creatinine clearance is more sensitive but is subject to inaccuracies related to urine collection. Autoantibodies (eg ANF, ANCA, AntiGBm) and complement may be indicated.

Urine examination Stick testing for protein, blood, glucose, ketones and pH. Microscopy for bacteria, WBCs and casts. Bacterial counts greater than 100 000/ml indicate significant infection in a proper MSU. Casts containing RBCs occur in conditions with glomerular inflammation; granular casts may indicate tubular damage while hyaline casts occur in chronic renal disease and in normal individuals after exercise. Urinary protein quantification from 24-hour urine collection.

Ultrasound This will assess kidney size and any dilatation of the proximal renal tract or bladder, indicating obstruction.

Radiology The plain abdominal film may identify the size, shape and position of the kidneys as well as radio-opaque calculi and nephrocalcinosis. Intravenous urography assesses the size of the kidneys, obstruction and to some extent renal function but may be nephrotoxic in acute renal failure and myeloma. Retrograde pyelography is used to identify the site and degree of ureteric obstruction. The micturating cystogram is invaluable in assessing vesicoureteric reflux.

Radionuclide scan This is useful in assessing asymmetrical renal function. Dynamic computer analysis allows assessment of renal blood supply as well as the degree and rate of excretion. It is particularly useful in differentiating acute tubular necrosis from renal ischaemia in renal transplants.

Renal biopsy This is essential for establishing the diagnosis when this is unclear and when renal size is normal, but carries a 1% risk of serious complications such as haemorrhage. Electron microscopy and immunohistochemistry have greatly increased its diagnostic sensitivity. Its value in those with bilateral small shrunken kidneys where management is unlikely to be influenced is limited.

Renal angiography Essential in demonstrating renovascular disease and may be intra-arterial or intravenous using digital subtraction techniques. When renal artery stenosis is detected angioplasty may be curative.

E ▶ ACUTE RENAL FAILURE (ARF) page 473

POLYCYSTIC RENAL DISEASE

Science basics This inherited disorder may be associated with cystic disease of other organs, eg liver and pancreas. Two main forms exist: • the infantile autosomal recessive variety and • the adult autosomal dominant form. Both kidneys are involved with cysts, primarily cortical, increasing in size with time.

Clinical features Renal angle pain, haematuria, hypertension and uraemia. Renal masses related to cysts or renal tumours may be palpable. Intracranial vascular malformation giving rise to bruit or CVA may be present.

Investigations • U&Es • Creatinine • Creatinine clearance • Abdominal US, IVU and retrograde pyelography.

> **Management box**
> ▶ Symptomatic with control of hypertension and treatment of renal failure with dialysis or transplantation when indicated.
> ▶ Screening of relatives over the age of 30 years by renal US should be undertaken in association with genetic counselling.

Prognosis End-stage renal failure develops in middle age. Death may be from cardiac failure or stroke as well as uraemia.

RENAL TUBULAR ACIDOSIS

Science basics This results from failure of acid secretion in the distal tubule or proximal bicarbonate absorption. It may be inherited or secondary (Table 7.1).

> **Management box**
> ▶ Removal of cause where possible.
> ▶ Bicarbonate supplements to maintain plasma bicarbonate >18 mmol/l.
> ▶ Potassium supplements for those with hypocalcaemia.
> ▶ Calcium and 1-α-hydroxycholecaliferol if osteomalacia.

Table 7.1
Types and causes of RTA)

Cause	Distal RTA (type I)	Proximal RTA (type II)
Primary	Autosomal dominant	Familial
Secondary		
Renal disease	Pyelonephritis	Nephrotic syndrome
	Medullary sponge kidney	Fanconi syndrome
	Hydronephrosis	Transplanted kidney
	Transplanted kidney	
Drugs	Lithium	Tetracycline
Metabolic	Hypercalcaemia	Hypercalcaemia
	Amyloidosis	Cystinosis
	Hyperglobulinaemia	Tyrosinosis
	Cryoglobulinaemia	Amyloidosis
Miscellaneous	Connective tissue disease eg PBC, SLE	Heavy metal poisoning

RENAL CALCULI

Science basics Renal stones affect 1% of the population and occur when solutes come out of solution, either because they are present in excessive quantities, the urine is over-concentrated or because of lack of inhibitors of crystallization. The majority are composed of calcium (75%), magnesium-phosphate mixtures (15%) or urate (5%).

Clinical features

Symptoms: may be asymptomatic especially if intra-renal. Loin pain, renal colic with pain radiating to groin, nausea and vomiting, strangury.

Signs: often few, haematuria, loin tenderness, pyrexia if associated infection.

Investigations To identify stone: • Plain abdominal X-ray (calcium and magnesium phosphate stones are radio-dense and urate stones radio-lucent) • Renal US • IVU • Collect and sieve urine. To identify cause: • History of dehydration, excessive calcium intake, diuretic or vitamin D therapy, gout or small bowel resection resulting in hyperoxaluria • U&E, plasma and urinary calcium, urinary pH and culture, plasma uric acid and bicarbonate • 24-hour urinary excretion of Ca^{2+},

PO_4 and urate • Cystinuria is rare but a family history of stones should prompt exclusion by urinary cystine measurement • IVU or US will identify causes such as medullary sponge kidney.

> **Management box**
> ▸ Analgesia: this usually requires opiates, eg pethidine 100 mg im, although NSAIDs such as indometacin 50 mg tid or diclofenac 50 mg bd/tid may also be useful providing patient is not dehydrated and renal function is normal.
> ▸ Antispasmodic agents such as Pro-Banthine 10 mg tid may be useful.
> ▸ High fluid intake, eg 250–500 ml/hour.
> ▸ Most stones pass spontaneously but intervention is necessary in those in whom infection and/or obstruction is identified. In such cases the stone may be extracted cystoscopically with a Dormia basket if in the distal ureter, operatively if proximal or be fragmented by ultrasonic lithotripsy.

Prevention of recurrence Attention to high fluid intake and avoidance of dehydration. Where a precipitating factor such as excessive calcium intake is suspected dietary modification is advisable.

RENAL TRACT TUMOURS

RENAL ADENOCARCINOMA (HYPERNEPHROMA)

This arises from renal tubular epithelium and is commonest in males in the 5th decade. Risk factors include smoking, renal cysts in dialysis patients and von Hippel-Lindau disease.

Clinical features

Symptoms: haematuria, loin pain, fever and fatigue.

Signs: include palpable mass, anaemia or polycythaemia.

Investigations • Urinalysis • Biochemistry for hypercalcaemia • Haematology for anaemia or polycythaemia • CXR for metastases • Renal and hepatic US, IVU • Angiography and CT scanning.

Management box
▶ Nephrectomy if no evidence of metastatic disease offers a 5-year survival of 70%. If spread is identified progesterone therapy may induce remission.
▶ Rarely resection of solitary metastases is indicated.

TRANSITIONAL CELL TUMOURS OF THE RENAL PELVIS

Risk factors include smoking and analgesic abuse. Presentation, diagnosis and treatment similar to hypernephroma.

BLADDER TRANSITIONAL CELL TUMOURS

These are commoner in males over 40 years. Risk factors include smoking, exposure to industrial chemicals, cyclophosphamide therapy and *Schistosoma haematobium* infection.

Clinical features Painless haematuria or symptoms of urinary retention.

Investigations • Urinary cytology and cystoscopy.

Management box
▶ Superficial disease can be adequately treated by endoscopic resection with follow-up surveillance.
▶ Intravesical chemotherapy may be useful.
▶ Advanced disease requires surgery and chemotherapy.

PROSTATIC CANCER

The third commonest malignancy in males, this occurs in the elderly and may be very slow growing.

Clinical features Urinary obstruction commonest although distant metastases, eg to vertebrae, may produce symptoms.

Investigations • PR may reveal a craggy gland with obliteration of the median furrow • Serum acid phosphatase or prostate specific antigen are commonly elevated when metastatic spread has occurred • Transrectal prostatic biopsy.

Management box
▶ Transurethral resection of prostate (TURP) relieves symptoms of prostatism.

▸ Diethylstilbestrol 1 mg/day or buserelin nasal spray, which suppresses gonadotrophin release, reduce tumour growth as does orchidectomy.
▸ Radiotherapy in selected cases.

Prognosis   Very variable from months to many years.

URINARY TRACT INFECTION

Science basics   Infection within the urinary tract can be conveniently divided into that affecting the kidney (pyelonephritis) or the bladder (cystitis). They are not mutually exclusive. UTI is particularly common and 50% of women will experience symptoms of UTI sometime during life. Bacteria involved are: *Enterobacteriaceae*, eg *Enterobacter* spp., *Escherichia coli*, *Klebsiella* spp., *Proteus* spp., *Serratia* spp; Pseudomonadaceae, eg *Pseudomonas aeruginosa*; Gram-positive cocci, eg *Enterococci*, *Staph.* spp., *Strep.* Group *B*, *D* and *G*, *Strep. viridans* and others, eg *Flavobacterium* spp.

Clinical features

Symptoms: may be none. Commonly dysuria, frequency, urgency, fever, incontinence and retention.

Signs: include haematuria and tenderness suprapubically (cystitis) or over the renal angle (pyelonephritis) and features of uraemia. Features of cystitis without evidence of infection occur in the urethral syndrome.

Investigations   • Urine analysis, microscopy and culture. Microscopic haematuria and proteinuria are common. More than 100 000 organisms/ml on a fresh MSU indicates UTI despite any lack of symptoms and should be treated in the elderly, children and during pregnancy. Pyuria without obvious organisms occurs with renal TB and with analgesic abuse • BP • plasma electrolytes and creatinine should be checked and • IVU considered particularly if infection is recurrent or in childhood • Radionuclide scanning to show scarring.

Management box
▸ Drink frequently, eg 3–4 l/day, administration of sodium bicarbonate 2 g qid to alkalinize the urine and avoid sexual intercourse. Careful perineal hygiene.
▸ Antibiotics ideally tailored according to sensitivity determined from urine culture. Most usually amoxicillin 250 mg tid or two 3 g sachets over 24 hours or trimethoprin 200 mg bd for 5 days. →

▶ Causes of failure to respond to treatment or relapse include failure to complete course of antibiotics, reinfection from septic site, eg renal calculi or bladder tumour, urinary retention, eg neurogenic bladder, resistant organisms and post-menopausal urethral atrophy.

CHRONIC RENAL FAILURE

Science basics This refers to the gradual permanent loss of renal function leading to uraemia.

Aetiology Diabetes mellitus, GN, pyelonephritis, hypertension, renal stones, chronic reflux nephropathy, bladder outlet obstruction, connective tissue diseases, polycystic kidneys, myeloma and hypercalcaemia.

Clinical features

Symptoms: patients may be asymptomatic in the early stages. Pruritus, nocturia, polyuria, anorexia, dyspnoea, confusion, neuropathy, vomiting and lethargy.

Signs: pallor, pleural effusions, pericarditis, pulmonary oedema, hypertension, bruising, ascites, peripheral oedema and increased pigmentation.

Investigations

Biochemistry: increased urea and creatinine, hyperkalaemia, hyponatraemia, hyperphosphataemia, hypocalcaemia and metabolic acidosis • Urine: microscopy for casts, analysis for protein, specific gravity and creatinine clearance (this may be significantly reduced with a normal serum creatinine especially in the elderly).

Radiology: • Plain film • US to demonstrate renal size and possible obstruction • Retrograde pyelography if ureteric obstruction is suspected • Renal biopsy only usually considered if renal size is normal.

Management box
▶ Dialysis should be considered in those with symptoms, uncontrolled fluid retention and creatinine > 500μmol/l or bicarbonate < 12 mmol/l and in asymptomatic patients with a serum potassium > 5 mmol/l; this may be either haemodialysis or chronic ambulatory peritoneal dialysis (CAPD).
▶ The choice of treatment must be tailored to the individual patient.

- Abdominal surgery or sepsis and poor patient motivation are contraindications to CAPD, while coagulopathy, HBV carriage and poor venous access are factors against haemodialysis. For patients fit for surgery renal transplant must be considered to improve the quality of life.
- Treatment of BP is vital in management of CRF. Aim is <130/80 mmHg; <120/70 mmHg in diabetes mellitus or proteinurea. Drugs used are metoprolol 50–100 mg/day and/or nifedipine 10–20 µg tid.
- Reduction of hyperphosphataemia with calcium carbonate in doses titrated to reduce phosphate to normal.
- Prevention of renal bone disease with 1 α vitamin D 0.25 µg/day.
- Avoidance of nephrotoxic drugs, eg tetracycline, aminoglycosides and potassium-sparing diuretics, eg spironolactone and amiloride.
- Low protein diets (0.8 mg/kg/day) and good BP control may delay the progression of renal failure.
- A restricted fluid intake is required in the majority both before and after dialysis.
- Low salt diet is indicated in some patients with hypertension.
- Erythropoietin to correct anaemia.

DIALYSIS AND RENAL TRANSPLANTATION

DIALYSIS

Treatment of acute and chronic renal failure is most commonly with dialysis in which the patient's blood is perfused across a semipermeable membrane against dialysis solution, thereby removing salt, water and low molecular weight solutes such as urea. The membrane may be synthetic as in haemodialysis or natural as in peritoneal dialysis. As well as treating acute and chronic renal failure, dialysis is indicated in the treatment of severe poisoning with lithium, aspirin, methanol and ethylene glycol.

Indications ARF when complicated by water overload, hyperkalaemia, acidosis or uraemia. CRF when symptoms of uraemia develop.

Haemodialysis access This is usually via a radiocephalic arteriovenous (Cimino) fistula although short-term dialysis is possible via large central veins (care should be taken to avoid cannulating the veins between wrist and antecubital fossa to allow for fistulae later). Haemofiltration, whereby large volumes of fluid can be removed, is possible via more peripheral veins.

Despite haemodialysis many of the manifestations of CRF, such as anaemia and lethargy, persist although erythropoietin therapy may be important in the future.

Complications Infection and thrombosis of vascular access, haemorrhage, hypotension, hypoxia, cramps, seizures, air embolism, haemolysis.

Peritoneal dialysis In ARF intermittent peritoneal dialysis is effective in removing fluid, solutes and balancing electrolytes. In CRF CAPD is an effective alternative to haemodialysis in cooperative patients. Its main advantages include freedom from the dialysis machine and lack of requirement for vascular access. The main disadvantage is peritonitis.

TRANSPLANTATION

Now an accepted therapeutic alternative which allows the patient to return to near-normal life. The donor and recipient should be blood-group matched and an attempt made to optimize HLA match, especially DR, although this is not always achieved. 5-year survival for an HLA identical kidney is approximately 75%. Immunosuppressive drugs, usually prednisolone, azathioprine and ciclosporin or tacrolimus, are necessary to prevent rejection. The transplanted kidney is usually sited in the right iliac fossa where subsequent biopsy is easy.

Complications Acute rejection, thrombosis, ATN, opportunistic infections, ciclosporin renal toxicity, chronic rejection, hypertension and increased risk of malignancy, eg lymphoma.

GLOMERULONEPHRITIS

Science basics Acute glomerulonephritis is characterized by haematuria, proteinuria, hypertension, oedema, uraemia and often oliguria. It is believed to be due to humoral immune mechanisms. Numerous causes are recognized and associated with different clinical features (Table 7.2).

Poststreptococcal GN

This is less common now than formerly. It is commonest in childhood developing 1–3 weeks after streptococcal laryngitis or skin infection. Diagnosis is by a positive skin or throat swab for Lancefield group A beta-haemolytic streptococci, rising ASO titre, reduced plasma C3 and biopsy showing diffuse proliferative GN. Treatment is supportive, correcting fluid and electrolyte imbalance and hypertension, bed-rest initially, 40 g protein and 100 mmol sodium diet and penicillin if streptococcal infection

Table 7.2
Causes of nephrotic syndrome

Glomerular disease (75%)
    Membranous GN
    Minimal-change GN
    Focal segmental glomerulosclerosis
    Membranoproliferative
    Mesangiocapillary
    SLE
Infections
    SBE, HBV infection, malaria (commonest worldwide), sickle
cell disease, syphilis, HIV
Metabolic
    Diabetes mellitus, amyloidosis
Drugs
    Penicillamine, gold, NSAID, captopril, tolbutamide, iv drug
abuse
Malignancy
    Lymphoma, leukaemia, GI and breast tumours, myeloma

still present. Haematuria and proteinuria may persist for 1–2
years but rarely progresses to CRF.

Postinfective GN
This is similar but often milder than poststreptococcal GN and
often resolves after adequate treatment of the underlying
infection.

Henoch–Schönlein purpura
This generalized vasculitis, commonest in children, is characterized by purpura, GN, abdominal pain and arthralgia. Serum
IgA is increased in 50%. Treatment is supportive and the value
of steroids is unproven. A variant of this (IgA nephropathy)
presenting with haematuria is found in young male adults.

Rapidly progressive GN
Characterized by a gradual onset of proteinuria, haematuria and
renal failure over a period of weeks or months. The cause may be
secondary to infection, eg subacute bacterial endocarditis and
hepatitis B, connective tissue disease, eg SLE, Goodpasture's
vasculitis, Wegener's granulomatosis, polyarteritis nodosa or
idiopathic. Renal biopsy shows crescents of fibrosis in Bowman's
capsule; linear IgG or immune complex deposits in the glomerular
basement membrane may or may not be present. Treatment
depends upon the underlying disease. In the idiopathic form

plasmapheresis, steroids and cytotoxic agents may be useful in some patients.

Membranous GN

This usually presents with proteinuria and often nephrotic syndrome (urinary protein >3 g/day with oedema and hypoalbuminaemia <30 g/l) (Table 7.2). Haematuria and hypertension are usually absent. Renal vein thrombosis is a common complication. Underlying conditions such as connective tissue disorders, neoplasia and drug reactions, eg penicillamine, may be present. Renal biopsy shows subepithelial IgG deposits with a thickened basement membrane. Steroids may reduce proteinuria but not the progression of disease which ends in uraemia in 30%. Outcome is improved with combined immunosuppression.

Mesangiocapillary GN

This usually affects young patients presenting with haematuria, hypertension, reduced GFR and hypocomplementaemia, progressing to renal failure over some years. Renal biopsy identifies two variants: type 1 with large subepithelial deposits and type 2 with deposition within the lamina densa of the basement membrane. Treatment with prednisolone in those with associated SLE and/or aspirin and dipyridamole may slow progression.

Minimal-change GN

This is commonest in childhood causing 80% of cases of nephrotic syndrome. It is responsible for 30% of nephrotic syndrome in adults. Renal biopsy reveals normal glomeruli on light microscopy although electron microscopy shows fusion of podocytes. Immune-complex deposition is not seen. The proteinuria is selective and is steroid-sensitive, although relapse is common.

Focal segmental glomerulosclerosis

This is a slowly progressive disease with hypertension, haematuria and reduced GFR. It may follow minimal change GN or be due to vesicoureteric reflux, iv drug abuse or HIV infection. Renal biopsy shows fibrosis of some of the juxtamedullary glomeruli. Approximately 50% respond to steroids.

8

Neurology

INVESTIGATIONS

More than in any other system, assessment of the nervous system relies upon thorough clinical examination. Further investigations to a large part serve to confirm or refute clinical suspicions.

Lumbar puncture (LP) Indications include suspected acute or chronic infection, inflammation, subarachnoid haemorrhage and malignancy. The pressure should be measured and CSF taken for naked eye examination, biochemical (including oligoclonal bands if suspecting MS), cytological (must reach lab within 4 hours) and bacteriological analysis. Complications include headache, introduction of infection and cerebellar herniation (in those with raised intracranial pressure (ICP)). LP should not be performed before CT if confusion, depression of consciousness, focal neurological signs, seizures, local infection or coagulopathy are present.

CT scan Readily available imaging of brain and CSF spaces for diagnosis of subdural and extradural haematoma, intracranial tumours, cerebral oedema and atrophy and hydrocephalus. Valuable in differentiating cerebral haemorrhage from infarction. Contrast CT scanning may identify large cerebral aneurysms and arteriovenous malformations.

Angiography Required for the accurate diagnosis of vascular occlusions, vasculitis, stenosis and aneurysms and to determine the vascular anatomy of tumours prior to surgery. Carotid Doppler and transcranial Doppler are useful in identifying abnormalities in blood flow in major intracranial and extracranial vessels.

Electroencephalography Primarily used in the diagnosis of epilepsy and encephalopathy.

Magnetic resonance imaging (MRI) More sensitive than CT and avoids X-ray exposure. Particularly useful for examining the posterior fossa and spinal cord and detecting demyelination.

Myelography Used for the visualization of the spinal canal and cord when MRI not available.

Evoked responses These measure electrical activity within the cortex from visual, auditory and tactile stimuli. Useful in detecting abnormalities within sensory pathways where structural lesions cannot be identified and for monitoring disease progression during surgery.

Electromyography Essential in distinguishing neuropathies from myopathies, indicating whether mononeuropathy, mononeuritis multiplex or polyneuropathy, axonal or demyelinating, sensory and/or motor.

Perimetry, audiometry and labyrinthine function tests   Used to confirm and quantitate sensory neurological deficit as in MS.

Brain biopsy   Rarely indicated other than for tissue diagnosis of suspected tumour.

Tensilon test   The administration of edrophonium (Tensilon) 8 mg iv (after 2 mg test dose) improves power after 90 seconds for 3–5 minutes in myasthenia gravis; perform blinded versus N-saline. Perform ECG prior to test to exclude conduction defects. Perform with atropine and resuscitation facilities to hand.

CEREBROVASCULAR DISEASE

Science basics   A stroke results from ischaemic infarction (85%) or haemorrhage within the brain. It affects 1–2/1000 per year and is the third commonest cause of death. Risk factors include age, hypertension, diabetes mellitus, smoking, hyperlipidaemia, the oral contraceptive pill and excessive alcohol.

Aetiology   Thrombosis, embolism, haemorrhage, vasculitis and hypoperfusion.

Clinical features   These depend upon the cause, eg thrombosis or haemorrhage and the vessel involved: thrombosis is commoner and symptoms develop over hours often during sleep, while cerebral haemorrhage usually presents abruptly during waking hours often with a premonitory headache. Strokes can be divided into: • completed stroke (rapid onset with persistent deficit) • stroke-in-evolution (gradual step-wise development) • transient ischaemic attack (symptoms resolve completely within 24 hours and usually within half an hour) • progressive diffuse disease (no major incidents but gradual deterioration in cerebral function leading to multi-infarct dementia with bilateral pyramidal signs).

Investigations   In all strokes • BP (frequently increased temporarily after stroke) • U&Es, LFTs, glucose and cholesterol • FBC to exclude anaemia, thrombocytopenia or polycythaemia • ESR • sickle-cell screen in Afro-Caribbean patients • CT scan to exclude other intracranial pathology and to distinguish infarct from haemorrhage • ECG • Consider blood cultures, syphilis serology, echocardiography, temporal artery biopsy, carotid Doppler studies +/– angiography • In young strokes (under 50) embolic sources should be rigorously excluded with trans-oesophageal echocardiography and carotid Doppler for carotid dissection • ANF, RF, anticardiolipin antibodies • Coagulation studies • Protein electrophoresis • ANCA • Thick film if from malaria region.

Management box
▶ Where possible in Stroke Units, as this reduces short- and long-term mortality by 20–25%.
▶ Major international trials are in progress on the role of aspirin, heparin and thrombolysis in the acute treatment of stroke. Warfarin is indicated for definite cardiac emboli.
▶ Other than in hypertensive encephalopathy (>230/130) or proven cerebral haemorrhage with markedly elevated BP, hypertension should not be treated acutely, though it is the most important remediable long-term risk factor for stroke.
▶ Aspirin (300 mg daily) should be given to patients with non-haemorrhagic strokes to prevent further vascular events.
▶ Carotid endarterectomy significantly improves survival in those with symptomatic carotid disease with stenosis of >75%.
▶ Multidisciplinary rehabilitation approach accelerates recovery and placement in community.

Prognosis (Table 8.1) Impaired conscious level, TACI and haemorrhage are predictive of early death. LACI, PACI and POCI have similar, better outcomes. PACI has a high risk of early recurrence and requires urgent investigation and consideration for carotid endarterectomy to prevent a more devastating event.

Table 8.1
Clinical subtypes of stroke

Type	Aetiology	Clinical presentation
Lacunar infarct (LACI)	Small penetrating arteries of basal ganglia, internal capsule, thalamus and pons Rarely embolic – microvascular	Pure sensory* *or* Pure motor* *or* Sensorimotor* *or* Ataxic hemiparesis (never dysphagia, visiospatial, predominantly proprioceptive sensory loss or impaired conscious level)
Total anterior circulation infarct (TACI)	Large cerebral haemorrhage or internal carotid/ middle cerebral occlusion, frequently embolic	*All* of cerebral dysfunction, haemorrhage, homonymous field deficit

Table 8.1
Clinical subtypes of stroke *(Cont'd)*

Type	Aetiology	Clinical presentation
Partial anterior circulation infart (PACI)	Lobar haemorrhage or branch of middle/anterior cerebral artery or boundary zone infarct, frequently embolic	Motor/sensory deficit at least two of face/arm/leg 2 of 3 of TACI or motor/sensory deficit more restricted than LACI
Posterior circulation infarct (POCI)	Basilar and posterior cerebral circulation thromboembolic or microvascular	Ipsilateral cranial nerve palsy with contralateral motor/sensory deficit

*at least two of face/arm/leg and if only two whole limb must be affected

E **SUBARACHNOID HAEMORRHAGE** → page 446

CEREBRAL TUMOURS

Science basics These account for 2% of deaths and although may be histologically malignant, primary tumours rarely metastasize outwith the brain. 50% of brain tumours are metastases from other sites, 25% gliomas, 20% meningiomas and 5% neuromas, pituitary adenomas and craniopharyngiomas.

Clinical features Progressive nature is important – gradual over years to subacutely over days, include headache, cognitive or personality change, unsteadiness, weakness, paraesthesia and also epilepsy and visual obscurations.

Signs: focal deficit or non-localizing due to raised intracranial pressure – drowsiness, lateral rectus palsy, increased blind spots. Examine for evidence of primary, eg breast, thyroid, abdominal, genital or rectal masses, lymphadenopathy, chest signs or skin lesions, bradycardia, papilloedema (if unilateral with optic atrophy in the other eye = Foster Kennedy syndrome), nystagmus, grasp reflex.

Investigations • CT scan with contrast and MRI scanning. If metastatic disease is suspected likely sources should be screened non-invasively, eg CXR, abdominal/pelvic US, HCG, CEA and αFP • CSF cytological examination provided there is no evidence of raised ICP • Stereotactic or open-brain biopsy.

Management box

▶ Chemotherapy shown to improve survival in lymphomas, leukaemias, testicular tumours and to a lesser extent malignant gliomas; palliative to reduce symptoms related to cerebral oedema and raised intracranial pressure. Dexamethasone 4 mg qid may produce dramatic improvement in symptoms. Less often larger doses and intravenous mannitol 20% are required. Some pituitary adenomas may be reduced in size by such drugs as bromocriptine.

▶ Surgical treatment valuable if causing focal signs and operation is unlikely to cause substantial further neurological damage, particularly for benign tumours where it may be curative, but increasingly also palliatively for gliomas and single metastasis. Ventriculoperitoneal shunt can relieve obstructive hydrocephalus.

▶ Radiotherapy improves survival from most tumour types with an additive effect to surgery and chemotherapy.

CENTRAL NERVOUS SYSTEM INFECTIONS

E▶ MENINGITIS → page 444

E▶ ENCEPHALITIS → page 446

PARKINSONISM

Science basics A clinical syndrome characterized by bradykinesia (slow movement), hypokinesia (reduced movement), rest tremor, rigidity and postural instability. The underlying pathology is dopamine depletion within the basal ganglia, the cause of which is usually idiopathic (Parkinson's disease). In multiple system atrophy there are additional features of pyramidal, cerebellar, eye movement or autonomic dysfunction – these have a poor prognosis and poor response to dopaminergic therapy. Less common causes include drugs, especially phenothiazines, cerebral tumours, Wilson's disease and rarely carbon monoxide poisoning, repeated head trauma and following encephalitis lethargica.

Clinical features Usually in subjects over 40 years, presenting with hypokinesia or slowness and delay in movement typified by difficulty with fine manipulation and a slow, shuffling gait. The rest tremor is slow and gives rise to the characteristic pill-rolling movement and is often made worse by stress and embarrassment. Rigidity on passive movement often 'cog-wheel' or lead-pipe in nature. Power is well maintained. Symptoms are unilateral initially.

Investigations The diagnosis is essentially clinical and the cause can usually be obtained from the history, eg drug therapy and examination.

Differential diagnosis Other causes of tremor such as essential tremor, thyrotoxicosis, anxiety, alcoholism and cerebellar disease are usually easily differentiated. Dementia and hypothyroidism may mimic the slowness and paucity of movement. Atherosclerotic dementia with bilateral spasticity may mimic Parkinsonism.

Management box
▶ For mild disability anticholinergic drugs, amantadine or selegiline may be sufficient but as disability progresses L-dopa and/or dopamine agonists are required. Treatment must be introduced at low dose and very gradually increased to reduce adverse effects such as nausea, vomiting and hypotension. Selegiline may also be useful in 'off' effect and is perhaps neuroprotective. Apomorphine SC infusion can reduce fluctuations.
▶ Physiotherapy, OT and speech therapy are important in advanced disease.

Prognosis This is variable and although drug treatment improves symptoms it does not reduce the underlying progression. However, lifespan is not substantially reduced in idiopathic Parkinson's disease. Cognitive and neuropsychiatric problems are common with chronic disease and 20–30% develop dementia.

MULTIPLE SCLEROSIS

Science basics This inflammatory demyelinating disorder affects 1 in 1000 of the population and is the most common cause of severe disability in young adults in the UK. The aetiology is unknown but risk factors include habitation in temperate zones of both the northern and southern hemispheres, HLA A3, B7 DW2/DR2 and a family history of the disease and probably has an autoimmune basis triggered by a virus.

Clinical features

Symptoms: very variable. Age of onset is usually 20–50 years, commoner in women. Focal inflammation can affect any area of the CNS but there is a predilection for the optic nerves (pain on movement and blurring), brainstem and cerebellum (diplopia, vertigo and ataxia) and spinal cord (weakness, paraesthesia and sphincter disturbance). Fatigue is common. Symptoms appear subacutely before resolving partially or completely over weeks. A hot bath may markedly, though temporarily, exacerbate motor symptoms. A relapsing-remitting course is typical though 15% have a chronic progressive form.

Signs: include decreased visual acuity, optic disc pallor, internuclear ophthalmoplegia, nystagmus, dysarthria, intention tremor, spasticity, hyperreflexia (including extensor plantars), sensory loss notably proprioceptive.

Investigations History consistent with tremors disseminated in time and space and clinical features are usually highly suggestive • Oligoclonal bands of IgG present in the CSF but not serum • MRI scanning identifies periventricular lesions in 95% of clinically definite cases. However this appearance is non-specific occurring in other inflammatory conditions and over the age of 45 years • Delayed auditory, visual and sensory evoked potentials are useful in detecting abnormalities when not clinically apparent.

Management box
High-dose steroid therapy (methylprednisolone 1 g iv for 3 days or a reducing course of 60 mg prednisolone) often reduces the duration and severity of relapse, but does not influence the natural history. Many other immunomodulators have been proposed, of which azathioprine or cyclophosphamide may reduce the relapse rate but are too toxic for general use. Interferon beta can be prescribed by Consultant Neurologists for patients who have had two or more relapses in the past 2 years and are ambulant.

EPILEPSY

Science basics This is defined as a periodic disturbance in neurological function, often with changes in consciousness; due to abnormal excessive electrical discharge within the brain. Numerous classifications exist but the most commonly used is that where seizures are divided into primary generalized or partial attacks. The former may be tonic/clonic (grand mal), tonic or clonic in isolation, myoclonic or associated with absence (petit mal). The latter may be divided into simple partial (motor or sensory) with retained awareness or complex partial with impaired awareness and secondarily may progress into generalized seizures.

Aetiology This varies with age, but majority idiopathic.

- Infants: hypoxia, metabolic disorders, infection.
- Adolescents: trauma, alcohol/drugs, infection, tumour.
- Elderly: cerebrovascular, degenerative, tumour, metabolic.

Clinical features 'Positive' phenomena, eg tonic-clonic movements, hallucinations, rather than 'negative' as in a cerebrovascular event, eg weakness, field loss. Generalized seizures result in disturbance of consciousness, the classical variety progressing through tonic, clonic and postictal phases, consisting of headache, confusion and drowsiness, often with tongue-biting and incontinence. In petit mal seizures cessation of mental activity occurs without prostration for less than 30 seconds, but this seldom persists over the age of 20. Complex partial seizures may present with motor (automatism: lip-smacking, plucking at clothes, hair), sensory (transient paraesthesia), autonomic (odd epigastric sensation, nausea, abnormal taste or smell) or psychic (unreality, *deja vu*, fear) features.

Signs: focal signs may reflect an underlying structural cause such as infarct or tumour. Gum hyperplasia is characteristic of phenytoin therapy, port-wine naevi in Sturge-Weber syndrome, cafe-au-lait spots in neurofibromatosis and adenoma sebaceum in tuberous sclerosis. Evidence of previous CVAs with long-tract signs may also be obvious.

Investigations • History crucial and witness invaluable in distinguishing from syncope (arrhythmia, vasovagal, postural hypotension) or less common hypoglycaemia, phaeochromocytoma, panic attacks and pseudoseizures • Biochemical tests including U&E, glucose, calcium, LFT are required in the young and in acute presentation in adults • CT and MRI scans may be necessary in those suspected of having focal neurological deficit • EEG may provide evidence of focal activity but a normal test does not exclude the diagnosis • Prolactin levels should show a substantial increase from baseline following a tonic-clonic seizure – this will be absent in pseudoseizures.

Management box

▶ Phenytoin, carbamazepine and valproate are equally effective for most seizure types other than myoclonic epilepsy and petit mal where valproate or ethosuximide is preferred. Compliance and side-effect profile may determine the most suitable choice, eg phenytoin has the advantage of once-daily dosing but should be avoided in women as it may cause hirsutism. Most patients can be controlled on monotherapy.

▶ Newer anticonvulsants such as lamotrigine, gabapentin and vigabatrin are useful as add-on therapy in routine epilepsy. The correct dosage for an individual is that which controls seizures without unacceptable side-effects, the so-called therapeutic ranges are useful only for ensuring compliance and confirming suspected dose-related side-effects and need not be routinely checked.

▶ Seizures refractory to medical therapy should be referred for consideration of surgery.

E▶ STATUS EPILEPTICUS → page 447

NEUROPATHY

Science basics This can be divided into abnormalities which affect individual nerves (mononeuropathy) or several peripheral nerves either symmetrically (polyneuropathy) or asymmetrically (mononeuritis multiplex).

Clinical features

Symptoms: weakness, paraesthesia, pain and muscle cramps.

Signs: fasciculation, wasting, hypotonicity, weakness, hyporeflexia, sensory impairment (variably affecting different modalities).

MONONEUROPATHY

Aetiology Trauma, chronic entrapment, diabetes.

Clinical features The commonest affected nerves involved in mononeuropathy, irrespective of the cause, include median nerve, ulnar nerve, radial nerve, sciatic nerve, lateral popliteal nerve and tibial nerves. Compression of the median nerve at the wrist (carpal tunnel syndrome) presents with pain and paraesthesia characteristically waking at night (can affect whole of hand and radiate to forearm and shoulder). Weakness of thumb abduction and typical sensory loss.

Investigations The cause of the underlying abnormality is usually apparent on clinical examination, though consider endocrine, simple obesity or rarely amyloid in entrapment neuropathy. EMG confirms site of nerve damage and useful in clinically distinguishing most lesions on basis of motor and sensory involvement (Fig. 8.1).

> *Management box*
>
> **Management of carpal tunnel syndrome**
> Management is conservative with wrist splints and/or local corticosteroid injection, or surgical with decompression if signs or symptoms persist.

MONONEURITIS MULTIPLEX

Aetiology Diabetes, collagen-vascular, alcohol, leprosy, AIDS, *Borrelia*, malignancy, sarcoidosis, familial tendency to pressure palsies.

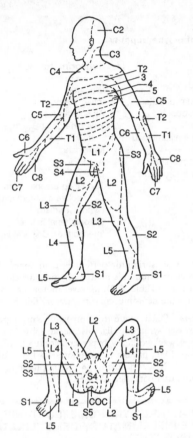

Fig. 8.1 Dermatomal anatomy.

Clinical features Involvement of two or more peripheral nerves.

Investigations • U&E, creatinine, glucose • FBC, ESR • RA/ANF/ANCA • protein electrophoresis • CXR • *Borrelia* serology • consider nerve biopsy, HIV, skin biopsy (leprosy).

POLYNEUROPATHY

This is a more generalized disturbance in peripheral nerves, typically starting distally giving rise to the 'glove-and-stocking'

Table 8.2
Causes of polyneuropathy

Motor	Sensorimotor
Guillain-Barré	Diabetes
Chronic demyelinating polyneuropathy	Inflammatory
Diphtheria	Alcohol abuse
Toxins, eg thallium, lead	Thiamine or vit B_{12} or E deficiency
Porphyria	Malignancy
HIV seroconversion	Amyloidosis
Hereditary neuropathies	Drugs
Botulism	Toxins, eg arsenic, gold
	Connective tissue disorders
	Hypothyroidism
	Chronic renal failure
	Infection, eg *Borrelia*, leprosy

distribution. A sensorimotor pattern is commonest but a pure motor, sensory or autonomic neuropathy may develop depending upon the cause (Table 8.2). Severe motor neuropathy may present with acute neuromuscular respiratory failure.

Investigations Differentiate from myopathy, myelopathy, motor neurone disease, syringomyelia, disease atrophy (no weakness), functional 'giveway' weakness, hyperventilation • U&E, creatinine, LFT, glucose, TFT, protein electrophoresis • FBC, ESR, plasma vitamin B_{12}, CXR, porphyrins • Neurophysiological studies • Nerve biopsy useful in selected cases.

GUILLAIN-BARRÉ SYNDROME (POST-INFECTIVE OR ACUTE INFLAMMATORY DEMYELINATING POLYNEUROPATHY)

This neuropathy commonly occurs 1–4 weeks after a diarrhoeal or respiratory infection, particularly *Campylobacter* or *Mycoplasma*.

Clinical features Rapidly progressive ascending motor weakness more marked proximally than distally. Respiratory muscle weakness may lead to ventilatory failure. The Miller-Fisher variant associated with antibodies to ganglioside GQ_{1b} presents with opthalmoplegia, areflexia and ataxia.

Investigations • Increased CSF protein content • Other causes of pure motor neuropathies should be excluded (eg lead poisoning).

Management box
▶ Regular monitoring of respiratory function with vital capacity and ABGs. Ventilatory support may be required. Plasma exchange and iv immunoglobulins shorten the duration of ventilation and improve prognosis if started within 14 days of the onset of symptoms. Steroids are ineffective.

MYOPATHY

Science basics Primary disorders of skeletal muscle are unusual and may have a wide range of causes.

Aetiology (Table 8.3)

Clinical features

Symptoms: most common is proximal weakness, eg difficulty washing hair, rising from chair, myalgia and cramps.

Signs: include proximal muscle wasting with waddling gait, tenderness and retained reflexes. In certain conditions characteristic associated features such as frontal baldness, ptosis, cataracts, sternomastoid muscle atrophy and testicular atrophy (in dystrophia myotonica) may be present.

Investigations • Biochemistry • U&E, glucose, calcium, magnesium, LFT, TFT, serum electrophoresis, CXR • FBC, elevated CK and ESR (particularly elevated in inflammatory myopathies) • EMG • Consider muscle biopsy, ANF, cortisol, HIV. The

Table 8.3
Causes of myopathy

Inherited	Acquired
Duchenne and Becker myotonic dystrophy	Alcohol
	Malignancy
Fascioscapulo-humeral dystrophy	Endocrine – thyroid, parathyroid, adrenal
Limb-girdle dystrophy	Drugs, eg cimetidine, zidovudine
Periodic paralysis	
Mitochondrial atrophy	Osteomalacia
Glycogen and lipid storage	Inflammatory – polymyositis, dermatomyositis, vasculitis
	Infection – viral (coxsackie, echo, influenzae, HIV), rarely bacterial and parasitic

muscle biopsy may however be normal in certain cases where obvious clinical disease exists due to often patchy involvement.

Management box

▸ For the inherited varieties no treatment exists and genetic counselling assumes high priority.

▸ In those acquired cases due to metabolic or toxic causes, correction of the metabolic defect or removal of the drug or toxin may result in rapid clinical improvement.

▸ Prolonged corticosteroid treatment is highly effective in poly-myalgia rheumatica.

MYASTHENIA GRAVIS

Science basics   In myasthenia gravis serum IgG antibodies are produced that cause loss of the postsynaptic acetylcholine receptors in the neuromuscular junction, blocking transmission of the action potential to the muscle. It is associated with thymic hyperplasia in 60%, thymoma in 10% and with other immune disorders, eg RA, SLE, thyroid disease.

Clinical features   Fatiguable muscle weakness causing ptosis, diplopia, dysphagia, dysarthria, 'myasthenic snarl' on smiling, difficulty holding up head, limb weakness proximal and distal. Varied presentation from purely ocular disease to acute respiratory failure.

Investigations   Clinical diagnosis, confirmed by positive Tensilon test (PS) with improvement in weakness. Acetylcholine receptor antibodies present in 85% of cases • EMG existence of detrimental response to repetitive stimulation • Thymoma should be excluded by CT.

Management box

▸ Mild forms may be controlled with acetylcholinesterase in-hibitors (eg pyridostigmine alone) but more often immuno-suppression (prednisolone and/or azathioprine) is required.

▸ In acute deterioration patency and vital capacity should be monitored and precipitants such as infection or drugs should be sought – plasma exchange is useful in severe disease.

▸ Thymectomy should be performed early in all under 45s and in those with thymoma.

▸ Drugs which may potentiate myasthenic weakness include aminoglycosides, tetracyclines, quinine, procainamide, and β-blockers.

MOTOR NEURONE DISEASE

Science basics   Largely sporadic progressive disorder of unknown cause affecting upper and lower motor neurones. Onset usually in elderly but can occur in younger adults with death in 3 years in around 50% from pneumonia secondary to respiratory failure and complications of immobility. Intellect is preserved.

Clinical features   Presentation depends on relative involvement of the anterior horn cells of spinal cord, cranial nuclei and corticospinal tract, ie primarily lower motor neurone, bulbar or pyramidal features – usually a combination of all three develop.

Symptoms: slurring of speech, drooling of saliva, dysphagia, fatigue, weakness, clumsiness, limb pain (secondary to cramps, immobility, spasticity), breathlessness.

Signs: dysarthria, dysphagia, wasting and fasciculation of tongue with back jaw jerk, neck weakness, characteristically prominent limb wasting and fasciculation with hyperreflexia in some muscle groups, normal sensation. Early on reflexes can be asymmetric.

Investigations   • Essentially clinical diagnosis preferably with EMG support if widespread chronic denervation. Important to exclude other potential diagnoses • CSF analysis for malignant or infective meningomyelitis • Syphilis serology • Imaging of cervical spine if no clear bulbar involvement • Causes of motor neuropathy (page 175) if predominantly lower motor neurone pattern.

> **Management box**
> Symptomatic treatment with analgesia, quinine, anticholinergics to reduce salivary production, orthotic splints, home support, consider percutaneous gastrostomy for feeding and antidepressants.

SPINAL CORD DISORDER

Science basics   In the adult, the spinal cord extends from the medulla at the foramen magnum to L1. From each segment dorsal (sensory) and ventral (motor) nerves reunite and exit via the corresponding intervertebral foramen. Disorders either affect the cord focally at a particular segment or systems throughout its length, eg dorsal column.

Aetiology   Compressive cord disorders occur with vertebral disease (trauma, acute disc prolapse, osteoporotic collapse (rheumatoid arthritis) meningeal disease (syphilis, TB, metastatic), intradural tumour or intraspinal infection (*Staphylococcus*). Non-compressive disorders include infection causing either transverse myelitis (eg syphilis, EBV, brucellosis, mycoplasma, *Borrelia*) or widespread disease (AIDS), MS, nutritional deficiency (vitamin B_{12}, or E), paraneoplastic and degenerative disease (motor neurone disease, hereditary myelopathies). Radiculopathies result from trauma, compression or infection (HSV, Guillain-Barré (GBS)).

Clinical features

Symptoms: onset may be acute or chronic • localized spinal pain worse on movement with disc or spondylosis, or at rest with tumour • radiating to the affected myotome is typical of radiculopathy • clumsiness, weakness, sensory loss and urinary symptoms (retention acutely, urgency in chronic disease) can occur. A family history or past medical history of malignancy (± spinal irradiation) is important to elicit.

Signs: the level of cord compression can be deduced from knowledge of root myotomes, reflex changes (hyporeflexia at the affected level with hyperreflexia below) and a sensory level from feet to below the corresponding dermatome (see page 173), in acute disorders with accompanying paraspinal tenderness. Pes cavus may be present in hereditary neuropathies. Root-involvement may be associated with myotomal weakness and wasting, dermatomal sensory loss and root irritation (eg straight leg raise).

Investigations • Plain spinal films – AP and lateral (plus oblique, flexion and extension in cervical spine) • MRI preferred to myelography ± CT • Consider bone scan of previous malignancy, angiography if suspected arteriovenous malformation. If compression excluded • Serum B_{12} • Syphilis, *Borrelia*, viral (± HIV) serology • CSF (malignancy or infection or oligoclonal bands) • EMG (MND or GBS).

Management box

▶ Recovery from cord compression depends on the extent of neurological impairment and the duration of compression. Early treatment within 24 hours for acute compression may allow the return of useful function. Extradural compression due to malignancy is responsive to radiotherapy and may not require surgical decompression. Complete paralysis and urinary involvement are poor prognostic signs. Radiculopathy secondary to disc prolapse is treated conservatively with bed-rest, strong analgesia and support (collar/corset). If persisting pain or worsening signs, surgical intervention may be appropriate.

9

Endocrinology and metabolism

THYROTOXICOSIS

Science basics The commonest cause in the UK is autoimmune (Graves' disease) due to stimulating antibodies to the TSH receptor. Less often, a toxic nodule within a multinodular goitre or a thyroid adenoma may over-produce thyroxine. Hyperthyroidism is sometimes seen in viral (de Quervain's) thyroiditis in the early stages. Treatment with amiodarone may cause thyrotoxicosis. Rarely, self-administered thyroxine may be the cause.

Clinical features Females outnumber males 5:1.

Symptoms: include sweating, heat intolerance, amenorrhoea, sleep disturbance, irritability, palpitations, weight-loss, increased appetite and anxiety.

Signs: tachycardia, atrial fibrillation, exophthalmos, lid-lag, proximal myopathy, fine tremor and goitre (sometimes with a bruit). Pretibial myxoedema and acropachy are found in 5% of Graves' disease.

Investigations • T3 is always raised, T4 or fT4 usually raised and TSH suppressed. Suppressed TSH may also be seen in those with multinodular goitres • Technetium isotope scan is useful to differentiate viral thyroiditis (low uptake) from other causes and to differentiate Graves' disease from multinodular goitre • Presence of thyroid autoantibodies suggests an autoimmune aetiology.

Management box

Three forms exist

▶ Antithyroid drugs, eg carbimazole 20 mg bd initially, reducing to 5–10 mg daily for 12–18 months, with β-blockers: for symptomatic relief. Relapse occurs in approximately 70% within 2 years and is commoner with large goitres and severe disease. Adverse reactions such as rashes and neutropenia are relatively common. Antithyroid drug regimens also include the 'block and replace' regimen, in which high-dose carbimazole (40 mg/day) is continued for 12–18 months, with thyroxine replacement to prevent hypothyroidism.

▶ Radioiodine has a high cure rate but is usually withheld in the UK in women of childbearing potential. Hypothyroidism is common after treatment, the frequency increasing with time after therapy, necessitating long-term surveillance. Some authorities advocate administration of a large dose with early thyroxine replacement.

▶ Surgery should only be undertaken once the thyrotoxic state has been controlled with propranolol and/or carbimazole. Hypothyroidism is common and relapse of thyrotoxicosis and →

hypoparathyroidism may occur. Damage to the recurrent laryngeal nerve is rare. Indications include medical failure in the young and large goitres causing stridor or dysphagia.

▶ Extrathyroid complications: Exophthalmos may benefit from treatment with high-dose corticosteroids but may require tarsorrhaphy and/or orbital decompression. Cardiac arrhythmias especially AF may respond poorly to digoxin and β-blockers are often required. Once the patient is euthyroid cardioversion should be considered. Thyrotoxic crisis, manifested by high-output cardiac failure, requires treatment with propranolol 80 mg qds, carbimazole 60–80 mg daily in divided doses followed by potassium iodide 15 mg 4–6 hourly, dexamethasone 2 mg qds and fluid replacement (usually with saline).

HYPOTHYROIDISM

Science basics The commonest cause worldwide is iodine deficiency but in the UK autoimmune disease (Hashimoto's disease if associated with a goitre) is commonest, followed by postoperative and post-^{131}I-therapy. Primary atrophic hypothyroidism, dyshormonogenesis, iodine excess and hypopituitarism are less common.

Clinical features

Symptoms: include weight-gain, cold intolerance, depression, tiredness, menorrhagia, constipation and slowing in mental function. In the elderly there may be no symptoms or the patient may present with dementia.

Signs: slow relaxation of tendon reflexes, myxoedema (deposition of subcutaneous mucopolysaccharide), hair-loss, hoarse voice, cold skin, bradycardia and slowness of movement.

Investigations • Low T4 with high TSH will identify the great majority • In hypopituitarism a low T4 is accompanied by a low TSH • Associated abnormalities include hypercholesterolaemia, anaemia and low voltage ECG complexes • Thyroid auto-antibodies are present in the autoimmune variants.

Management box
▶ Thyroxine replacement starting at a low dose such as 50 μg/day and increasing to 100 or 200 μg/day. The biochemical aim of replacement therapy (with T4) is to achieve a free T4 at the upper limit of normal, with TSH in the normal range. In patients with angina, replacement should be very slow and β-blockers may need to be introduced concomitantly. One should aim for a normal fT4 and slightly high TSH (5–10).

THYROID CANCER

Science basics   Thyroid cancer is rare but is important as some types have a good prognosis if treated early. The main types are:

Papillary (75%):   all age-groups, presents with a slow-growing nodule and sometimes metastasizes to cervical lymph nodes.

Follicular (10%):   middle-age commonest, tends to metastasize via the bloodstream to bones and lung.

Anaplastic (10%):   old-age, presents with a rapidly growing, firm thyroid mass resulting in stridor, vocal-cord paralysis and weight-loss.

Medullary (5%):   presents as solitary nodule often with spread to cervical nodes and the mediastinum. About 20% are associated with multiple endocrine neoplasia (MEN). The tumours may secrete calcitonin, serotonin, ACTH and other peptides causing intractable diarrhoea and flushing.

Lymphoma (<1%):   rare.

Investigations   Patients are usually euthyroid • US shows a solid mass within the thyroid which is 'cold' on isotope scan • Fine-needle aspiration is increasingly used for histological typing • Calcitonin levels are high in medullary carcinoma.

Management box
▶ Papillary and follicular tumours are usually treated by sub-total thyroidectomy followed by radioactive iodine, with long-term thyroid replacement therapy and further radio-iodine for recurrences.
▶ Medullary carcinoma is not radiosensitive and is usually treated surgically.
▶ Anaplastic tumours have a poor prognosis irrespective of therapy.

DIABETES MELLITUS

Science basics   This group of disorders is characterized by persistent hyperglycaemia due to deficiency of endogenous insulin or resistance to insulin action. A random blood glucose >14 mmol/l is diagnostic as is a fasting glucose >7 mmol/l. In equivocal cases a 75 g oral glucose tolerance test (OGTT) is indicated. A blood glucose >11.1 mmol/l 2 hours after the glucose load is diagnostic of diabetes mellitus (DM). Higher early glucoses which normalize (<7 mmol/l) at 2 hours (lag storage curve) may result in glycosuria and occur in situations associated with rapid gastric emptying.

Classifications Type 1 (insulin-dependent) DM which commonly presents in the young with ketosis and type 2 (non-insulin-dependent) DM, more characteristic of the obese, older subject. These clinical characteristics are by no means universal as a few diabetic children do not require insulin while many older subjects do.

Aetiology Although the cause of diabetes remains unclear, an autoimmune aetiology is likely in type 1 DM, perhaps triggered by viral infection, while type 2 DM has a significant genetic component and is strongly related to obesity. Other factors which may induce or precipitate DM are drugs, eg steroids, thiazides, pancreatic disease, stress, eg trauma or surgery and endocrine disorders, eg Cushing's syndrome and acromegaly. Gestational diabetes (transient diabetes during pregnancy) is an important complication of pregnancy.

Clinical features These vary in type 1 and 2 DM.

Type 1: weight-loss, dehydration, ketonuria, short duration of symptoms and hyperventilation.

Type 2: obesity and an insidious onset.

Common to both types: polyuria and polydipsia, lethargy, boils, pruritus vulvae and infections.

Investigations • Random blood glucose is usually diagnostic; otherwise fasting and 2-hour post-prandial blood glucose will establish the diagnosis in the majority • Glycosuria without hyper-glycaemia occurs in those with a low renal glucose threshold and in those with a lag-storage curve • Ketonuria occurs in type 1 DM and in fasting patients • In those in whom ketoacidosis is considered, blood glucose, U&E, blood gas analysis, CXR, MSU and blood cultures are indicated • Long-term monitoring of diabetic control as assessed by home blood-glucose measurements supplemented by regular clinic measurements of HbA1c • 'Target' levels for HbA1c (not achievable by all patients) are <7.5% in type 1 and <7.0% in type 2 • Screening for compli-cations includes regular serum creatinine, cholesterol and HDL measurements, measurement of microalbuminuria (as a marker of early renal disease) as well as funduscopy, attention to foot care, the peripheral circulation and detection of peripheral neuropathy and hypertension.

Management box

▶ **Type 1:** if ketoacidosis is present, immediate and aggressive treatment with iv fluids and insulin is indicated (see p 452). In those without ketosis but who have hyperglycaemia associated with weight-loss, rapid onset of symptoms and dehydration, insulin therapy is also indicated. Many different regimens of insulin administration exist but the majority employ short-acting insulin before meals (eg Humalog, Actrapid) with long-acting at bedtime (eg Monotard, Humulin I); alternatively a twice-daily mixture may be given (eg Mixtard 30). Approximately 0.5 units insulin per kg body weight is required per day. Pumps delivering continuous insulin infusions are occasionally used but require special training and highly specialized management. Dietary control and patient education are essential for good diabetic control and patient confidence.

▶ **Type 2:** many patients respond well to dietary treatment to reduce weight and restrict carbohydrate intake. In obese subjects who cannot or will not lose weight the addition of metformin 1000–2550 mg/day in divided doses often improves control. In others in whom dietary treatment alone does not provide adequate control sulphonylurea agents, eg glipizide 5–10 mg tid or gliclazide 80–320 mg daily are useful. A number of type 2 patients require insulin to achieve adequate glycaemic control. There is a major risk of weight-gain in this group.

Complications DM may result in damage to almost any organ. Poor diabetic control accelerates organ damage and good control reduces the risk. CNS damage may also accrue from frequent episodes of hypoglycaemia which may accompany overzealous attempts at achieving normoglycaemia.

Kidneys: the earliest manifestation of damage is micro-albuminuria which indicates risk of development of frank proteinuria due to diffuse glomerulosclerosis, chronic pyelo-nephritis or papillary necrosis but may be reversible in its early stages and responds to control of BP (and glycaemia). Some centres give ACE inhibitors to type 1 patients with micro-albuminuria even if BP is normal. Microalbuminuria is also a marker for increased vascular risk.

Eyes: Background: microaneurysms (dots) and haemorrhages (blots). Proliferative: infarction (cotton wool spots), exudates and neovascularization. Vitreous haemorrhage, rubeosis (new vessel formation on the iris) and cataracts are other complications.

Heart: IHD is more common, and there is a specific diabetic cardiomyopathy.

Circulation: large vessel disease due to atheroma may result in intermittent claudication or stroke. Small vessel disease may produce distal gangrene in the presence of good peripheral pulses.

Skin: abnormalities may develop at the site of insulin injection, including fat hypertrophy and scarring. Repeated injection in the latter results in highly variable blood glucoses.

Nervous system: peripheral neuropathy in a glove-and-stocking distribution is common. Mononeuropathy, eg VI nerve palsy is well recognized, as is autonomic neuropathy which may manifest as impotence, postural hypotension, diarrhoea, vomiting and cardiac arrhythmias.

Prognosis The standard mortality rate of DM is greater than the general population, the excess mortality in type 1 being due to renal disease and in type 2 due to cardiovascular and cerebrovascular disease. Evidence exists that good diabetic control involving a multidisciplinary team reduces the rate of development of complications.

E▶ **HYPOGLYCAEMIA** → page 452

E▶ **KETOACIDOSIS** → page 452

E▶ **HYPEROSMOLAR NON-KETOTIC COMA**
→ page 454

PITUITARY DISEASE

Science basics The anterior pituitary gland secretes the gonadotrophins FSH and LH, growth hormone, prolactin, ACTH and TSH. The posterior pituitary secretes antidiuretic hormone (ADH) and oxytocin.

HYPOPITUITARISM

This is complete or partial deficiency of anterior or posterior pituitary hormones.

Aetiology Most commonly due to anterior pituitary tumours, other causes include craniopharyngioma, metastatic tumour, autoimmune, granulomatous disorders, eg sarcoidosis, and postpartum haemorrhage (Sheehan's syndrome). Surgery and radiotherapy for pituitary tumours may result in hypopituitarism. Trauma to the head, often several years before, may cause hypopituitarism.

Clinical features

Symptoms: apathy, reduced libido, infertility, amenorrhoea, myxoedema, depression, symptoms of hypoglycaemia.

Signs: hypotension, small testes, reduced body hair, fine wrinkled skin, bitemporal hemianopia.

Investigations • CT scan or MRI • Glucose, T4 and TSH levels, prolactin, gonadotrophins, testosterone and cortisol • Absence of the normal increases in gonadotrophins, TSH, GH and cortisol after gonadotrophin-releasing hormone (GnRH), TRH and insulin-induced hypoglycaemia. This test should only be undertaken under medical supervision and with iv glucose available to reverse hypoglycaemia. It must not be performed in those with IHD or epilepsy • Glucagon or corticotropin-releasing hormone (CRH) can be used as an alternative to hypoglycaemia.

Management box
▶ Replacement therapy with deficient hormones, hydrocortisone 10 mg am, 5 mg at lunch and 5 mg in the evening, thyroxine 0.2 mg/day, testosterone 250 mg im 3-weekly in men and the combined oral contraceptive pill for pre-menopausal women.
▶ In many patients growth hormone replacement is offered to improve mood and muscle strength and to increase lean body mass.

DIABETES INSIPIDUS

Inability to produce concentrated urine due to complete or partial deficiency of ADH (cranial DI) or renal resistance to the antidiuretic action of ADH (nephrogenic DI).

Aetiology

Cranial DI: idiopathic (50%) and head injury commonest. Also post hypophysectomy, craniopharyngioma, sarcoidosis, post meningitis and inherited.

Nephrogenic DI: drugs (lithium commonest), hypokalaemia, hypercalcaemia, renal disease and glycosuria.

Clinical features Polyuria, nocturia and polydipsia. If deprived of water, dehydration and confusion develop.

Investigations • 24-hour urine output to confirm polyuria • Exclude DM and renal failure • Water deprivation test: if after 12 hours of fluid deprivation the urine osmolality is >800, DI is excluded; if below, administer desmopressin 2 µg im – if urine osmolality increases to >800 = cranial DI, if not = nephrogenic

DI • In difficult cases plasma ADH levels can be measured during hypertonic saline infusion.

Management box
▶ Cranial DI: treatment of the underlying cause may cure the DI, if not administer desmopressin 300–600 µg/day orally or 10–20 µg bd intranasally.
▶ Nephrogenic DI: treat the underlying cause. In refractory cases thiazide diuretics 5–10 mg/day may be beneficial.

PITUITARY TUMOURS

These are usually adenomas and can be divided into those which secrete hormones; eg acidophilic adenomas which secrete growth hormone or prolactin, and basophilic adenomas which secrete ACTH; and non-functional tumours, usually chromophobic adenomas.

Clinical features These may be due to local pressure effects, eg bitemporal, quadrantic or hemianopia, cranial nerve palsy, optic atrophy and hypothalamic disturbance, eg sleep and eating disturbance. Other effects may be due to hormone secretion which results in:

Acromegaly: characterized by insidious onset with headaches, coarsening of features, enlargement of extremities, prognathia, enlarged tongue, sweating, hypertension, cardiac failure and glucose intolerance.

Hyperprolactinaemia: characterized by amenorrhoea, infertility, galactorrhoea and impotence.

Cushing's disease: with mood changes, central distribution of fat, abdominal striae, 'moon face', proximal myopathy, hirsutism, osteoporosis, bruising, hypertension and oedema. Features of hypopituitarism may develop due to pituitary compression.

Investigations CT or MRI scan, visual-field assessment. Acromegaly is diagnosed by high GH levels which do not suppress during a 75 g OGTT. Prolactin levels >4000 mU/l (normal <400 mU/l) suggest a prolactinoma. For diagnosis of Cushing's disease → p 189. It is important to measure gonadotrophins, sex hormones, T4, TSH and to perform a short Synacthen test to screen for associated hormone deficiency.

Management box
▶ Deficient hormones must be replaced prior to surgery, which should be covered with iv hydrocortisone.
▶ Acromegaly should be treated with hypophysectomy followed by pituitary irradiation; post-operatively DI and hypopituitarism may develop. Octeotide therapy can also be used.
▶ Prolactinomas can be successfully treated with cabergoline 0.25–2 mg/week, although radiotherapy and surgery may be indicated.
▶ Non-secreting tumours are best treated by hypophysectomy to relieve local pressure effects on the optic chiasm and cavernous sinus.
▶ Post-operative pituitary function testing gives an indication as to the requirement for replacement therapy.
▶ Cushing's disease may be managed by pituitary surgery or, in a few cases, by bilateral adrenalectomy and pituitary irradiation.

ADRENAL INSUFFICIENCY

Science basics Adrenal insufficiency may be primary (Addison's disease), when adrenal disease occurs following autoimmune destruction (80%), TB, metastatic disease or intra-adrenal haemorrhage or secondary due to pituitary, hypothalamic disease or withdrawal of chronic corticosteroid therapy.

Clinical features

Symptoms: acute adrenal insufficiency, usually due to sudden cessation of steroid therapy or failure to increase dosage during stress, results in shock, nausea, abdominal pain and bowel disturbance. Chronic adrenal insufficiency presents with lethargy, weakness, weight-loss, postural dizziness, anorexia, nausea, constipation and amenorrhoea.

Signs: include hypotension, vitiligo (suggests autoimmunity), hyperpigmentation of mucous membranes and those areas exposed to light or pressure.

Investigations • Careful history, eg of steroid therapy • BP • U&E usually reveal hyperkalaemia, hyponatraemia, elevated urea and hypoglycaemia • In adrenal insufficiency secondary to pituitary or hypothalamic disease (in which aldosterone secretion is mostly preserved) hyponatraemia is usually milder and serum potassium and urea are normal • CXR and abdominal film to identify evidence of TB • Serum cortisol levels are low and do not increase following parenteral Synacthen (→ p 187) • ACTH levels are high in Addison's disease and low in secondary adrenal failure • Adrenal antibodies may be positive.

Management box
- If this follows withdrawal of corticosteroids immediate replacement therapy is essential, although gradual withdrawal over weeks may allow endogenous corticosteroid synthesis to resume. In other cases corticosteroid therapy is required indefinitely.
- Therapy of choice is hydrocortisone: 10 mg mane, 5 mg at lunch and 5 mg in the evening is the usual dose. Serum cortisol levels before and after oral administration should be checked. Cortisol therapy should be increased at times of stress, eg surgery and during acute illness.
- The majority of patients with Addison's disease also require mineralocorticoid replacement with fludrocortisone 0.05–0.2 mg/day.
- Mineralocorticoid therapy is not usually required in secondary adrenal insufficiency.

▣ ACUTE ADRENAL CRISIS → page 454

CUSHING'S SYNDROME

Science basics Prolonged exposure to abnormally high serum cortisol levels causes Cushing's syndrome. Causes other than iatrogenic can be divided into: ACTH-dependent, eg pituitary-dependent disease (Cushing's disease 60%), ectopic ACTH from tumours, eg small cell bronchial carcinoma (20%); and non-ACTH-dependent, eg adrenal adenoma (10%), adrenal carcinoma (5%) and alcohol-induced pseudo-Cushing's (5%).

Clinical features Often same as for Cushing's disease (p 187). Additional features may be present due to associated pathology, eg bronchial carcinoma. Pigmentation is prominent in ectopic ACTH syndromes but absent in non-ACTH-dependent causes. In ectopic Cushing's due to malignancy the patient may be pigmented and wasted rather than obese.

Investigations • U&E may show hypokalaemia, glucose intolerance may be present, as may hypertension • CXR to exclude bronchial carcinoma • Failures to suppress 09:00 hour serum cortisol to <170 nmol/l after overnight (23:00 hour) dexamethasone 2 mg, elevation of 24-hour urinary free cortisol and loss of diurnal variation in serum cortisol levels are useful screening tests • ACTH levels are high in pituitary disease, very high in ectopic ACTH syndromes and low in adrenal disease • A high-dose dexamethasone suppression test 2 mg qid will help differentiate pituitary-dependent Cushing's from ectopic Cushing's or adrenal disease • MRI scan of the pituitary and CT of adrenals may identify a tumour and inferior petrosal sinus sampling for ACTH may localize pituitary tumours.

> **Management box**
> ▶ Surgery is indicated for most pituitary and adrenal tumours and may be appropriate for some cases of ectopic ACTH syndrome, although pituitary radiotherapy is also used for Cushing's disease.
> ▶ The use of metyrapone, ketoconazole and aminoglutethimide, which inhibit cortisol production, are necessary preoperatively, and may produce benefit in cases not amenable to surgery.
> ▶ Iatrogenic Cushing's syndrome responds to reduction in steroid dosage when possible. Drugs such as azathioprine may be used in conjunction with steroids to enable lower doses to be used to control the underlying disease.

PHAEOCHROMOCYTOMA

Science basics   This a rare catecholamine-secreting benign (90%) tumour usually arising in the adrenal medulla. Other sites include chromaffin tissues of the sympathetic nervous system, eg para-aortic ganglia.

Clinical features   These depend upon the relative amounts of adrenaline (epinephrine) and noradrenaline (norepinephrine). Features may be episodic and include weight-loss, hypertension, tachycardia, pallor, sweating, headache, anxiety and nausea. Hyperglycaemia may exist.

Investigations • 24-hour urine for metanephrines or free catecholamine excretion with fractionation • Location of the tumour by CT scanning and venous sampling for noradrenaline (norepinephrine) if necessary • Isotope scanning with MIBG is also useful.

> **Management box**
> ▶ Surgical excision under α- and β-blockade using phenoxy-benzamine and propranolol. These should be given for at least 3 days preoperatively.
> ▶ Special care necessary during surgery because of blockage of sympathetic nervous system.

HYPERALDOSTERONISM

Primary hyperaldosteronism (Conn's syndrome)
This is a condition where high aldosterone levels exist independent of the renin-angiotensin system. It is rare and due either to an adrenocortical adenoma (most common) or to bilateral adreno-cortical hyperplasia.

Clinical features Often asymptomatic. Hypertension, lethargy and muscular weakness due to hypokalaemia.

Investigations • Hypokalaemia (<3.5 mmol/l) in patients not taking diuretics, steroids, laxatives, potassium • Plasma renin and aldosterone levels taken in the early morning before the patient moves from the supine position • Measurement of renin and aldosterone after standing for 4 hours will differentiate adrenal hyperplasia from adenoma • CT scan may identify an adrenal mass.

Management box
▶ Surgery to remove the adenoma after 4–6 weeks' spironolactone 300 mg/day.
▶ Surgery may not reverse established hypertension. If due to adrenal hyperplasia spironolactone therapy alone is usually sufficient.

Secondary hyperaldosteronism

This is said to exist when high aldosterone levels are present due to activation of the renin-angiotensin system. Causes include renal artery stenosis, decompensated liver disease, accelerated hypertension, cardiac failure and nephrotic syndrome.

Management box
▶ Remove the underlying cause if possible.

PARATHYROID DISEASE

PRIMARY HYPERPARATHYROIDISM

Science basics High levels of PTH occur in primary hyperparathyroidism, usually due to a • parathyroid adenoma • hyperplasia, less commonly and • carcinoma, rarely. Hyperparathyroidism is the commonest component of the multiple endocrine neoplasia syndromes.

Clinical features These may be absent and many cases are detected by identifying hypercalcaemia on routine blood screening. Hypercalcaemia may cause thirst and polyuria, anorexia, weakness, constipation, vomiting and confusion. Renal colic, backache, hypertension, nephrolithiasis, nephrogenic DI, pseudogout, pancreatitis and peptic ulceration are also well recognized. Corneal calcification is rare.

Investigations • Ionized calcium if available, otherwise serum calcium avoiding the use of a tourniquet and correcting for hypo-albuminaemia • Other causes of hypercalcaemia, eg malignancy, myeloma and vitamin D excess require exclusion • Serum phosphate is usually low in primary hyperparathyroidism as is plasma bicarbonate, with high plasma chloride • X-rays of the hands and skull may reveal subperiosteal erosions of the phalanges or a 'pepper-pot' skull in primary hyperparathyroidism, while an abdominal film may reveal renal stones or nephrocalcinosis • US of the neck may identify a parathyroid adenoma as may a radio-active thallium-technetium subtraction scan • Immunoassays for PTH can differentiate primary hyperparathyroidism (high PTH) from the hypercalcaemia of malignancy (low PTH).

Management box

▶ Surgery to remove a parathyroid adenoma is highly successful, although in elderly asymptomatic patients conservative therapy may be indicated.

▶ In those with parathyroid hyperplasia, resection of all four glands with subsequent transplantation of parathyroid tissue to the forearm is also successful.

▶ Treatment of severe hypercalcaemia requires adequate rehydration with iv saline (4 l/day) along with iv pamidronate disodium. Steroid therapy and the use of calcitonin are seldom effective for the hypercalcaemia due to hyperparathyroidism but may be useful in hypercalcaemia of malignancy.

SECONDARY/TERTIARY HYPERPARATHYROIDISM

Science basics This occurs following prolonged hypocalcaemia, eg associated with renal failure or malabsorption, which stimulates PTH secretion in order to correct the hypocalcaemia. Occasionally PTH secretion may become autonomous in these circumstances leading to hypercalcaemia (tertiary hyperparathyroidism).

Management box
▶ Correct the underlying cause.

HYPOPARATHYROIDISM

Science basics This may be either primary (autoimmune, associated with hypothyroidism and Addison's disease) or secondary, usually after thyroid surgery.

Clinical features   If acute this may give rise to tetany, peri-oral and peripheral paraesthesiae, cramps and fits. Occult tetany may be revealed by Trousseau's and Chvostek's tests. If chronic it is associated with abnormalities of nails, teeth and hair. Cutaneous moniliasis is more common in the autoimmune variant. Less often cataracts and rarely papilloedema are found.

Investigations   • Low serum calcium, increased phosphate and normal alkaline phosphatase • Skull X-ray may reveal basal ganglia calcification • Plasma PTH levels low • Decreased urinary excretion of cyclic AMP which rises following PTH infusion.

Management box
▶ In acute cases of hypocalcaemia give 10–20 ml 10% calcium gluconate iv.
▶ If hypomagnesaemia exists iv magnesium chloride should be given.
▶ Long-term management requires therapy with alfacalcidol.
▶ Calcium supplements are not usually required to maintain normal serum calcium levels.

PSEUDOHYPOPARATHYROIDISM

Science basics   This is a rare inherited disorder with resistance to PTH. Similar biochemical features to hypoparathyroidism are found in association with short stature, mental retardation, short 4th and 5th metacarpals, a 'moon' face, cerebral calcification and hypothyroidism. Pseudo-pseudohypoparathyroidism has the same phenotypic features but these are biochemically normal.

OSTEOMALACIA/RICKETS

Science basics   Failure of organic bone matrix (osteoid) to mineralize normally produces rickets during bone-growth and osteomalacia following epiphysial closure.

Aetiology
- Low dietary vitamin D_2.
- Lack of sunlight – reduced level of vitamin D_3.
- Malabsorption/impaired absorption of vitamin D_2/D_3 – coeliac disease, bowel resection, biliary cirrhosis, excessive aluminium hydroxide.
- Renal disease (hereditary or acquired).
- Resistance to vitamin D_3.
- Drugs – phenytoin.

Clinical features

Symptoms: skeletal pain, proximal muscular weakness, lethargy.

Signs: bony tenderness, swelling of distal ends of radius and ulna, rickety rosary (costochondral swelling), delayed dentition, waddling gait, tetany, spontaneous fractures, knock-knees, bow legs.

Investigations • Hypocalcaemia, hypophosphataemia, raised alkaline phosphatase, low vitamin D • Bone biopsy shows incomplete mineralization • Radiology (pseudofractures in pubic rami, scapula, upper ends humerus and femur, cupped and ragged metaphysial surfaces in rickets).

Management box
▶ Replace deficient vitamin D (dose depends on aetiology).
▶ Treat any underlying condition.
▶ Monitor calcium level.

MULTIPLE ENDOCRINE NEOPLASIA (MEN)

May occur spontaneously or familially (autosomal dominant).
MEN I (Werner's syndrome):
  Pancreatic endocrine tumour (insulinoma, gastrinoma, vipoma, glucagonoma)
  Parathyroid adenoma
  Pituitary adenoma (eg prolactinoma)
  Associated with carcinoids, adrenal cortical tumours, lipomas
MEN IIa (Sipple's syndrome):
  Parathyroid adenoma
  Medullary carcinoma of the thyroid
  Phaeochromocytoma
MEN IIb:
  Medullary carcinoma of the thyroid
  Phaeochromocytoma
  Mucosal neuromas
  Marfanoid habitus

HYPERLIPIDAEMIA

This term is applied to a group of disorders in which the blood contains high levels of cholesterol or triglyceride (TG) or both.

• Cholesterol and TG are both insoluble in water and are therefore transported in the blood in complexes called lipoproteins, which consist of a lipid-rich core surrounded by phospholipid and specific proteins called apoproteins.

- Dietary fat contains both cholesterol and TG, the latter being hydrolysed to glycerol and free fatty acids in the intestine. These are absorbed and recombined into TG in the wall of the small intestine; this TG is the main constituent of chylomicrons, the lesser components of which are cholesterol and certain apoproteins.
- Chylomicrons deliver TG to muscle and to fat stores, the depleted residues, called remnant particles, being taken up by the liver.
- The liver makes another type of TG-rich lipoprotein called very low density lipoprotein (VLDL) which, after various metabolic exchanges between the liver and the peripheral tissues, may be converted into low density lipoprotein (LDL).
- LDL is the only lipoprotein to deliver cholesterol to the peripheral tissues, including the arterial wall, and is closely involved in atherogenesis, especially when oxidized.
- High density lipoprotein (HDL), made in the liver and in the gut, acts as a scavenger of cholesterol from peripheral tissues; low levels therefore place the individual at increased risk of atherosclerosis.

Clinical significance The incidence of atherosclerosis is clearly linked to levels of total cholesterol. More recent studies have shown, however, that the closest links are with the cholesterol/HDL ratio and with levels of LDL, especially oxidized LDL. Hypertriglyceridaemia is weakly linked to atherosclerosis; its clinical significance is greatest in relation to pancreatitis. Thus, from the point of view of clinical management of the patient and family the laboratory measurements required are • levels of total cholesterol • HDL • LDL • TG • Total cholesterol (TC) and HDL may be measured in the non-fasted state • LDL and TG measurement require the subject to fast.

Classification of types

Familial hypercholesterolaemia (FH) and familial combined hyperlipidaemia (FCH): both monogenic disorders linked to an increased risk of atherosclerosis. Tendon xanthomata (Achilles, patellar or triceps tendon) and palmar xanthomata may be seen if the TC level is very high; corneal arcus and xanthelasmata may also be seen but these can occur in subjects with a normal serum cholesterol. Heterozygotes for FH usually have LDL levels >9 mmol/l and early vascular disease; homozygotes tend to have even higher levels (>15 mmol/l). In FCH the degree of hypercholesterolaemia is less.

Polygenic hypercholesterolaemia: much commoner than FH. TG levels may be normal or elevated. Tendon xanthomata are not seen.

Familial hypertriglyceridaemia: increases the risk of pancreatitis and may cause eruptive xanthomata on the elbows, knees, back and buttocks. The risk of atherosclerosis is not increased.

Secondary hyperlipidaemia: may occur as the result of hypothyroidism (TC and LDL), diabetes, obesity (in both conditions: ↑TC, LDL and TG, ↓HDL), liver disease (especially with cholestasis; ↑LDL), nephrotic syndrome (↑LDL and TG), alcohol abuse (↑TG; risk of pancreatitis). Oral oestrogens may also increase TC and a mild elevation may be seen with thiazide diuretics.

Assessment of vascular risk Hyperlipidaemia interacts with other risk factors for vascular disease: smoking, hypertension, obesity, presence of diabetes, physical inactivity. In primary prevention, overall vascular risk is best assessed using a table or chart which takes account of all of these factors (eg the Joint British Guidelines or Sheffield Tables). An estimated 10-year vascular risk of 30% or more indicates the need to treat modifiable risk factors, including hyperlipidaemia. In secondary prevention vigorous treatment of risk factors is indicated, including an attempt to lower TC to less than 5.0 mmol/l and LDL to less than 3.0 mmol/l.

Management box

▶ Diet: for hypercholesterolaemia, should be high in complex carbohydrate, low in total fat and low in saturated fat, with most fat being mono- or polyunsaturated. Dietary treatment will not lower TC by more than about 10%, so people with moderate or severe hypercholesterolaemia or in whom strict control of lipids is required will often need medication as well as diet. Dietary treatment of hypertriglyceridaemia is based on weight reduction, reduction of fat intake and restriction of alcohol; increasing exercise should also be recommended.

▶ Statins: these should be prescribed for anyone with established vascular disease whose TC is > 5 mmol/l, especially those who have had a recent MI. People who, on risk charts, have an estimated 10-year vascular risk of 30% or above should also receive a statin if the TC/HDL ratio is > 5.0.

▶ Fibrates are useful in those with a low HDL and in some people with combined hyperlipidaemia. They may be combined with statins but there is a risk (especially with earlier fibrates) of myalgia or a myositis-like picture.

▶ Resins (colestyramine and colestipol) are effective in lowering TC and LDL but their use is limited by gastrointestinal side-effects. They may be combined with statins in the treatment of FH.

▶ Fish oils (omega-3 marine oils) and acipimox are used in the treatment of hypertriglyceridaemia.

10

Haematology

INVESTIGATIONS

Full blood count: RBC, WBC and platelet counts; RBC morphology; WBC differential.

Blood film: RBC, WBC and platelet morphology.

Erythrocyte sedimentation rate (Table 10.18, p 221).
  Normal range (mm in first hour)   1–5 in adult males
                                     1–8 in adult females.

Bone marrow (BM)/aspiration/trephine/culture

Serum protein estimation: protein electrophoresis, immuno-globulins, plasma viscosity, haptoglobins, haemopexin.

Bence Jones protein: free immunoglobulin light chains in the urine.

Surface marker studies: rosetting techniques, immunofluorescence.

Haemoglobin studies: sickle cell screening, haemoglobin electro-phoresis, oxygen dissociation curves, methaemoglobin detection, 2, 3-DPG quantification, G-6-P dehydrogenase assay.

Isotope studies: red cell mass, plasma volume, red cell survival, iron absorption.

DEFINITIONS

Microcytosis: reduction in average volume of RBC MCV < 78 fl.

Macrocytosis: increase in average volume of RBC MCV > 98 fl.

Hypochromia: red cells contain less than the normal amount of haemoglobin and so appear pale, mean cell haemoglobin concentration (MCHC) < 30 g/dl.

Poikilocytosis: irregularity of RBC shape.

Anisocytosis: variation in size of RBCs.

Elliptocytosis: elliptical RBCs.

Ovalocytosis: oval RBCs.

Spherocytosis: spherical RBCs (loss of normal biconcave disc of RBC), loss of central pallor, eg congenital haemolysis.

Dimorphic: dual population of RBCs in the peripheral circulation, eg sideroblastic anaemia.

Reticulocytosis: the presence of immature anucleate RBCs in the peripheral blood.

Polychromasia: blue tinge to RBCs in the blood film due to the presence of a reticulocytosis.

Nucleated RBC: indicates overactive erythropoiesis, eg leukaemia, marrow infiltration.

Blast cells: nucleated precursor cells, eg leukaemia.

Schistocytes: red cell fragments secondary to mechanical trauma, eg prosthetic heart valves, DIC.

Punctate basophilia (basophilic stippling): indicates damaged RBCs, eg severe anaemia, lead poisoning, β-thalassaemia.

Leucocytosis: increase in total circulating WBCs ($>11.0 \times 10^9$/l), eg pyogenic infection.

Leucopenia: decrease in total circulating WBCs ($<4.0 \times 10^9$/l), eg TB, overwhelming infection.

Eosinophilia: increase in total circulating eosinophils, eg parasitic infection, lymphoma, worms, drug reactions, allergies and skin diseases.

Monocytosis: increase in circulating monocytes, eg TB and malaria.

Leucoerythroblastic: blood film containing nucleated RBCs and immature WBCs, usually in association with tumour infiltration of the bone marrow (BM).

Thrombocytopenia: decrease in circulating platelets ($<150 \times 10^9$/l), eg marrow suppression or drug reaction.

Thrombocytosis: increase in circulating platelet count ($>350 \times 10^9$/l).

Extramedullary erythropoiesis: production of RBCs outside the bone marrow, eg liver, spleen.

Burr cells: irregularly shaped RBCs seen in uraemia.

Howell–Jolly bodies: nuclear remnants seen in the RBCs in post-splenectomy cases, leukaemia, megaloblastic anaemia.

Target cells: RBCs with central staining surrounded by a ring of pallor and an outer ring of staining, eg thalassaemia, severe liver disease.

Heinz bodies: denatured haemoglobin in RBCs.

Haemolysis: excessively rapid red-cell breakdown.

Left shift: increase in immature white cells, eg infection.

Right shift hypersegmented polymorphs, eg uraemia, liver disease and megaloblastic anaemia.

ANAEMIA

Science basics Anaemia exists if the haemoglobin level is less than that which is expected when both age and sex are taken into account. The haemoglobin level at birth is high (20 g/dl), but falls during the first 3 months of life to a nadir (10 g/dl) before rising again to the adult value (>12 g/dl in females and >13 g/dl in males).

Aetiology (→ Table 10.1).

Table 10.1
Aetiology of anaemia

Loss of blood	Acute or chronic

Impaired RBC formation	Congenital:
	    marrow aplasia,
	    red cell aplasia
	Nutritional deficiencies:
	    iron, B_{12}, folate, vitamin C,
	    protein (kwashiorkor)
	Immune dysfunction:
	    SLE, RA
	Infection:
	    viral – EBV, HIV, TB
	Bone marrow invasion:
	    leukaemia, carcinoma, fibrosis
	Endocrine abnormalities:
	    hypothyroidism, hypoadrenalism,
	    hypopituitarism, hypogonadism
	Drugs/toxins:
	    antibiotics – sulphonamides,
	    chloramphenicol
	    antimalarials – pyrimethamine
	    anti-inflammatory – gold salts,
	    indometacin, phenylbutazone
	    antithyroid – carbimazole
	    anticonvulsants – phenytoin
	    antidepressants – chlorpromazine
	    cytotoxics – dose-dependent
	    ionizing radiation
	    solvents – benzene
	Thalassaemia
	Sideroblastosis
	Porphyria: erythropoietic
	Hepatic failure
	Renal failure

Table 10.1
Aetiology of anaemia *(Cont'd)*

Loss of blood	Acute or chronic

Haemolysis	Congenital red cell defects:
	    membrane defects – spherocytosis
	    enzyme defects – G6PD
	    defects in Hb structure – sickle
	    cell anaemia
	Acquired: B_{12}/folate deficiency
	    infections: malaria
	    trauma: prosthetic valve
	    chemicals: drugs
	    antibodies: autoimmune,
	    isoimmune toxins, tumours

Clinical features These depend on the degree of anaemia present and on the speed of its development.

Symptoms: lethargy, malaise, headache, increasing breathlessness, palpitations, dizziness, syncope, and angina.

Signs: include pallor of the conjunctivae, mucous membranes and skin, tachycardia, systolic flow murmurs, koilonychia, glossitis, angular stomatitis and peripheral oedema. Hypotension may be present. Splenomegaly, pigmented gallstones and jaundice may be present in haemolytic anaemia. Leg ulceration in hereditary haemolysis. Papilloedema and retinal haemorrhages may occur rarely.

Investigations • FBC: red cell indices often give a pointer to the underlying aetiology.

Microcytic anaemia (MCV < 76 fl, MCH < 27 pg, MCHC < 30 g/dl): iron deficiency (Table 10.2), inherited sideroblastic anaemia, thalassaemia, chronic disease.

Normocytic anaemia: haemolytic conditions, following haemorrhage, aplastic anaemia, combined deficiencies, eg iron and folate, chronic disease, eg RA, uraemia, infection, malignancy.

Macrocytic anaemia (MCV > 96 fl): megaloblastic erythropoiesis (Table 10.3): B_{12} deficiency, folate deficiency; normoblastic erythropoiesis: reticulocytosis, marrow infiltration/suppression, aplastic anaemia, hypothyroidism, hypopituitarism, alcoholism, liver disease.

• Peripheral blood film • ESR • bone marrow (BM) examination • Iron binding capacity • Serum iron • Ferritin • Vitamin

Table 10.2
Causes of iron-deficiency anaemia

Inadequate diet	
Malabsorption	Coeliac disease
Blood loss/bleeding diathesis	GI malignancy, ulceration, varices, gastritis, menorrhagia, haematuria, hookworm, inflammatory bowel disease, diverticulitis, haemorrhoids
Achlorhydria	
Previous gastric surgery	
Increased physiological demand	Pregnancy, growth
Intravascular haemolysis	Paroxysmal nocturnal haemoglobinuria, RBC fragmentation due to prosthetic valves
Delayed weaning from the breast	

Table 10.3
Causes of megaloblastic anaemia

Vitamin B_{12} deficiency:	Inadequate diet < 1–2 µg/day Alcohol abuse Malabsorption: – intrinsic factor deficiency – pernicious anaemia, previous gastric surgery, congenital absence, atrophic gastritis, Zollinger-Ellison Syndrome Terminal ileal disease: – ileal resection, Crohn's disease, ulcerative colitis, tropical sprue Infection: – blind loop syndrome, fish tapeworm Pancreatic insufficiency Drug-induced: – neomycin, colchicine, metformin Increased requirements: – pregnancy, hyperthyroidism, increased erythropoiesis, transcobalamin II deficiency

Table 10.3
Causes of megaloblastic anaemia *(Cont'd)*

Folate deficiency:	Inadequate diet Malabsorption: – coeliac disease, jejunal resection, tropical sprue, Crohn's disease, Whipple's disease, GI lymphoma Increased requirements: – pregnancy, lactation, puberty, prematurity, dialysis, increased erythropoiesis, psoriasis, severe dermatitis Anti-folate drugs: – alcohol, methotrexate, trimethoprim, isoniazid, OCP Congenital enzyme deficiency: – dihydrofolate reductase
Pyridoxine deficiency Thiamine deficiency Myelodysplastic syndrome Lesch–Nyhan syndrome	

B_{12} and folate levels • Schilling test, and ↑ reticulocyte count
• Tests for haemolysis include increased bilirubin, increased
urinary urobilinogen, reduced or absent serum haptoglobin,
haemoglobinuria, reticulocytosis, haemosiderinuria, methaemalbuminaemia, RBC morphology – spherocytes, elliptocytes,
fragmentation, target cells • Reduced RBC survival can be
assessed using labelled 51Cr, and antibodies against RBC by
direct anti-globulin test (Coombs' test).

Management box
▶ Treat the underlying cause.
▶ Remove any provoking drugs.
▶ Blood transfusion may be required.
▶ Replace vitamin or mineral deficiencies, eg oral ferrous
  sulphate 200 mg 3 ×/day, parenteral iron is only rarely needed,
  vitamin B_{12} as im hydroxycobalamin 1 mg 2 × during the first
  week followed by 1 mg weekly until the blood count is normal.
  B_{12} injections may be needed 3-monthly for life. Folate 5 mg
  tid for treatment and 5 mg/day maintenance therapy.

→

▶ Never give folate alone in pernicious anaemia as subacute combined degeneration of the spinal cord may be provoked.
▶ Steroids (40–60 mg/day initially) or splenectomy may be needed in haemolytic anaemia.

PERNICIOUS ANAEMIA

Science basics Disorder characterized by megaloblastic change in the bone marrow and anaemia, often with neurological abnormalities. It is due to a failure of secretion of gastric intrinsic factor and has an autoimmune basis. F>M, usually presents at 45–65 years. Higher incidence in people with blood group A. Achlorhydria and atrophic gastritis are present. Bone marrow morphology reflects failure of DNA synthesis with maturation arrest of RBC, granulocyte and platelet precursors. Haemolysis occurs.

Clinical features Insidious onset and a profound degree of anaemia may be present at the time of diagnosis. Weight-loss and diarrhoea are common, mild pyrexia, jaundice due to haemolysis and pallor give the skin a lemon-yellow tinge. The tongue is smooth, atrophic and may be tender. Splenomegaly may be present. Degenerative changes in the posterior and lateral tracts of the spinal cord may cause subacute combined degeneration which presents with 'glove-and-stocking' impairment of superficial sensation with loss of both proprioception and vibration sense. The tendon reflexes may be brisk but the ankle jerks are often lost. The plantar reflex is extensor. Ataxia and a toxic confusional state may be present. Dementia may occur.

Differential diagnosis Any cause of megaloblastic anaemia (Table 10.3). Exclude any other coexisting autoimmune diseases, eg vitiligo, DM, hypothyroidism, ovarian failure, myasthenia gravis.

Investigations • FBC shows macrocytic anaemia • Anisocytosis, poikilocytosis and RBC fragmentation may be present. Low reticulocyte count. Leucopenia and hypersegmentation of neutrophils are common. Platelet count is usually normal • BM aspiration confirms a megaloblastic picture • Serum vitamin B_{12} level is low (<160 ng/l), serum folate is not reduced • Schilling test shows lack of B_{12} absorption (but it is not necessary to perform a Schilling test in the presence of a low vitamin B_{12} level and a positive intrinsic factor Ab) • Autoantibodies may be detected, eg intrinsic factor (50%) or parietal cell (80%) • Atrophic gastritis.

Management box

▶ im hydroxycobalamin as for any case of B_{12} deficiency. Reticulocytosis may be > 50% by the 10th day. Iron (ferrous sulphate 200 mg 8-hourly) and potassium (KCl 1.2 g 8-hourly) supplements may be needed.

▶ Blood transfusion if the degree of anaemia is critical but should be given slowly with diuretic cover to avoid precipitating cardiac failure.

AUTOIMMUNE HAEMOLYTIC ANAEMIA

Science basics Antibodies are formed against RBC antigens leading to premature destruction of the cells (normal life-span 120 days). Two types of antibody exist based on thermal characteristics: 'warm' IgG (occasionally IgA or IgM) antibodies are most active at 37°C; 'cold' IgM antibodies at 4°C.

Aetiology ($\rightarrow$ Table 10.4).

Clinical features

'Warm' type: insidious onset, lethargy, jaundice, splenomegaly, fever and rarely renal failure, F>M.

'Cold' type: anaemia precipitated by cold conditions, Raynaud's

Table 10.4
Causes of autoimmune haemolytic anaemia

'Warm' antibody type	Idiopathic, SLE, lymphoma, chronic lymphatic leukaemia, Evans' syndrome, drugs, eg methyldopa
'Cold' antibody type	Cold haemagglutinin disease, paroxysmal cold haemoglobinuria (PCH), mycoplasma pneumonia, lymphoma, infectious mononucleosis, viral infections, chronic lymphatic leukaemia
Drug-related	Drug absorbed onto RBC surface: penicillin, cephalosporins Immune complex-mediated: sulphonamides, quinidine
Immune disease of the newborn	
Secondary to blood transfusion	

phenomenon, cyanosis, acrocyanosis and non-specific symptoms of any anaemia.

Investigations • FBC shows spherocytosis • Demonstrate evidence of antibody attack against RBC by direct antiglobulin test (Coombs' test) at various temperatures to classify the responsible antigen • Reticulocytosis • Evidence of excessive RBC destruction (rise in unconjugated bilirubin and LDH, fall in concentration of haemoglobin scavenger levels – haptoglobin and haemopexin – free haemoglobin may bind to albumin-methaemalbumin, or spill over into the urine with haemoglobinuria or haemosiderinuria) • Donath–Landsteiner IgG antibody is present in PCH. Look for underlying cause.

Management box

▸ 'Warm' type: prednisolone 40–60 mg/day initially reducing slowly after 4 weeks. If this fails splenectomy or other immunosuppressive agents may be needed, eg azathioprine (50–100 mg/day). Transfuse if necessary. Folate supplements, thymectomy may be useful occasionally in infants.

▸ 'Cold' type: keep extremities warm, avoid transfusions if possible (always pre-warm), steroids and splenectomy are less successful.

APLASTIC ANAEMIA

Science basics Decrease in haemopoietic bone marrow with resultant pancytopenia.

Aetiology (→ Table 10.5)

Table 10.5
Causes of aplastic anaemia

Congenital	Fanconi's	(autosomal recessive)
Acquired	Drugs	gold salts
		cytotoxias
		chloramphenicol
		thiazide diuretics
	Infections	viral
	Chemicals	benzene
	Radiation exposure	
	Paroxysmal nocturnal haemoglobinuria (PNH)	
	Pregnancy	

Clinical features M>F, peak incidence around 30 years. Insidious onset, symptoms are due to the deficiency of RBCs, WBCs and platelets with anaemia, bleeding and increased susceptibility to infection. Purpura, epistaxis, GI bleeding and haematuria are common. Skin and mucous membrane ulceration and infection.

Investigations • FBC: anaemia (normocytic or macrocytic), reduced reticulocyte count, granulocytopenia, monocytopenia, lymphopenia, thrombocytopenia • BM is hypocellular (multiple site biopsies) • Elevated erythropoietin • Radioactive iron studies show reduced clearance from the blood with poor marrow uptake.

Management box

▶ Remove any identifiable cause, eg drugs. Support with replacement therapy: RBC, granulocyte and platelet transfusions.

▶ Treat infections: antibiotics, antiviral agents and antifungal agents as required.

▶ Folate supplements if folate deficiency is confirmed.

▶ Stimulate haemopoiesis: androgenic steroids (testosterone, oxymetholone, nandrolone deconate or fluoxymesterone), glucocorticoids (methylprednisolone), allogenic BMT may be needed.

▶ Immunosuppressive agents (ciclosporin and antilymphocyte globulin) as the disease may have an immune basis in some cases, but this is not without risk.

Prognosis Only 50% 1-year survival.

HAEMOGLOBINOPATHIES

Science basics The haemoglobinopathies are a group of conditions in which the structure/production of haemoglobin has been altered in some way (Table 10.6).

**Table 10.6
Classification of haemoglobinopathies**

Structural haemoglobin variants
   HbS: the sickle cell syndromes
   Methaemoglobins
Defective haemoglobin synthesis
   Thalassaemias
Persistence of fetal haemoglobin

SICKLE CELL ANAEMIA

Science basics Widespread disease in equatorial Africa in which an inherited mutation in the gene sequence leads to an abnormal amino-acid structure in the β-globin chain of haemoglobin. The normal glutamine amino acid at position six is replaced by valine. When the sickle cell haemoglobin molecule (haemoglobin S-HbS) is deoxygenated, aggregations of fibrils are produced which distort the RBC into a characteristic 'sickle' shape. This polymerization is initially reversible when reoxygenation occurs, but the distortion of the RBC membranes may become permanent if excessive hypoxia or acidosis is present. This condition is inherited in an autosomal fashion, the homozygote having sickle cell disease and the heterozygote sickle cell trait, which is usually asymptomatic and confers resistance to *falciparum* malaria. The coexisting presence of other haemoglobinopathies, eg HbA or HbF, reduces the concentration of HbS and makes sickling less likely.

Clinical features The two major problems are haemolytic anaemia due to reduced RBC survival and vascular occlusions by sickled cells. Symptoms begin during the second 6 months of life when HbF levels are falling and HbS levels rising. Severe anaemia occurs, with lethargy, growth retardation, delayed puberty, increased susceptibility to infection, leg ulceration and hyperplasia of the BM leading to bossing of the skull. The anaemia is due to marrow hypoplasia, haemolysis, splenic sequestration and folate deficiency. Vaso-occlusive crises produce pain because of infarction in bones, fingers (dactylitis), lungs, spleen, kidneys, bowel, liver and retina. They are precipitated by dehydration, infection or cooling but may appear spontaneously and are characterized by fever, malaise, pain and prostration. Splenomegaly may be present in infancy and early childhood, but autosplenectomy due to recurrent infarcts with reduction in spleen almost always occurs.

Investigations • FBC, blood film shows sickle-shaped cells (not in sickle cell trait) • Affected cells will sickle within 20 minutes when mixed on a slide with 2% sodium metabisulphate • Haemoglobin electrophoresis.

Management box

▶ Avoid precipitating factors, eg treat infections, prevent cold, hypotension, acidosis, hypoxia and dehydration. Special care is needed in pregnancy and during anaesthesia. Folate supplements if indicated.

▶ Treat crisis by hydration, warmth, antibiotics, analgesia (usually opiates), transfuse if necessary.

▶ Pneumococcal, meningococcal and haemophilus vaccines and prophylactic penicillin have proven useful in those with evidence of splenic dysfunction.

Prognosis Without treatment few children survive into adulthood.

THALASSAEMIAS

Science basics Inherited disorders in which the rate of synthesis of one or more globin chains is reduced or absent, producing haemolysis, ineffective erythropoiesis and anaemia. β-chain production is most commonly affected. Both heterozygote and homozygote states exist. Commonly found in Africa, the Orient, Middle East, Asia and Mediterranean.

β-thalassaemia

This is due to failure to synthesize β chains. Heterozygote form (minor) is mild and may be asymptomatic and produce no signs. Homozygotes (major) are unable to synthesize normal amounts of adult haemoglobin A and retain production of the much less effective haemoglobin F.

Clinical features There are symptoms of severe anaemia after the first 2 months of life, anorexia, failure to thrive, developmental delay and early death. Marrow hyperplasia leads to head bossing and mongoloid appearance. Hepatosplenomegaly and leg ulceration occur.

Investigations

Minor: • iron-deficiency anaemia-like picture, but ferritin normal • haemoglobin electrophoresis shows increased HbA_2 to 4–6% (normal 1.5–3%) and slight, if any, elevation of HbF levels (2–5%).

Major: • profound hypochromic anaemia with RBC dysplasia, erythroblastosis, absent HbA and raised HbF levels • radiology shows expanded marrow cavity, eg skull and phalanges, and 'hair-on-end' appearance to skull vault.

Management box
▶ Transfuse to maintain Hb > 10 g/dl. This inevitably leads to iron overload but subsequent haemochromatosis with cardiac failure may be prevented/delayed by treatment with the iron chelating agent desferrioxamine. This should be administered to all patients receiving regular transfusions. Treat folate deficiency with supplements.
▶ Splenectomy may be needed for hypersplenism with preceding vaccine against pneumococcus, meningococcus and haemophilus and subsequent prophylactic administration.

ACUTE LEUKAEMIAS

Science basics These are characterized by uncontrolled proliferation of malignant cells derived from one of the haemo-poietic precursor cells with resulting replacement of the normal bone marrow. There is often systemic involvement. They are usually progressive and ultimately fatal due to overwhelming infection, haemorrhage or anaemia. Aetiology is usually unknown but may be related to ionizing radiation, cytotoxic drugs, viral infection, chromosome changes or chemical exposure, eg benzene.

There are many different forms of this disease, each arising from a separate stem-cell component. In acute leukaemia the disease tends to be aggressive with a short life expectancy and many primitive blast cells are seen in the blood film. The presence of Auer rods in the cytoplasm of blast cells indicates a non-lymphoblastic type. Acute lymphoblastic leukaemia (ALL) has a dual demographic distribution with peaks in children and the elderly while acute myeloid leukaemia (AML) is commonest in young adults and the middle aged (Table 10.7).

Clinical features This often appears as a flu-like illness with fatigue, fever, malaise, rapidly progressing anaemia, persistent bacterial, viral or fungal sepsis (mouth, throat, anorectal or tongue ulceration) in the absence of pus formation. Purpura, bruising, bleeding from the gums, nose and GI tract. DIC may be present in type M_3. Lymphadenopathy and hepatosplenomegaly are present in ALL. Gum hypertrophy and diffuse skin involvement are features of the monocytic type of AML. CNS involvement with cranial nerve palsies may occur. Muscle and joint pain are common.

Table 10.7
Classification of acute leukaemia

Lymphoblastic (ALL):	T-Cell
	B-Cell
	Null
	Common
Myeloid (AML):	M0: Undifferentiated
	M1: Poorly differentiated
	M2: Myeloblastic
	M3: Promyelocytic
	M4: Myelomonoblastic
	M5a: Monoblastic
	M5b: Monocytic
	M6: Erythroleukaemia
	M7: Megakaryoblastic

ACUTE MYELOID LEUKAEMIA

This is a group of aggressive neoplastic diseases involving myeloid stem cells (Table 10.7). They can arise de novo or following myelodysplastic syndromes. The various subtypes are classified on the basis of peripheral blood and BM morphology, cytochemical staining, immunophenotyping and cytogenetic studies.

Management box

▶ Aggressive combination chemotherapy involving a series of individual pulses of treatment at monthly intervals allowing marrow recovery between.

▶ Allogenic bone marrow transplant in first remission (< 45 years) from an HLA-matched sibling donor may be used.

▶ The adverse reactions of chemotherapy are numerous and include anaemia, total alopecia, gastrointestinal mucositis with diarrhoea and infections secondary to immuno-suppression. The patient requires intensive red cell support, reverse barrier nursing with iv antibiotics, platelet support and nutritional support for several weeks after each pulse of treatment. Long-term consequences of treatment are less well defined: rashes are common and the risk of secondary neoplasia is increased.

▶ There is an increasing role for peripheral blood stem-cell harvesting.

Prognosis Chemotherapy achieves an initial remission rate of 80% though long-term cure is probably only around 30% with chemotherapy alone. Allogenic BMT improves long-term remission to 50%.

ACUTE LYMPHOBLASTIC LEUKAEMIA

Presentation is usually with bone marrow failure although generalized lymphadenopathy and splenomegaly are common.

Management box

▶ Involves intensive combination chemotherapy with inductive, early and late consolidative and maintenance phases.

▶ CNS relapse is a significant problem and prophylactic cranial radiotherapy and intrathecal chemotherapy are given. An allogenic transplant may be performed in first remission in adults.

Table 10.8
Good prognostic indices in ALL

WBC: $< 10 \times 10^9/l$
Age: 2–10 years
Sex: Female
Cell markers: common ALL Ag
Remission: early (within 4 weeks)

Prognosis 70% 5-year survival in children with good prognostic indices (Table 10.8).

MYELODYSPLASTIC SYNDROMES

Science basics The myelodysplastic syndromes comprise a spectrum of disorders including those that used to be regarded as 'preleukaemic states' (Table 10.9). There is progressive marrow failure leading to anaemia, leukopenia and thrombocytopenia. Approximately 30% of patients develop an acute leukaemia. An allogenic BMT should be considered in young patients. No other specific treatment is available other than supportive measures.

MYELOPROLIFERATIVE DISORDERS

Science basics Neoplastic diseases involving a proliferation of the myeloid stem cell or its derivatives (Table 10.10). A degree of

Table 10.9
Classification of the myelodysplastic syndromes

Refractory anaemia
Refractory anaemia with ring sideroblasts
Refractory anaemia with 'excess blasts' in transformation
Chronic myelomonocytic leukaemia (CMML)

Table 10.10
Classification of myeloproliferative disorders

Chronic myeloid leukaemia
Polycythaemia rubra vera
Essential thrombocythaemia
Myelofibrosis/Myeloid metaplasia

overlap exists between these various disorders. Patients are often diagnosed following a routine FBC although some present with symptoms of marrow failure or hyperviscosity (retinal haemorrhages, infarcts, papilloedema, renal failure, TIAs, cerebral infarction or intermittent claudication).

CHRONIC MYELOID LEUKAEMIA

Science basics   A less aggressive neoplastic disorder than AML involving more differentiated myeloid cell lines.

Clinical features   Some patients have few, if any, symptoms at presentation. When symptoms develop they may have insidious onset: lassitude, weight-loss, arthralgia, myalgia, epistaxis, priapism, gout, sweating, recurrent infections. Lymphadenopathy is not a prominent feature. Massive splenomegaly is characteristic.

Investigations   • Elevation of the WBC count with a predominance of mature neutrophils but a spectrum of less mature cells is often present in the peripheral blood • BM aspiration and trephine biopsy with chromosome analysis demonstrates the Philadelphia chromosome in 90% of cases (translocation of the long arm of chromosome 22 to another site, usually chromosome 9; the residual chromosome 22 is the Philadelphia chromosome) • Monoclonal immunoglobulin bands may be present • Serum urate may be elevated.

Management box

▶ Control of the elevated WBC using hydroxyurea. Interferon may be used. New drugs (signal transduction inhibitors) may revolutionize treatment in the near future. The disease can often be controlled for some time before some patients develop related myeloproliferative disorders, eg myelofibrosis or an elevated platelet count. Inevitably the disease transforms to an acute leukaemia with a poor prognosis.

▶ Allogenic BMT is the only available treatment and is offered to patients < 45 years of age. GVH reactions may complicate the transplant and is due to the cytotoxic effect of donor lymphocytes which become sensitized to the tissues of the recipient which they regard as foreign. Acute GVH disease may occur and is characterized by mucositis, diarrhoea, hepatitis and dermatitis. It may respond to corticosteroids, ciclosporin or anti-thymocyte globulin. Chronic GVH disease mimics diffuse connective disease and may respond to corticosteroids and azathioprine.

POLYCYTHAEMIA

Science basics   Polycythaemia may be true (primary = polycythaemia rubra vera, or secondary) or apparent.

POLYCYTHAEMIA VERA

Science basics   Excessive production of red cells occurs despite the presence of low levels of erythropoietin. The disease often terminates in acute leukaemia (15%) or myelofibrosis (30%). Polycythaemia indicates an increase in red cell mass in the peripheral blood. Apparent polycythaemia is caused by a reduction in plasma volume, true polycythaemia reflects a real increase in red cell mass (Table 10.11).

Clinical features   M>F and usually occurs in middle age. Dizziness, lethargy, headache, visual disturbance, pruritus, poor concentration, blackouts, dyspepsia, thrombosis and gout. Patients are plethoric, hypertensive, have engorged retinal veins and hepatosplenomegaly.

Investigations   • FBC: Hb >18 g/dl in males and 16 g/dl in females, RBC $8-12 \times 10^{12}$/l, raised PCV, WBC is usually raised, thrombocytosis in 50%, • ESR usually low • BM usually hypercellular • Isotope studies provide a measure of red cell mass and plasma volume: red cell mass is increased and plasma volume normal • Whole blood viscosity raised • Neutrophil alkaline phosphatase (NAP) score elevated • Urate often high • Serum vitamin B_{12} often raised, folate normal • Exclude secondary causes (CXR, ABG, Hb electrophoresis, IVU).

Table 10.11
Causes of polycythaemia

Primary	Polycythaemia vera
Secondary (increased erythropoietin)	
Appropriate (hypoxia):	cardiac disease, pulmonary disease, altitude, obesity, sleep apnoea, methaemoglobinaemia, sulphaemoglobinaemia
Inappropriate:	smoking, tumours (kidney, cerebellum, uterus, adrenal, liver)
Spurious	'Stress' (Gaisböck syndrome), dehydration

Management box
▶ Repeated venesection.
▶ Iron supplements are withheld to curb erythropoiesis.
▶ Hydroxyurea

Prognosis   Average survival exceeds 10 years.

MYELOID METAPLASIA AND MYELOFIBROSIS

Science basics   Both are myeloproliferative disorders (Table 10.10, p 213). Myeloid metaplasia is the appearance of marrow stem cells in abnormal sites, eg liver and spleen. The BM contains increased amounts of fibrous tissue (myelofibrosis). Unknown aetiology.

Clinical features   Fatigue, malaise, weight-loss, heat intolerance and night sweats. Gross splenomegaly is present. Bone pain and dyspepsia are common.

Investigations   • Blood film is leukoerythroblastic and characteristic 'tear-drop' poikilocytes are present • Thrombocytosis occurs • NAP score is elevated as is the serum urate level • BM aspiration often produces a 'dry' tap due to the extensive fibrosis, but the trephine biopsy is helpful.

Management box
▶ Supportive with transfusions, androgens for ineffective erythropoiesis, allopurinol for gout and folate if required. Splenectomy may be needed.
▶ Radiotherapy for bone pain or for hypersplenism. Chemotherapy is rarely useful.

Prognosis   Usually progressive disease with a mean survival of 5 years. Death is usually due to acute leukaemia or marrow failure.

LYMPHOPROLIFERATIVE DISORDERS

Table 10.12
Classification of lymphoproliferative disorders

Chronic lymphatic leukaemia
Hodgkin's lymphoma
Non-Hodgkin's lymphoma
Waldenström's macroglobulinaemia

Table 10.13
Staging of CLL

Stage	Features
0	Peripheral blood lymphocytosis
1	Generalized lymphadenopathy
2	Splenomegaly
3	Anaemia
4	Thrombocytopenia

CHRONIC LYMPHATIC LEUKAEMIA

Science basics   CLL is a chronic lymphoproliferative disorder in which the predominant early feature is that of peripheral blood lymphocytosis though features of BM failure, generalized lymphadenopathy and splenomegaly develop in more advanced disease (Table 10.13). An associated autoimmune haemolytic anaemia and thrombocytopenia may occur.

Management box
▶ Symptomatic patients with a high peripheral white count can usually be controlled using a combination of chlorambucil and prednisolone.
▶ Death usually occurs due to BM failure or intercurrent infection.

HODGKIN'S LYMPHOMA

Science basics   Usually arises in a group of lymph nodes and spreads to other adjacent nodes before metastasizing to non-lymphoid tissues. Uncommon before puberty but reaches a peak

Table 10.14
Histological classification of Hodgkin's lymphoma (Rye)

		Prognosis
Nodular sclerosing		Good
Non-sclerosing	Lymphocyte predominant	Good
	Mixed cellularity	Good
	Lymphocyte depleted	Poor

incidence at 20–40 years and peaks again in the elderly. M>F. Unknown aetiology but viral infection may be important. The malignant cell is the Reed-Sternberg giant cell with paired mirror-imaged nuclei and prominent nucleoli ('owl's eyes appearance'). A classification is given in Table 10.14.

Clinical features Non-tender, rubbery discrete lymphadenopathy (commonly cervical initially) which extends to involve other nodes. The enlarged nodes compress adjacent structures producing dysphagia, dyspnoea, stridor, SVC obstruction, paraplegia, nerve-root compression or jaundice. Splenomegaly may occur. Alcohol-induced lymph node pain can occur. General features include intermittent pyrexia (Pel-Ebstein fever), pruritus, weight-loss, night sweats and lethargy.

Investigations • FBC: normochromic, normocytic anaemia, eosinophilia, autoimmune haemolysis, thrombocytopenia, increasing lymphocyte depletion is a poor prognostic sign • BM involvement is uncommon initially • Lymph node biopsy is diagnostic • Staging includes inspection of Waldeyer's ring, CXR, liver and spleen isotope scan, CT scan of thorax and abdomen, bone scan, gallium scan, IVU, and lymphangiogram (Table 10.15) • Whole body CT scanning has superceded staging laparotomy.

Differential diagnosis Infectious lymphadenopathy (TB, chronic bacterial infection, infectious mononucleosis, syphilis, HIV infection), leukaemia, Non-Hodgkin's lymphoma, sarcoidosis, connective tissue disease and secondary malignancy.

Table 10.15
Staging of Hodgkin's lymphoma (Ann-Arbor)

Stage I	Single lymph node region/extra-lymphatic site
Stage II	Two or more node regions on one side of the diaphragm/one node region plus one extralymphatic site on the same side of the diaphragm
Stage III	Node regions on both sides of the diaphragm +/– extra-lymphatic or splenic involvement
Stage IV	Disseminated involvement of one or more extra-lymphatic tissues

Each stage can be divided into separate categories (A or B) according to the absence or presence of systemic symptoms. The poorer 'B' group have: weight-loss > 10% in 6 months, fever > 38°C, night sweats. Pruritus does not merit a 'B' category.

> **Management box**
> ▶ Depends on the stage of the disease.
> ▶ Radiotherapy: stages I–IIIA, using a 'mantle' field supra-diaphragmatically and an 'inverted Y' field subdiaphragmatically.
> ▶ Chemotherapy: stages IIIB–IV and cases relapsing after radiotherapy. Combinations of chlormethine (mustine), vincristine, procarbazine and prednisolone (MOPP) are used monthly and achieve remission in 80%. Adverse reactions are common: vomiting, alopecia, lethargy, marrow suppression with haemorrhage, anaemia and increased susceptibility to infection, peripheral neuropathy and constipation.

Prognosis Good prognostic factors: category A disease, nodular sclerosing and lymphocyte predominant histologies, and normal Hb level. 5-year survival for stage IA exceeds 90% but for stage IIIB is 50%.

NON-HODGKIN'S LYMPHOMA

Science basics Malignant proliferation of lymphoid cells (usually B cells). M>F, pre-adolescent peak followed by a nadir in incidence with a gradual rise thereafter. Unknown aetiology but certain predisposing factors may exist (Table 10.16).

Many different classification systems exist but the most important distinction is whether or not the nodular (follicular) structure of the lymph node is preserved. The nodular forms have a better prognosis than the more aggressive diffuse forms (Table 10.17).

Clinical features Painless lymphadenopathy, lassitude, weight-loss, fever, sweating and anorexia. Spread occurs both via lymphatic channels and the bloodstream, thus the disease may be widely disseminated at the time of diagnosis. Hepato-splenomegaly may occur.

Table 10.16
Possible predisposing factors to NHL

Viruses: Epstein-Barr
Radiation
Chemicals
Immunodeficiency: post transplant, SLE, HIV infection, primary immunodeficiency states
Chromosomal abnormalities: translocation of Ch 9

Table 10.17
Classification of NHL

Low-grade:	small lymphocytic
	follicular types
Intermediate grade:	diffuse types
High-grade:	large cell
	lymphoblastic
Miscellaneous:	mycosis fungoides,
	Burkitt's lymphoma

Investigations • Lymph-node biopsy is essential • FBC shows anaemia, neutropenia and thrombocytopenia secondary to marrow involvement or hypersplenism • Autoimmune haemolytic anaemia may be present • Hypoalbuminaemia and hyper-gammaglobulinaemia are common • BM aspiration and trephine to define marrow involvement • Cell membrane receptor studies help to classify the disease (immunopherotyping) • Staging investigations as for Hodgkin's lymphoma can be performed but most patients are in stages III or IV at diagnosis • HIV serology.

Management box
▶ Depends on the grade of the disease. Low grade may be simply observed unless symptomatic, as treatment at an early stage probably has little effect on survival. Intermediate or high-grade disease should be treated immediately as they are rapidly fatal.
▶ Combination chemotherapy is employed, eg cyclo-phosphamide, doxorubicin, vincristine, bleomycin and prednisolone in pulses, but the disease is often difficult to control.
▶ Radiotherapy can also be used and often produces good local control.

Prognosis Mean survival of follicular forms is about 8 years but the diffuse forms only have a mean survival of 2 years.

MULTIPLE MYELOMA

Science basics A disease characterized by neoplastic B lymphocyte proliferation within the BM. The predominant cell type is the plasma cell and monoclonal immunoglobulins are secreted with an associated immunoparesis. Myeloma may be diagnosed if two of the following are present: monoclonal band in serum, urine, or both; BM plasmacytosis; osteolytic lesions on

X-ray. In some cases only the light chains are produced and appear in the urine as Bence Jones proteins. IgG paraprotein is produced in >50%, IgA and Bence Jones in 20% each and IgD, IgE and IgM in the remainder. M>F, peak incidence from 60–70 years. There is usually progressive replacement of the BM by abnormal plasma cells. Rarely a solitary plasmacytoma may occur in either soft tissue or bone.

Clinical features Bone involvement: pain due to osteoporosis, erosion and stress fractures, nerve root compression. Hypercalcaemia leads to thirst, polyuria, constipation, abdominal pain and confusion. Haemopoietic dysfunction produces anaemia, leucopenia, and thrombocytopenia (bleeding). Hyperviscosity causes lethargy, dizziness, headaches, gangrene, fundal haemorrhages. Renal failure may occur.

Investigations • Elevated ESR with rouleaux formation (Table 10.18) • BM shows a plasmacytosis >10% • Skeletal radiographs show osteoporosis; crush fractures and lytic lesions ('pepper-pot' skull) • Hypoalbuminaemia and hypergammaglobulinaemia • Plasma protein electrophoresis shows a monoclonal band (usually >10 g/l) with a reduction in the concentration of other immunoglobulin (immune paresis) • Bence Jones protein may be present • Urea, creatinine clearance, calcium, phosphate, alkaline phosphatase and urate • Occasionally plasma cells spill over into the peripheral blood producing plasma cell leukaemia.

Table 10.18
Causes of abnormal ESR

Increased	Pregnancy
	Advanced age
	Infection
	Multiple myeloma
	Collagen diseases
	Malignancy
	Cold agglutinin disease
	Injury
	Anaemia
Decreased	Polycythaemia
	Reduced plasma volume
	Newborn
	Sickle cell disease
	Clotted blood
	Cryoglobulinaemia

Management box
▶ Radiotherapy for skeletal problems.
▶ Chemotherapy (melphalan alone or in combination with cyclophosphamide, vincristine and prednisolone).
▶ Hypercalcaemia is treated with rehydration, furosemide (frusemide), corticosteroids and biphosphonates.
▶ Plasmapheresis for hyperviscosity.
▶ RBC transfusion if needed.
▶ Solitary plasmacytomas can be treated by surgery or irradiation.

Prognosis Mean survival is about 2 years. Poor prognostic factors are urea >10 mmol/l, Hb <7.5 g/dl.

WALDENSTRÖM'S MACROGLOBULINAEMIA

Science basics Rare B cell malignancy with monoclonal IgM production and hyperviscosity. M>F, usually in the elderly.

Clinical features Lethargy, haemorrhage, headaches, dizziness, vertigo, confusion, increased susceptibility to infection, Raynaud's phenomenon, thromboses, weight-loss, lymphadenopathy and cardiac failure.

Investigations • Increased plasma viscosity resulting from the IgM paraprotein • FBC: normocytic anaemia, normal WBC and platelet counts • Elevated ESR • BM shows infiltration with lymphocytes and plasma cells • IgM monoclonal band on protein electrophoresis.

Management box
▶ Plasmapheresis, chlorambucil, cyclophosphamide and corticosteroids.

Prognosis Mean survival is 5 years.

AMYLOIDOSIS

Science basics Group of disorders characterized by tissue infiltration by eosinophilic material which demonstrates emerald-green birefringence with Congo red stain. The classification is given in Table 10.19.

Clinical features Protean depending on the tissue involved, eg peripheral neuropathy, carpal tunnel syndrome, macroglossia, malabsorption, arthropathy, cardiomyopathy, haemorrhage, nephrotic syndrome, hepatosplenomegaly and confusion.

Investigations • Tissue biopsy (usually subcutaneous fat, rectum, kidney) • monoclonal gammopathy • search for underlying condition.

Table 10.19
Classification of amyloidosis

Type	Associated disease	Nature of deposit
Immunocytic	myeloma, Waldenström's	AL amyloid fibrils similar to monoclonal light chains
Reactive	RA, systemic infections, hypernephroma, lymphoma	AA amyloid fibrils, formed from serum precursor SAA (induced by interleukin 1)
Hereditary	familial Mediterranean fever, other familial types	AA amyloid fibrils AF amyloid fibrils (similar to prealbumin)
Senile	Senile cardiac amyloid	AS amyloid fibrils
Endocrine	MEN II tumours	Hormones, eg calcitonin (AEmct fibril)

Management box
▸ Supportive, eg cardiac or renal failure, and treat the underlying condition.
▸ Colchicine in familial Mediterranean fever.

BLEEDING DISORDERS

Science basics Normal haemostasis involves a complex series of steps including spasm of small vessels in response to injury, formation of platelet plugs on the damaged endothelial surface and finally the triggering of the coagulation cascade mechanism (→ p 225) to arrest the haemorrhage. There are thus many ways in which haemostasis can be adversely affected with resultant haemorrhage. The site of bleeding varies with different abnormalities.

Cutaneous/mucosal bleeding: vessel/platelet disorder.

Skin ecchymoses/haemarthroses: coagulation disorder The classification is given in Table 10.20.

General investigations • FBC, blood film, bone marrow and trephine, template bleeding time (2–7 min) • Platelet studies

Table 10.20
Classification of bleeding disorders

Blood vessel defect	vascular purpuras:
	– drugs: aspirin, NSAIDs,
	  furosemide (frusemide)
	– infections: meningococcus,
	  typhoid, SBE
	– anaphylactoid:
	  Henoch–Schönlein
	– metabolic: uraemia, liver
	  failure
	– scurvy
	hereditary haemorrhagic
	telangectasia

Platelet defect	thrombocytopenia: – idiopathic, secondary thrombocythaemia thrombasthenia

Coagulation cascade defect	hereditary:
	– haemophilia A, haemophilia B,
	  von Willebrand's disease
	acquired:
	– oral anticoagulants, liver
	  disease, vitamin K deficiency,
	  malabsorption, DIC

(count, adhesion and aggregation) • Coagulation screen extrinsic system and intrinsic system (p 226) • Assay of specific coagulation factors (eg VIII). Fibrinogen level and FDPs are measured if DIC is suspected. Inhibitors of haemostasis (antithrombin III) can also be estimated.

THROMBOCYTOPENIA

Thrombocytopenia can occur for a number of different reasons (Table 10.21).

Idiopathic thrombocytopenic purpura
This follows a viral infection and is characterized by a severe reduction in the number of circulating platelets. Probably due to IgG antibody attack. Acute form M=F, peak incidence in childhood. Chronic form F:M, 3:1, usually occurs in adults. The normal platelet count is $150–350 \times 10^9$/l, if the count falls below 50×10^9/l the patient will have a bleeding diathesis and if the

Table 10.21
Causes of thrombocytopenia

Decreased marrow production	Fanconi's syndrome, marrow infiltration, lymphoproliferative disorders, alcoholism, uraemia, viral infection
Decreased platelet survival	ITP, SLE, drugs (thiazides, NSAIDs, rifampicin, sulphonamides), post incompatible transfusion
Increased platelet consumption	DIC, haemolytic uraemic syndrome, drugs (heparin), infections (meningococcus, SBE, EBV)
Platelet sequestration	hypersplenism
Platelet dilution	massive transfusion

count falls below $20 \times 10^9/l$ there is a high risk of spontaneous intracranial haemorrhage.

Clinical features Skin bleeding (purpura, ecchymoses), epistaxis, GI and intracranial bleeding and haematuria. Headache and dizziness. The spleen is often enlarged but not usually palpable.

Investigations • BM: normal or increased numbers of mega-karyocytes • Normal Hb and WBC levels • Thrombocytopenic on blood film • Platelet antibodies can be demonstrated • Exclude cirrhosis.

Management box
▶ Usually self-limiting in childhood and seldom needs active treatment. In adults prednisolone 60 mg/day initially.
▶ Splenectomy may be needed. Post-splenectomy patients are more vulnerable to infection with encapsulated Gram-positive organisms (eg pneumococci) thus prophylactic penicillin is needed and/or vaccination against pneumococci meningo-coccus and haemophilus before splenectomy (iv IgG is useful in some cases).
▶ In resistant cases immunosuppressives (cyclophosphamide, azathioprine, chlorambucil or vincristine) can be used.

COAGULATION CASCADE

Consolidation of the platelet plug is achieved through the

formation of cross-linked fibrin polymers (Fig. 10.1). The coagulation protein precursors (zymogens) are converted into active proteases by the action of their predecessors in the cascade system. This produces rapid amplification of the clotting process producing a stable fibrin mesh. The system is held in check by inhibitory factors which neutralize the activated factors rapidly (eg antithrombin III, C_1 esterase inhibitor, proteins C and S and α_1-antitrypsin). The fibrin polymer is destroyed by the fibrinolytic system (Fig. 10.2).

The extrinsic system requires tissue thromboplastin for activation, which is released by damaged tissues. The extrinsic and common pathways are reflected in the INR and are affected by warfarin (warfarin works by blocking the post-ribosomal γ-carboxylation of factors II, VII, IX and X, which are then released in an inactive form into the circulation). The INR is used to monitor warfarin activity. The intrinsic system requires factor XII activation through contact with subendothelial tissues or enzymes such as kallikrein. The intrinsic and common pathways are reflected in the partial thromboplastin time with kaolin (PTTK). Heparin acts by augmenting the effect of

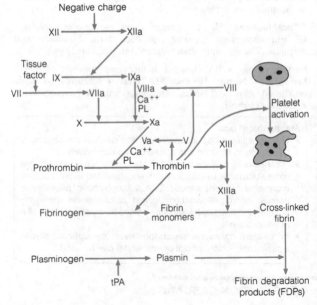

Fig. 10.1 Coagulation cascade.

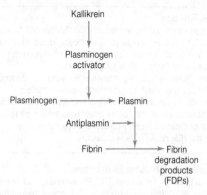

Fig. 10.2 Fibrinolytic system: iv vitamin K will reverse the bleeding diathesis within 24–48 hours but makes the patient refractory to further warfarinization for 1–2 weeks. Heparin overdosage can be reversed by protamine.

antithrombin III and control is best measured by PTTK or activated partial thromboplastin time (APPT). Warfarin overdosage can be reversed in the short term by FFP.

HAEMOPHILIAS

The haemophilias are a group of genetic disorders giving rise to deficiency of one of the coagulation pathway factors.

Haemophilia A

X-linked recessive disorder affecting males and carried by females and characterized by a deficiency of one subunit of factor VIII (factor VIII C). Factor VIII:VWF (von Willebrand's factor) level is normal. If >5% of the factor is present the disease is mild, 1–5% moderate and <1% severe. Occasionally no genetic link can be established and the disease is then thought to arise by mutation.

Clinical features Excessive bruising and haemarthroses from the time of crawling. Pain, swelling, heat and eventually deformity occur in the affected joints. Bleeding into muscles often occurs. Intra-abdominal, retroperitoneal and intracranial bleeding may all occur. Hepatitis B, and C and HIV infection can complicate this disease following transfusion of blood products.

Investigations • Clinical history • Factor VIII C assay • Prolonged PTTK • Bleeding time is normal.

Management box
▶ Early treatment, eg at home, is vital. Factor VIII levels can be elevated by the administration of freeze-dried or recombinant factor VIII concentrate. Repeated administration is needed as the half-life of factor VIII is only 8 hours.
▶ Oral antifibrinolytics, eg tranexamic acid or desmopressin, can reduce the need for factor VIII administration.
▶ Factor VIII inhibitors can develop and large doses of factor VIII or plasmapheresis may be needed to overcome them.
▶ Early mobilization helps prevent contractures.
▶ Antenatal diagnosis is now possible.

Haemophilia B: Christmas disease
X-linked deficiency of factor IX. Five times less common than haemophilia A. Clinical features are identical to haemophilia A. Treatment is by factor IX replacement.

Von Willebrand's disease
Autosomal dominant inheritance, M=F. There is both defective platelet function and a deficiency or abnormality of factor VIII:VWF.

Clinical features Skin/mucous membrane bleeding, eg after tooth extraction. Haemarthroses are uncommon.

Investigations • Family history • Prolonged bleeding time • Normal platelet count but abnormal function (poor aggregation by ristocetin and impaired adherence to glass beads) • Reduced factor VIII: VWF level.

Management box
▶ Factor VIII concentrate or DDAVP.

DISSEMINATED INTRAVASCULAR COAGULATION

Science basics The process in which coagulation and fibrinolysis occur simultaneously in the circulation.

Aetiology (Table 10.22).

Clinical features Extensive bruising, oozing from venepuncture sites, mucosal bleeding. Patient is usually gravely ill (hypotensive, hypoxaemic, pyrexial, confused).

Investigations • Thrombocytopenia • Red cell fragmentation may be present on blood film • Prolongation of PTR, PTTK and thrombin time • Reduced fibrinogen level • Raised FDPs.

**Table 10.22
Causes of DIC**

Bacterial toxins	Septicaemia – meningococcal, Gram negative
Parasitaemia	Malaria
Viral infection	Yellow fever
Acute pancreatitis	
Shock	Hypovolaemic, anaphylactic, burns
Major surgery	
Heart–lung bypass	
Incompatible blood transfusion	
Pulmonary embolism	
Fat embolism	
Obstetric	Amniotic embolism, placental abruption, intrauterine death, eclampsia
Malignancy	Leukaemia, hepatoma, renal, breast, lung, GI tract, prostate
Diabetic ketoacidosis	
Aortic aneurysm	
Snake venom	
Vasculitis	

Management box
▶ Identify and treat the underlying cause, supportive measures, eg oxygen, antibiotics, fluid expansion.
▶ Replace coagulation factors to stem haemorrhage (FFP, cryoprecipitate, platelets).
▶ Rarely antifibrinolytic agents, eg tranexamic acid or heparin, are employed.

BLOOD PRODUCTS AND THEIR USAGE

Science basics 450 ml of blood is usually collected from donors at each donation. The collection pack consists of two or three separate bags so that fractionization can be undertaken with minimal external interference, thus reducing the risk of introducing infection (Fig. 10.3, p 230).

AVAILABLE BLOOD PRODUCTS

Whole blood
Only occasionally used for the rapid restoration of red cells

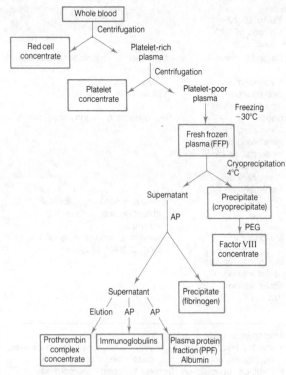

Fig. 10.3 Blood fractionation.

following massive haemorrhage. The viability of whole blood declines rapidly with storage: after 4–5 days the platelet and coagulation factor components have deteriorated.

Red cell concentrate

The preparation of choice for the management of active bleeding and for the elective correction of chronic anaemia. A single unit of RCC contains approximately 300 ml of fluid with a haematocrit of 70%. The red cells are stored in an optimal additive solution to release the plasma for other uses.

Platelet concentrate

Prepared by centrifugation of platelet-rich plasma. Each unit contains approximately 50×10^9 platelets, 5 units are usually given at each transfusion. Some individuals develop antibodies to platelet-derived HLA antigens, and should be provided with single-donor platelets.

White cell concentrate

Only used rarely as it is difficult to give sufficient quantities of leucocytes to combat infection ($t_{1/2}$ is only 8 hours). Neutrophils express HLA- and leucocyte-specific antigens very strongly and development of antibodies with non-haemolytic transfusion reactions are very common. Most patients with sepsis and leucopenia respond to broad spectrum antibiotics.

Plasma products

Do not contain cells and do not require cross-matching but blood grouping is required.

Fresh frozen plasma: platelet-poor plasma can be stored at $-30°C$ with a shelf-life of 3–6 months. FFP contains all the components of normal plasma and is particularly useful in situations where replacement of several factors is required, as in DIC, massive red cell transfusion or replacement of coagulation factor deficiencies due to liver failure or warfarin overdosage.

Cryoprecipitate: prepared from FFP by allowing it to thaw slowly at $+4°C$. A precipitate is formed which is rich in factor VIII, VWF, fibrinogen factor XII and factor XIII. The precipitate can be refrozen and stored for 3–6 months.

Factor VIII concentrate: prepared by further fractionation of cryoprecipitate and specifically indicated for haemophilia A. Plasma from a large number of donors is pooled in the preparation and in the past suboptimal sterilization techniques have led to a high viral infection rate in haemophiliacs, especially with hepatitis B and C and HIV. Current sterilization techniques involve heat-treatment of the lyophilized product.

Prothrombin complex concentrate: contains factors II, VII, IX and X and is indicated in haemophilia B.

Human immunoglobulin: non-specific immunoglobulin is used in congenital and acquired immunodeficiencies and in the treatment of severe ITP. Specific immunoglobulins are used after exposure to certain serious viral infections by a non-immune patient, eg hepatitis B, rubella (in pregnant women), herpes zoster, rabies, tetanus and measles (in the immunosuppressed).

Albumin containing solutions: a number of products are available with various degrees of albumin purity, eg PPS, human albumin solution. These are useful in two clinical situations – as plasma expanders in a patient with acute haemorrhage while awaiting blood, and to maintain plasma albumin levels in patients with severe malnutrition, liver failure, or a protein-losing state. Salt-poor albumin is expensive and usually only used in liver failure.

BLOOD TRANSFUSION → also page 519

TISSUE TYPING

RBC membranes contain a number of surface antigens including ABO, rhesus, Lewis, P and Ii which are autosomally inherited. The function of these antigens is unknown but they may help to maintain the integrity of the membranes. Red cell antibodies are present in the serum and are produced in response to stimulation by the appropriate antigen on the RBC membrane but may also be present in bacteria and in certain foodstuffs. For prevalence of various blood groups (Table 10.23). Blood group O are universal donors for red cells and AB are universal recipients.

Approximately 85% of the European population contain the D antigen on the RBC surface and are known as rhesus (Rh) positive.

HLA SYSTEM

Human leucocyte antigens are important in producing the immune response which rejects foreign tissues including tissue allografts. They are genetically determined and coded for by an area on chromosome 6 known as the MHC. HLAs are found on cells in most tissues and can be divided into types: HLA-A, HLA-B, HLA-C, HLA-D, HLA-DR and HLA-DW. Certain genotypes are associated with disease (Table 10.24). HLA tissue typing is performed before organ transplantation (except liver) as matched tissue has the best chance of survival.

Table 10.23
Occurrence of ABO blood groups and serum antibodies in the UK

Blood group	Serum antibody	UK frequency(%)
A	Anti-B	42
B	Anti-A	8
AB	None	3
O	Anti-A/anti-B	47

Table 10.24
Association of HLA and disease

Rheumatoid arthritis	– DR4
Addison's disease	– B8, DW3
Seronegative arthritis	– B27
Thyrotoxicosis	– B8, DR3
IDDM	– B8, B15, DR3, DR4
Myasthenia gravis	– A8
Haemochromatosis	– A3, B14
Multiple sclerosis	– DRW2
Coeliac disease	– D8

11

Rheumatology

RHEUMATOID ARTHRITIS

Science basics A chronic inflammatory, erosive and symmetrical polyarthritis associated with systemic disturbance, many extra-articular lesions and the presence of circulating antiglobulin antibodies (rheumatoid factors). Evidence points to persistent immune overactivity, autoimmunity and the presence of immune complexes at sites of articular and extra-articular lesions. Circulating antibodies to IgG (rheumatoid factors) are produced in response to some unknown antigen and the immune system is triggered with resulting inflammation and tissue destruction. The joint synovial membrane becomes swollen and congested with lymphocytes, neutrophils, plasma cells and macrophages. It has the histological appearance of granulation tissue and is known as 'pannus'. This pannus destroys the articular cartilage and sub-chondral bone producing bony erosions. Fibrosis and bony ankylosis are produced, joint effusions occur and adjacent muscles atrophy. Subcutaneous nodules contain fragmented collagen fibres, cellular debris and exudate and are surrounded by pallisades of mononuclear cells.

Aetiology and pathogenesis Unknown aetiology, adult prevalence approximately 1%, commonly commences in early adult life and associated with a significant increase in HLA-D4 and HLA-DR4. There is also an increase in urban dwellers suggesting that environmental factors may be important. F:M = 3:1. Disease remission often occurs during pregnancy and relapse may occur following the menopause.

Classification The revised American College of Rheumatology (ACR) criteria are used to clarify RA. At least four of the following seven criteria must be present: • Morning stiffness • arthritis ≥ three joints • arthritis of hand joints • rheumatoid nodules • symmetrical arthritis • radiographic change (eg erosions) • serum rheumatoid factor.

Clinical features Insidious onset of symmetrical joint pain, stiffness and swelling which is most marked in the mornings and usually affects the hands, feet and wrists first. However, a sudden onset ('explosive') variant is recognized. Swelling of the proximal (PIP), but not the distal (DIP) interphalangeal joints gives the fingers a 'spindled' appearance and swelling of the metatarsophalangeal joints (MTP) produces 'broadening' of the forefoot. As the disease progresses other joints become involved including the elbows, shoulders, knees, ankles, tarsal joints, cervical spine and temperomandibular joints. The hips are usually spared. Systemic features including fever, malaise, night sweats and weight-loss may also be present. Popliteal cysts (Baker's cysts) may be produced and mimic DVT. Joint

Table 11.1
Extra-articular manifestations of RA

Anorexia
Weight-loss
Malaise
Lethargy
Myalgia

Rheumatoid nodules over bony prominences — eg elbows, occiput, scapulae, Achilles tendon, flexor tendons of the fingers (cause 'triggering')

Vasculitic lesions — nail bed or finger pulp infarcts, skin necrosis, pyoderma gangrenosum

Raynaud's phenomenon
Lymphadenopathy
Osteoporosis

Eye signs — keratoconjunctivitis sicca, episcleritis, scleromalacia, nodular scleritis, scleromalacia perforans

Cardiac — pericarditis, myocarditis, conduction defects, endocarditis, aortic regurgitation, cardiomyopathy

Pulmonary — pleural effusions, interstitial fibrosis, pneumothorax, bronchitis, nodules, pleurisy, stridor due to cricoarytenoid arthritis, obliterative bronchiolitis, pulmonary vasculitis, rheumatoid pneumoconiosis (Caplan's)

Neurological — mononeuritis multiplex, entrapment neuropathy, distal sensory neuropathy cervical myelopathy

Haematological — anaemia – normochromic, normocytic, iron deficiency due to GI blood loss or defective utilization, Coomb's +ve haemolytic, Felty's syndrome (splenomegaly, leg ulcers, neutropenia), macrocytic (folate deficiency), hyperviscosity, thrombocytosis

Renal — proteinuria, amyloid, glomerulonephritis

Tenosynovitis
Bursitis

destruction occurs causing increasing joint instability, subluxation, ankylosis and decreasing mobility.

Characteristic deformities are produced and include: ulnar deviation of the fingers due to subluxation at the metacarpo-phalangeal joints; loss of finger function due to hyperextension of the PIP joints with fixed flexion of the DIP joints; 'swan necking' or fixed flexion of the PIP joints with hyperextension of the DIP joints; 'boutonniere' or Z deformity of the thumb. Rupture of the extensor tendons of the hand can occur secondary to either tenosynovitis or stretching over a prominent ulnar styloid process. Foot involvement leads to clawing of the toes and a painful sensation of 'walking on pebbles' due to exposure of the metatarsal heads. Severe cervical pain may be present and the potentially fatal complication of atlantoaxial subluxation may occur. For other manifestations see Table 11.1.

Investigations • FBC, ESR • C-reactive protein, low albumin level, hypergammaglobulinaemia, increased fibrinogen level, circulating complement levels are usually normal (synovial fluid levels low) urinalysis for protein • Arthroscopy and synovial biopsy • Rheumatoid factor titre. Rheumatoid factor may however be negative during the early stages of the disease and indeed may remain negative in up to 30% cases. False-positive values also occur (Table 11.2). Radiological features are listed in Table 11.3.

Differential diagnosis Gout, SLE, polyarteritis nodosa, rheumatic fever, dermatomyositis, mixed connective tissue disease, infective arthritis, eg TB, bacterial or viral, Reiter's syndrome, hypertrophic osteoarthropathy, sarcoidosis,

---

Table 11.2
Causes of a false-positive rheumatoid factor

Scleroderma
SLE
SBE
Chronic active hepatitis
TB
Leprosy
Syphilis
Sarcoidosis
Paraproteinaemia, eg multiple myeloma
Sjögren's syndrome
Mixed connective tissue disease
Chronic juvenile arthritis
Malaria

Table 11.3
Radiological features of RA

Early	soft tissue swelling
	periarticular osteoporosis
	periostitis
	erosions – periarticular, subarticular cysts
Late	narrowed joint spaces
	articular surface irregularity
	osteoporosis
	subluxation
	ankylosis
	secondary osteoarthritis

osteoarthritis, psoriatic arthropathy, arthritis due to inflammatory bowel disease, polymyalgia rheumatica, seronegative arthritides.

Management box

The principles are:
▶ Maintain normal function.
▶ Relieve pain.
▶ Prevent deformity.
▶ Patient education, physiotherapy; exercise, occupational therapy and drugs are all used.
▶ *Early disease*: NSAIDs (aspirin, mefenamic acid, indometacin, naproxen) stimulate the cyclooxygenase (COX) enzyme system involved in the production of prostaglandins. Intra-articular corticosteroid (methyl-prednisolone or triamcinolone) may be useful. Joint splinting may be required for severe acute episodes. If poor response, proceed to disease-modifying anti-rheumatoid drugs (DMARDs).
▶ *Progressive disease*: DMARDs slow disease progress. Sulfasalazine gives a response in 1–3 months. Intramuscular gold is more effective than oral preparations. These drugs may have serious side-effects (Table 11.4). In severe cases systemic corticosteroids may be useful. Steroid requirement may be reduced by the use of immunosuppressants (eg methotrexate, azathioprine, cyclophosphamide, chlorambucil).

Prognosis Most patients follow a chronic course with remissions and relapses. After 10 years 25% will have complete remission, 40% moderate impairment, 25% severe impairment and 10% will be crippled by their disease. Poor prognostic factors include insidious onset, progressive disease without periods of remission,

Table 11.4
Adverse reactions of disease-modifying rheumatoid drugs

Penicillamine	Rashes, loss of taste, fever, nausea, vomiting, glomerulonephritis, Goodpasture's syndrome, SLE-like syndrome, myasthenic syndrome, thrombocytopenia, pancytopenia, mouth ulcers
Gold	Mouth ulcers, nephrotic syndrome, pruritic rash, enterocolitis, aplastic anaemia, proteinuria
Sulfasalazine	Bone marrow suppression, rashes, nausea
Chloroquine	Diarrhoea, ocular toxicity – reversible corneal deposits on drug withdrawal, permanent retinopathy, haemolytic anaemia

high titres of rheumatoid factor, rheumatoid nodules, and the development of extra-articular manifestations.

SERONEGATIVE SPONDARTHRITIDES

Science basics A group of conditions characterized by inflammatory asymmetrical oligoarthritis, sacroiliitis, anterior uveitis, high incidence of HLA-B27 but negative rheumatoid factor tests.

Types: • Ankylosing spondylitis • Psoriatic arthritis • Behçet's syndrome • Reiter's syndrome • Reactive arthritis • Whipple's disease • Enteropathic arthritis • Juvenile chronic arthritis.

ANKYLOSING SPONDYLITIS

A disease of young men M:F = 9:1, teenage peak age-of-onset. Unknown aetiology but strong link with HLA-B27 (50% risk of transmitting this Ag to their children and 33% of developing the disease). Sporadic disease (80%) may be more severe than familial cases.

Clinical features Initially low back pain and stiffness >3 months, especially in the mornings, bilateral sacroiliitis, progressing to thoracic backache, thoracic kyphosis. Loss of lumbar lordosis. Achilles tendinitis and pain over iliac crest. Anterior uveitis, aortic regurgitation, apical pulmonary fibrosis, osteoporosis, myopathy, amyloidosis, atlanto-axial subluxation.

Investigations • FBC (leucocytosis), high ESR • C-reactive protein, hypergammaglobulinaemia • Negative rheumatoid factor

• HLA-B27 • Radiology (sacroiliitis, 'bamboo spine', erosions, sclerosis and ankylosis).

> **Management box**
> ▶ Maintain mobility.
> ▶ Physiotherapy.
> ▶ Hydrotherapy.
> ▶ NSAIDs.
> ▶ Pulsed intravenous corticosteroid in severe disease.
> ▶ Rarely radiotherapy or surgery.
> ▶ Genetic counselling.

PSORIATIC ARTHRITIS

This affects 7% psoriatic sufferers. Various types exist: DIP joint involvement with nail changes, seronegative RA, arthritis mutilans with digit destruction, ankylosing spondylitis and asymmetrical disease affecting the hands and feet. May be triggered by stress, trauma or infection.

Clinical features Think of the diagnosis when psoriasis co-exists with arthritis. Nail pitting common in DIP joint disease. 'Opera glass' fingers may occur with extensive bone resorption (arthritis mutilans).

Investigations As for ankylosing spondylitis • Radiology shows asymmetrical disease, DIP joint involvement and little periarticular osteoporosis.

> **Management box**
> ▶ NSAIDs.
> ▶ Methotrexate in severe disease.
> ▶ Low-dose ciclosporin.
> ▶ Avoid chloroquine derivatives (can produce an acute psoriatic skin reaction).
> ▶ Sulfasalazine, azathioprine or gold may be tried.

BEHÇET'S SYNDROME

An association of arthritis, iritis and recurrent oral and genital ulceration. Commoner in Eastern Mediterranean and Japan. M>F. Associated with HLA-B5. Unknown aetiology.

Clinical features As above. Vasculitis, eg erythema nodosum, thrombophlebitis, synovitis, meningitis, encephalitis, pericarditis, and sacroiliitis may also be present.

Investigations As for ankylosing spondylitis.

Diagnosis Usually clinical.

> **Management box**
> ▸ Symptomatic to oral and genital ulcers, eg local anaesthetic cream.
> ▸ NSAIDs.
> ▸ Systemic corticosteroids and immunosuppressives for severe disease, especially if the eyes are involved.
> ▸ Azathioprine and ciclosporin may have a role in the future.

REITER'S SYNDROME

A triad of conjunctivitis, urethritis and seronegative lower limb oligo-arthritis. Two forms exist.

The genital form: occurs in 1% of patients with non-specific urethritis.

The intestinal type: follows enteric infection with *Shigella*, *Salmonella*, *Yersinia* or *Campylobacter* in genetically predisposed individuals. M:F = 20:1 (but urethritis is often asymptomatic in females).

Clinical features As above, usually affects the knees 1–4 weeks after exposure, may be recurrent although the urethritis may not always be recurrent. Backache, heel pain (due to calcaneal spur enthesopathy), tender fingers. Skin lesions are common, eg circinate balanitis, keratoderma blenorrhagica, macules, papules, pustules, nail dystrophy and scales. Rarely pleurisy and pericarditis.

Investigations As for anklosing spondylitis, the diagnosis is suggested by the classical presentation.

> **Management box**
> ▸ Usually self-limiting although 80% continue to have active disease at 5 years.
> ▸ NSAIDs.
> ▸ Local joint corticosteroid injection.
> ▸ Antibiotics for urethritis (eg tretracycline or erythromycin).
> ▸ Steroid eyedrops for conjunctivitis.
> ▸ In severe cases corticosteroids or immunosuppressive agents may be needed.

REACTIVE ARTHRITIS

This is an arthritis with a similar pattern to that of Reiter's disease, but without the extra-articular features.

WHIPPLE'S DISEASE (intestinal lipodystrophy)

A rare disease, M>F, caused by infection with *Tropheryma whippleii*

Clinical features Malabsorption, weight-loss, lymphadenopathy, abdominal pain, migratory polyarthritis (usually knee or ankle), sacroiliitis, pyrexia and increased skin pigmentation.

Investigations • Negative rheumatoid factor • Small intestinal biopsy shows PAS-positive staining macrophages.

> ***Management box***
> ▶ NSAIDs.
> ▶ Tetracycline 1 g daily for at least a year.

ENTEROPATHIC ARTHRITIS

This is the association of a seronegative arthritis with either infection or inflammatory bowel disease, eg ulcerative colitis or Crohn's disease, or with intestinal bypass operations performed for obesity.

Clinical features Acute and often migratory oligo-arthritis of weight-bearing joints or sacroiliitis which classically follows exacerbations of bowel disease. Aphthous ulceration, erythema nodosum or uveitis may be present.

Investigations As for ankylosing spondylitis • Bowel investigations as indicated, eg barium studies, endoscopy.

> ***Management box***
> ▶ NSAIDs.
> ▶ Physiotherapy
> ▶ Treat the underlying bowel disease, eg corticosteroids or sulfasalazine.

JUVENILE CHRONIC ARTHRITIS

Disease onset before 16 years. Various types: Still's disease (systemic juvenile chronic arthritis), polyarticular juvenile chronic arthritis, seropositive polyarticular disease and pauci-articular juvenile chronic arthritis.

Clinical features These depend on the type but may include fever, malaise, lymphadenopathy, myalgia, arthralgia, pleurisy, pericarditis, weight-loss, growth retardation and polyarthritis which may affect large or small joints and the spine. The eyes may be affected.

Investigations As for any seronegative arthritis.

Management box
▸ Bed-rest during acute exacerbations.
▸ Continue education, physiotherapy, hydrotherapy.
▸ NSAIDs.
▸ Try to avoid corticosteroids because of growth retardation secondary to adrenal suppression.
▸ Intra-articular corticosteroids may be useful.
▸ Disease-modifying drugs, eg gold, penicillamine or chloroquine derivatives can be used as long as the patient is closely monitored for possible adverse reactions.
▸ Surgery may be needed in severe cases.

POLYMYALGIA RHEUMATICA

Science basics   Related to giant-cell arteritis (p 316) this condition is characterized by pains and stiffness in proximal muscles particularly in the morning. Anorexia, malaise, and low-grade fever may occur. F:M = 3:1. The ESR is usually raised.

Management box
▸ Prednisolone (15 mg) is effective with a view to reducing dose after 6–8 weeks and stopping treatment after 2 years.

OSTEOARTHROSIS

Science basics   A disorder which is the end result of a variety of conditions which produce joint destruction. It is characterized by destruction of articular cartilage, and proliferation of new bone, cartilage and fibrous supporting tissue. Extremely common condition affecting in excess of 80% of people older than 65 years, although not all of these cases are symptomatic. Primary is commoner in females. Damp environmental conditions are associated with increased symptoms.

Aetiology and pathogenesis   (Table 11.5). This is unknown but two main theories exist. The first considers that the initial feature is fatigue fracture of the collagen support network underlying the articular cartilage. This leads to an increased level of hydration of the cartilage with subsequent unravelling of the proteoglycans. The alternative hypothesis suggests that the initiating event in joint destruction is the development of microfractures in the subchondral bone whose healing produces increased stress on the overlying cartilage with subsequent fracture of its surface exposing the underlying bone. The joint is eventually destroyed with loss of normal function.

Table 11.5
Aetiology of osteoarthrosis

Primary	Unknown cause	
Secondary	Traumatic	malaligned fractures
		excessive wear and tear
	Metabolic	haemochromatosis,
		chondrocalcinosis,
	Endocrine	acromegaly,
		hypothyroidism
	Inflammatory	gout, alkaptonuria
	Aseptic necrosis	corticosteroids,
		sickle cell disease
	Paget's disease	
	Developmental	slipped femoral epiphysis
		Perthe's disease
	Neuropathic	Charcot's joint,
		diabetes mellitus
	Haemophilic arthritis	
	Pyrophosphate arthroplasty	

Clinical features These may be asymptomatic. Pain which is usually worse on activity and eased by rest, joint swelling, stiffness, limitation of movement and muscle wasting. Crepitus may be elicited. Deformity due to articular cartilage damage and bony remodelling may be present. Heberden's nodes are gelatinous cysts or bony outgrowths on the dorsal aspects of the DIP of the hands and are characteristic of primary OA. Bouchard's nodes are similar but occur at the proximal interphalangeal joints. The joints which are characteristically involved are weight-bearing, eg hips, knees and spine, MTP joint of the great toe, DIP joints in the hands, carpometacarpal of the thumb, temporomandibular and sternoclavicular joints.

Investigations • Radiology: joint-space narrowing, subchondral sclerosis, osteophytes, cysts, erosions, chondrocalcinosis • FBC and ESR are both normal • RF is negative unless the initiating condition is RA • Synovial fluid aspiration/microscopy • Serum uric acid if gout is considered.

Management box
▶ Symptomatic, eg bed rest, weight reduction, NSAIDs, heat or US.
▶ TENS.
▶ Intra-articular corticosteroids.
▶ Treat the underlying condition.
▶ Joint replacement.

CRYSTAL DEPOSITION DISEASES

GOUT

Metabolic disorder of purine metabolism characterized by hyper-uricaemia and recurring attacks of arthritis, due to the deposition of microcrystals of sodium urate monohydrate (uric acid). In the later stages of the disease chronic arthritis, tophi and renal failure may develop. Commonest in middle age and may be inherited in an autosomal dominant manner in some cases. Predisposing factors are listed in Table 11.6.

Clinical features

Acute attack: acute monoarthritis affecting MTP of the great toe in 60% of cases. May also affect the ankle, knee, small joints of the feet and hands, wrist or elbow, sometimes in a spreading fashion. Joint is hot, tender, and swollen with shiny overlying skin. Fever, nausea and mood-swings may be present. Attacks last 2–10 days and resolution may be accompanied by pruritus and local desquamation. The attack can be precipitated by dietary excess, alcohol, trauma, uricosuric drugs or during initiation of allopurinol therapy.

Table 11.6
Factors predisposing to hyperuricaemia and gout

1. *Impaired excretion of uric acid (75%)*
   Undefined genetic defect
   Drugs – low-dose salicyclates, thiazides, alcohol,
     sulphonamides, pyrazinamide, ciclosporin, nicotinic acid
   Chronic renal failure
   Lactic acidosis – alcohol, exercise, starvation, toxaemia of
     pregnancy
   Hypothyroidism
   Down's syndrome
   Hyperparathyroidism
   Lead poisoning
   Cystinuria
   Glucose-6-phosphatase deficiency.

2. *Increased production of uric acid (25%)*
   Myeloproliferative disorders – chronic lymphatic leukaemia,
     polycythaemia rubra vera
   Psoriasis
   Enzyme deficiencies – HGPRT, glucose-6-phosphatase

Chronic gout: produces progressive joint destruction with deformity. Tophi may be produced in the cartilage of the ear, bursae and tendon sheaths. They are composed of monosodium urate, cholesterol, calcium and oxalate. Urate urolithiasis occurs in 10% and rarely chronic urate nephropathy with renal failure.

Differential diagnosis Septic arthritis, RA, trauma, cellulitis, bunion, chondrocalcinosis, seronegative arthritis.

Investigations • Serum urate (serum uric acid level >0.42 mmol/l in adult males or >0.36 mmol/l in adult females) is usually raised but may be normal • Aspiration and polarized light examination of synovial fluid (negative birefringence of needle-shaped particles) • Radiology shows osteoporosis, 'punched out' erosions, secondary osteoarthritic changes • Leucocytosis and raised ESR during an acute attack.

Management box

▸ NSAIDs should be used as early as possible during an acute attack, eg naproxen 250 mg 6-hourly.

▸ Alternatively colchicine 1 mg stat followed by 0.5 mg 2-hourly may be used but it may be poorly tolerated due to vomiting and diarrhoea.

▸ Once the acute attack is controlled long-term prophylaxis can be considered if attacks are frequent, there is joint damage, or tophi are present using allopurinol 300–900 mg daily to reduce the serum urate level. Lower doses of allopurinol should be used in renal impairment. Allopurinol should not be started until several weeks after the last acute attack.

▸ Avoid precipitating factors, eg alcoholic binges, and reduce weight if obese.

▸ Uricosuric drugs can also be used as prophylaxis, eg probenecid 0.5–1.0 mg bd together with colchicine 0.5 mg bd, but must be avoided in renal failure, urate urolithiasis and in gross uricosuria.

▸ If urate calculi are present push fluids and alkalinize the urine to pH > 6.

PYROPHOSPHATE ARTHROPATHY

Calcium pyrophosphate dihydrate crystals are deposited in cartilage (chondrocalcinosis), where they are associated with degenerative changes. Shedding of the crystals into the joint space produces acute synovitis and a clinical picture which resembles acute gout. It is associated with a number of underlying conditions, eg metabolic diseases (hyperparathyroidism, hypothyroidism, haemochromatosis, Wilson's disease, oxalosis, gout, OA, dialysis and long-term steroid use). M = F incidence.

Clinical features   Various forms exist.

Pseudogout: mimics an acute attack of gout.

Polyarticular attacks: multiple joint involvement with subacute attacks.

Chronic arthropathy: osteoarthritic like.

Chronic destructive arthropathy: produces a neuropathic joint.

Polymyalgic type: generalized muscle aches.

Asymptomatic form: noticed on X-ray.

Investigations • Radiology shows linear opacification of articular cartilage • Synovial fluid examination under polarized light reveals positively birefringent rhomboid crystals • Arthroscopy shows 'microtophi' on the synovial membrane • Identify possible underlying conditions.

> **Management box**
> ▶ NSAIDs.
> ▶ Joint aspiration and injection of steroids.
> ▶ Colchicine.

CONNECTIVE TISSUE DISEASE

SYSTEMIC LUPUS ERYTHEMATOSUS

Systemic disease of unknown aetiology characterized by the presence of non-organ-specific autoantibodies. F:M = 9:1, occasionally familial, associated with HLA-A1, B8 and DR3, and much commoner in the Black population. May be precipitated by a variety of drugs, eg phenytoin, isoniazid, OCP, hydralazine and penicillamine. Commonest during childbearing years and exacerbations can occur during pregnancy and also during menstruation. There may be a past history of spontaneous abortion and thrombosis (antiphospholipid antibody syndrome).

Clinical features   (Table 11.7)

Investigations • FBC (normochromic normocytic anaemia, leukopenia, thrombocytopenia, haemolytic anaemia, prolongation of INR in the presence of lupus anticoagulant) • Elevated ESR • C-reactive protein (usually normal in the absence of infection), cold agglutinins, hypergammaglobulinaemia, low albumin, raised fibrinogen, cryoglobulins • Low serum complement, raised immune complexes • antinuclear antibodies (ANF, anti-double-stranded DNA, anti-histone, anti-extractable nuclear antibodies: anti-RNP,

Table 11.7
Clinical features of SLE

General	Fever, malaise, lethargy
Locomotor	Arthralgia, arthritis, Jaccoud's arthropathy in 50%, tenosynovitis, myalgia
Skin	'Butterfly rash', erythematous or maculopapular rash, vasculitis, purpura, Raynaud's phenomenon, alopecia, livido reticularis, chillblains, oral ulceration
Cardiovascular	Pericarditis, myocarditis, endocarditis (Libman-Sacks), lupus anticoagulant with recurrent venous or arterial thrombosis, thrombophlebitis
Pulmonary	Pleurisy, pleural effusions, atelectasis, breathlessness due to pulmonary fibrosis, 'shrinking lung syndrome'
Renal	Nephrotic syndrome, nephritis
Nervous system	Peripheral neuropathy, transverse myelitis, hemiparesis, seizures, psychosis, meningitis, cranial nerve palsies, dementia
Gastrointestinal	Ulceration, protein-losing enteropathy, abdominal pain, pancreatitis
Haematological	Haemolytic anaemia
Ophthalmic	Cystic bodies in retina, episcleritis, soft exudates
Hepatic	Jaundice, abnormal LFTs
Lymphadenopathy	
Splenomegaly	

anti-Sm, anti-SSA, anti-SSB • False-positive RF • False-positive tests for syphilis (VDRL or TPHA) • Renal function tests (urea, electrolytes, creatinine clearance, 24-hour urinary protein, urinary casts or RBCs) • Synovial fluid examination (absence of crystals and infection) • Radiology may show changes indistinguishable from RA • Biopsy of skin or renal tissue.

Differential diagnosis Systemic sclerosis, polyarteritis, RA or mixed connective tissue disease, SBE, infective arthritis.

Management box
▶ Mild cases need rest, NSAIDs and removal of any precipitating causes, eg drugs or sunlight.
▶ Severe cases need systemic corticosteroid therapy, eg 40–60 mg prednisolone daily initially, or 'pulse' therapy using methyl-prednisolone 1 g daily for 3 days to gain control of the disease. →

▶ As the disease comes under control the dose of steroids can be gradually reduced to an alternate day regime if possible.
▶ Antimalarials, eg chloroquine derivatives, are useful in skin and joint disease.
▶ Immunosuppressive agents (eg azathioprine) or plasmapheresis are reserved for those cases which cannot be controlled with steroids alone.
▶ Dialysis may be needed in renal failure.
▶ Anticoagulants are used when the lupus anticoagulant is present and there is a history of thrombosis. Otherwise low-dose aspirin is sufficient.

Prognosis Poor prognosis is indicated by childhood onset of disease, high urea, persistent proteinuria, evidence of arteritis, CNS and cardiopulmonary involvement and requirement for long-term corticosteroids. The overall 5-year survival for this disease is now in excess of 90%.

PROGRESSIVE SYSTEMIC SCLEROSIS

Generalized connective tissue disorder characterized by fibrosis. The skin is the predominant organ to be affected but the gut, heart, lungs and kidneys may also be involved. Unknown aetiology, associated with HLA-A1, B8' and DR3 haplotypes. F:M = 4: 1 and an increased incidence is present among miners.

Clinical features (Table 11.8)

Table 11.8
Clinical features of systemic sclerosis

Skin	Severe Raynaud's phenomenon, non-pitting shiny digital oedema, 'sausage shaped' fingers, atrophy and ulceration of finger tips, subcutaneous calcinosis, loss of hair follicles and sweat glands, sclerodactyly, puckering around mouth, 'pinched' nose, telangiectasia, localized morphoea
Musculoskeletal	Arthralgia, myositis, non-erosive arthritis
Gastrointestinal	Reflux oesophagitis, dysphagia, bowel dilatation causing abdominal pain, diarrhoea, malabsorption
Pulmonary	Lung fibrosis, cor pulmonale, alveolar cell carcinoma
Renal	Hypertension, renal failure
Cardiac	Pericarditis, myocarditis, cardiomyopathy

Investigations • FBC (normochromic, normocytic anaemia)
• Raised ESR • Positive ANF in 50% (nucleolar or speckled
staining pattern), antibodies to single-stranded RNA are more
specific: RF may be false-positive • Complement levels are
normal • Radiology reveals soft tissue calcification, resorption of
the tufts of the terminal phalanges, pulmonary fibrosis and
barium studies may show a hiatus hernia, oesophageal stricture
or dysmotility.

Differential diagnosis CREST syndrome (calcinosis,
Raynaud's phenomenon, oesophageal involvement, sclerodactyly
and telangiectasia), morphoea, eosinophilic fasciitis, amyloid,
acromegaly, myxoedema.

> **Management box**
> ▸ None arrests the disease.
> ▸ Keep the hands and feet warm, treat infections, hypertension
>   and dysphagia.
> ▸ Corticosteroids and cyclophosphamide may be helpful.
> ▸ NSAIDs for joint symptoms
> ▸ 5-year survival is approximately 70%.

DERMATOMYOSITIS AND POLYMYOSITIS

Inflammatory conditions of unknown aetiology affecting the skin
and striated muscle. Linked with HLA-B8 and DR3. Five
categories exist:

- Primary (idiopathic) polymyositis
- Primary dermatomyositis
- Dermatomyositis associated with malignancy
- Dermatomyositis associated with collagen disease
- Childhood dermatomyositis.

Clinical features The adult forms typically affect middle-aged
females and present with difficulty rising from the seated position. Examination reveals limb-girdle weakness. The pharyngeal,
laryngeal and respiratory muscles may also be involved leading to
dysphagia, dysphonia and respiratory failure. Arthralgia, myalgia,
Raynaud's phenomenon, swelling of the fingers, purple
discolouration on the face and knuckles ('heliotrope rash'), and
subcutaneous calcinosis may all occur. An underlying tumour
of the breast, lung, ovary, prostate, GU tract or GI tract may
be present in 3% of cases of polymyositis and 15% of
dermatomyositis. In children the presenting features are usually
muscle weakness, calcification, contractures and the heliotrope
rash.

Investigations • FBC (normochromic, normocytic anaemia, leucocytosis) • Raised ESR • Raised serum muscle enzymes (CPK, aldolase) • Autoantibodies are often positive (ANF, RF and extractable nuclear antigen PM-1) • EMG • Muscle biopsy.

Management box
▶ Prednisolone 40–60 mg/day initially to produce remission, reducing slowly to a maintenance dose of 5–15 mg/day.
▶ Immunosuppressive agent, eg azathioprine, can be used as a steroid-sparing agent.
▶ Splinting and physiotherapy are important.
▶ Treatment directed at any underlying tumour can produce some improvement in the condition.

MIXED CONNECTIVE TISSUE DISEASE

Combines the features of two or more connective tissue disorders, eg SLE, scleroderma or dermatomyositis. High incidence of Raynaud's phenomenon, arthralgia, erosive arthritis, myositis, oesophageal motility problems and hypergammaglobulinaemia. Low titres against DNA but high titre against an extractable nuclear antigen (ENA – ribonuclear protein). There is characteristically a good response to steroids.

INFECTIVE ARTHRITIS

Science basics Relatively rare in normal joints except when the joint space is breached by a foreign body, eg nail, splinter or rose thorn.

Table 11.9
Causes of infective arthritis

Bacterial	Viral	Fungal
Staphylococci	Rubella	Histoplasmosis
Streptococci	Mumps	Coccidioidomycosis
Gonococci	Hepatitis A, B	Blastomycosis
Syphilis	CMV	Spirotrichosis
Tuberculosis	Coxsackie B	Aspergillosis
Meningococci	Parvovirus	Actinomycosis
Enteric fever	Arbovirus	
Brucellosis	Varicella	
Leprosy	HIV infection	
Lyme disease		
Chlamydia		

Table 11.10
Predisposing factors to joint infection

Septicaemic spread from infective focus elsewhere:
Abscess, bronchiectasis, enteric fever
Previous joint damage: OA, RA
Immunosuppression: Leukaemia, lymphoma, steroids,
   cytotoxics
General debility: Elderly, neonates, malignancy, diabetes,
   alcohol
Sickle cell disease
iv drug abuse
Operations: Orthopaedic procedures, eg arthroplasty
Trauma
Neuropathic joint: Diabetes, syphilis

Aetiology   (Tables 11.9 and 11.10).

Clinical features   Pyrexia, lethargy, rigors. Affected joint is painful, swollen, hot and stiff with limitation of movement. Spinal infection may present as backache. The physical signs may be extremely subtle if the patient is immunosuppressed. Macular patches may be present in gonococcal disease.

Investigations   • Multiple blood cultures before initiating antibiotic therapy • FBC shows leucocytosis with a 'left shift' • ESR • C-reactive protein • Synovial fluid aspiration (culture, microscopy, Gram stain, examination for crystals and rheumatoid factor) • ASO titre • Radiology shows soft-tissue swelling acutely and in the chronic state some peri-articular osteoporosis and loss of cartilage may be present • If tuberculosis is suspected a tuberculin test, eg Mantoux, CXR, and specific culture for AAFB, should be undertaken.

Differential diagnosis   Trauma, haemarthrosis, monoarticular arthritis (RA, gout, seronegative arthritis), osteomyelitis or battered baby syndrome.

Management box
▶ Rest, analgesia, joint splintage and prompt iv antibiotic therapy following multiple blood cultures and joint aspiration.
▶ Surgical drainage may be needed (Table 11.11).

Table 11.11
Management of infective arthritis

Organism producing joint infection	Antibiotic
Staphylococcus	flucloxacillin 500 mg 6-hourly
	fusidic acid 500 mg 8-hourly
Streptococcus	ampicillin 500 mg 6-hourly
	benzylpenicillin 0.6 g 6-hourly
Haemophilus influenzae	ampicillin
Pseudomonas, E. coli	aminoglycoside, eg gentamicin (dose depends on weight, age and renal function)
	cephalosporin, eg ceftazidime 1 g 8-hourly
	cefuroxime 750 mg 8-hourly
Neisseria gonorrhoeae	ampicillin, benzylpenicillin
Neisseria meningitides	ampicillin, benzylpenicillin
Salmonellae	ampicillin, co-trimoxazole 960 mg 12-hourly
Mycobacterium tuberculosis	rifampicin + isoniazid + ethambutol +/– pyrazinamide
Viral	symptomatic
Fungal	amphoteracin

DISEASES OF BONE

OSTEOMYELITIS

Denotes infection of bone and is usually bacterial in origin. Organisms reach the bone to produce infection by one of three routes: • haematogenous spread • direct extension from a contiguous source of infection or • direct introduction of organisms by trauma (including operations). Most common in children. The organisms most commonly involved are staphylococci, streptococci, salmonellae and *Mycobacterium tuberculosis*.

Clinical features   Fever, malaise, nausea, vomiting, severe pain at the site of infection. An effusion may occur if the infection is close to a joint. The affected area is hot and tender.

Investigations   • FBC • ESR • Multiple blood cultures • Glucose • Radiology shows bony destruction with radiolucent areas, radio-opaque sequestrae and involucrum formation but changes do not occur for some days or weeks • Radioisotopic bone scans are useful.

Management box
▶ Early appropriate antibiotic therapy (as for infective arthritis, see Table 11.11).
▶ Surgical decompression may be needed.

PAGET'S DISEASE

Bone disorder of unknown aetiology characterized by increased osteoclastic bone absorption followed by disorderly, excessive osteoblastic new bone formation. This leads to softening, painful enlargement and bowing of the affected bones. The disease affects certain bones preferentially: skull, vertebrae, pelvis and long bones. It may be asymptomatic. Affects approximately 3–4% of the population over 50 years old rising to 10% in the 85+ age group. M>F.

Clinical features Bone pain (often at night), tenderness, compressive symptoms, eg deafness, blindness, nerve entrapment, slowly progressive paraparesis, pathological fractures, high-output cardiac failure and rarely the development of osteogenic sarcoma.

Investigations • Normal FBC • ESR may also be normal • Serum calcium and phosphate levels are usually normal unless the patient is immobilized, when the calcium level can rise • Alkaline phosphatase (bony isoenzyme) is raised and reflects increased osteoblastic activity • Urinary hydroxyproline and collagen breakdown products (e.g. N-telopeptide) are also elevated and reflect increased osteoclastic activity • Acid phosphatase is normal • Hyperuricaemia may be present • Radiology reveals osteolytic lesions (cortical resorption), areas of osteosclerosis and bony distortion, stress fractures, and osteoporosis circumscripta in the skull (osteolytic but no osteosclerotic lesions) • Bone scan is positive at an early stage of the disease.

Management box
▶ None is necessary in asymptomatic cases.
▶ Diphosphonates, eg disodium etidronate and pamidronate: synthetic analogs of pyrophosphate which act by stabilizing the bony matrix hydroxyapatite crystals thus decreasing bony turnover. Main adverse reaction is the development of osteomalacia.
▶ Calcitonin (human or salmon), 50–100 u sc per day can be used but may cause allergic reactions.
▶ NSAIDs for analgesia and physiotherapy are useful.
▶ Surgery is occasionally needed.
▶ Radiotherapy is rarely used.

OSTEOPOROSIS

Reduction in bone mass per unit volume. Histologically there is loss of bone matrix with secondary loss of bone mineral. The resultant bone is weak and apt to fracture. This loss of bone occurs with age and is linked to androgen/oestrogen deficiency and is greatest in post-menopausal women. Clinically significant osteoporosis is rare in men.

Aetiology (Table 11.12)

Table 11.12
Causes of osteoporosis

Ageing	post-menopausal
Endocrine	thyrotoxicosis, hypogonadism, Cushing's syndrome, hyperparathyroidism
Nutritional	calcium deficiency
Hereditary	Marfan's syndrome, osteogenesis imperfecta
Inflammatory arthritis	RA
Bone marrow replacement	lymphoma, leukaemia, myeloma, glycogen storage disease
Chronic renal disease	
Malabsorption	
Post-gastrectomy	
Chronic liver disease	
Immobility	
Drugs	steroids, thyroxine, heparin

Clinical features Bone pain, backache, crush vertebral fractures, kyphosis, fractures with minimal trauma (distal radius and neck of femur). Bones are not particularly tender.

Investigations • Serum biochemistry is normal (calcium, phosphate and alkaline phosphatase), unless a fracture is present or

Management box
▶ Correct underlying cause.
▶ Analgesia and physiotherapy.
▶ Calcium and vitamin D supplements.
▶ Diphosphonates and oral calcium in cyclical courses.
▶ HRT
▶ Selective oestrogen-receptor modulators eg raloxifene

osteomalacia coexists • Radiology may reveal reduced bone density, fractures and vertebral wedge collapse • Assessment of bone density (CT scan, neutron activation analysis or photon densitometry) • A bone biopsy may be needed to confirm the diagnosis.

Prevention HRT, exercise, calcium supplementation (1.0–1.5 g/day)

12

nfectious diseases

No attempt has been made to cover tropical diseases in any detail in this chapter.

History This is vital and should include detailed questions about exposure to possible infection (occupation, travel, immunization (Table 12.1)), date of onset, place of onset,

Table 12.1
UK immunization schedule

Age	Vaccine
2 months	DTP, polio, Hib
3 months	DTP, polio, Hib
4 months	DTP, polio, Hib
12–18 months	MMR
4–5 years	Booster DT
10–13 years	BCG (tuberculin negative)
	Rubella to girls if no previous MMR
15–19 years	TT, polio booster

DTP = diphtheria, tetanus, pertussis, DT = diphtheria, tetanus, TT = tetanus toxoid, Hib conjugate = *Haemophilus influenzae B*, MMR = measles/mumps/rubella

Table 12.2
Causes of pyrexia of unknown origin (PUO)

Infections	Tuberculosis, infective endocarditis, localized abscesses, brucellosis, HIV, relapsing fever, EBV, CMV, cholangitis, enteric fever
Malignancy	Hypernephroma, lymphoma, hepatoma, myxoma, leukaemia
Connective tissue diseases	RA, SLE, temporal arteritis
Drugs	Virtually any drug
Endocrine	Hypothalamic lesions, thyrotoxicosis, phaeochromocytoma
Myocardial infarction	
Pulmonary embolism	
Familial Mediterranean fever	
Vasculitis	
Munchausen's syndrome	

animal contact, recent operations and sexual history. The cause of fever may be unknown (PUO) (Table 12.2).

Examination Must be complete and include eyes, ears, mouth, nose, sinuses, lymph glands, skin, anus, vagina and external genitalia.

INVESTIGATIONS

These will be guided by the above and include: • FBC • ESR • C–reactive protein • LFTs • Immunoglobulins • Protein electrophoresis • Multiple blood cultures before starting antibiotics • Sputum Gram stain and culture • MSU • Autoantibody profile (RF, ANF) • Mantoux test • CXR • Plain abdominal X-ray • Serology (paired acute and convalescent samples) • CT scans • MRI • US • Bone scans • Indium labelled WBC scans may be useful in localizing the site of sepsis.

E **SEPTICAEMIA** → page 450

BACTERIAL INFECTIONS

STAPHYLOCOCCAL

Staph. aureus produces a variety of suppurative conditions including wound infections, boils, carbuncles, abscesses, bone and joint infections, cavitating pneumonia and endocarditis. The toxic shock syndrome is commonly due to toxins released following *Staph. aureas* infection of the female genital tract in association with tampon use. Clinical features include shock, a sunburn-like rash followed by desquamation, diarrhoea, myalgia, and headache. Treatment must include removal of tampon. Multi-system involvement is common in this condition and includes vomiting, diarrhoea, renal failure, hepatitis, thrombocytopenia, DIC, rash and encephalopathy.

Management box

▶ Flucloxacillin (500 mg 6-hourly oral or iv), if penicillin allergy erythromycin (500 mg 6-hourly oral or iv and/or fusidic acid 500 mg 8-hourly oral or iv).

▶ More severe infections may require vancomycin, clindamycin or teicoplanin.

STREPTOCOCCAL

Streptococci produce a number of toxins and can rapidly produce septicaemia and disseminated infection (Table 12.3).

Scarlet fever
Strep. pyogenes infection involving the throat, tonsils and skin. Incubation period 2–4 days.

Clinical features Sudden-onset fever, sore throat, headache, vomiting, cervical lymphadenopathy, yellow friable tonsillar exudate, erythematous rash affecting the arms, legs and behind the ears and furred tongue (white or red 'strawberry' tongue). Rarely rheumatic fever and nephritis.

Investigations Throat swab, antistreptolysin O titre (ASO).

Management box
▶ Ampicillin (500 mg 6-hourly orally or iv).
▶ Amoxicillin (500 mg 8-hourly orally or iv).
▶ Erythromycin (500 mg 6-hourly orally or iv if penicillin allergy).

Pneumococcal pneumonia (p 77)
Erysipelas (p 318)
Impetigo (p 318)
Cellulitis (p 318)
Endocarditis (p 51)

Table 12.3
Streptococci and disease

Variety	Disease
Group A (pyogenes)	Scarlet fever, impetigo, erysipelas, tonsillitis, cellulitis, necrotizing fasciitis
Group B	Neonatal infection
S. pneumoniae	Pneumococcal pneumonia, meningitis
S. faecalis	Pyelonephritis, endocarditis, wound infection
S. viridans	Endocarditis
Anaerobic	Abscesses

ANAEROBIC

Anaerobic bacteria are responsible for many different infections due to both tissue invasion and their ability to produce a variety of toxins (Table 12.4).

Clinical features   Anaerobic organisms produce putrid-smelling pus at the site of sepsis, eg gingivitis, dental abscess, mastoiditis, sinusitis, cellulitis, intra-abdominal infection, peritonitis, bone and joint infection, bites and diabetic foot ulcers. There is often synergistic infection with aerobic organisms.

Investigations   • Gram stain and culture of pus in a medium containing 10% CO_2.

Management box
▸ Surgical exision of necrotic material.
▸ Metronidazole (500 mg hourly iv, 1 g 8-hourly PR, 400 mg 8-hourly orally).

TETANUS

Infection due to *Clostridium tetani* which exists as a gut commensal as well as in the soil. The Gram-positive bacilli remain localized at the portal of entry but they produce an exotoxin which acts on the CNS. Not transmissible. Incubation period 1–15 days.

Clinical features   Fever, trismus ('lockjaw') due to masseter muscle spasm, myalgia, apprehension, alert, hypertonia, rigidity

---

Table 12.4
Anaerobes and disease

Variety	Disease
Clostridium perfringens	Gas gangrene, foot ulcers, necrotizing enterocolitis, food poisoning, abscesses, endocarditis, intra-abdominal infection
Clostridium difficile	Pseudomembranous colitis
Clostridium botulinum	Food poisoning
Clostridium tetani	Tetanus
Actinomyces	Actinomycosis
Borrelia vincenti	Acute necrotizing gingivitis

of face, neck and trunk muscles ('risus sardonicus' and opisthotonos). Muscle spasm may occur in response to noxious stimuli (unexpected noise or touch) and can produce asphyxia. Autonomic instability occurs with cardiac arrhythmias, sweating and swings in BP. Umbilical sepsis is an important source in the Third World.

Investigations • Usually a clinical diagnosis. Isolation of the organism is rare.

Differential diagnosis Hysteria and phenothiazine dystonia.

Management box
▸ Prevent the disease if possible: active immunization (Table 12.1, p 261) and adequate wound toilet following injury.
▸ Treat as soon as the disease is suspected: prevent further toxin absorption by wound toilet, iv/im human tetanus anti-toxin, iv benzylpenicillin 600 mg 6-hourly or metronidazole 500 mg 8-hourly iv, nurse in a quiet room and prevent muscle spasms with diazepam, or paralyse the patient if necessary with d-tubocurarine or pancuronium following intubation and artificial ventilation.
▸ Ensure adequate nutrition and hydration.

DIPHTHERIA

Acute epidemic notifiable disease caused by *Corynebacterium diphtheriae* spread by droplets. It is preventable by active immunization. Rare in the UK nowadays but still important in underdeveloped countries. Incubation period 2–4 days. Organisms remain localized in the throat but produce an exotoxin which damages the heart and brain.

Clinical features Sore throat with classical tonsillar appearance: oedematous yellow/haemorrhagic membrane with a well-defined edge which may extend onto the faucial pillars and the palate. In severe cases the neck may become swollen 'bull-neck diphtheria'. Marked tachycardia, mild pyrexia, husky voice and nasal discharge. Rarely solitary skin ulcers in tropical climates. In severe cases laryngeal obstruction, stridor, circulatory collapse and death may occur.

Investigations • Clinical diagnosis confirmed by culture of throat swab.

> **Management box**
> ▸ Give diphtheria anti-toxin im immediately on clinical suspicion (anaphylaxis may occur as horse serum is used so adrenaline (epinephrine), chlorphenamine (chlorpheniramine), salbutamol and hydrocortisone should be available).
> ▸ Penicillin or erythromycin should be given for 2 weeks to eliminate *C. diphtheriae* from the throat.
> ▸ The disease should be prevented by active immunization of children aged 3–12 months (Table 12.1, p 261).
> ▸ Carriers should be identified in any outbreak and treated with a week of penicillin or erythromycin and kept in isolation until six daily throat swabs are negative.

Complications Neurological involvement includes palatal paralysis, extrinsic eye-muscle paralysis, peripheral neuropathy and diaphragmatic weakness. Myocarditis with resultant arrhythmias and cardiac failure may occur.

PERTUSSIS (WHOOPING COUGH)

Gram-negative bacillus *Bordetella pertussis*, spread by droplets. Highly infectious. Usually affects pre-school children. Incubation period 7–14 days.

Clinical features

Catarrhal stage: rhinitis, conjunctivitis, unproductive cough.

Spasmodic stage: staccato coughing bouts, vomiting, exhaustion. Bronchial hyperactivity may remain for many months.

Investigations   • Clinical diagnosis confirmed by culture of perinasal swabs. Lymphocytosis is common in early stages.

> **Management box**
> ▸ Prevent by active immunization of pre-school children (Table 12.1, p 261).
> ▸ The risk of vaccination-induced brain damage is small and can be minimized if the vaccine is not given to babies with a history of birth injury, CNS damage, previous convulsions or a family history of such or a previous reaction to the vaccine.
> ▸ The established disease is treated with erythromycin during the catarrhal stage.
> ▸ Cough suppressants are useful.
> ▸ Adequate hydration and nutrition must be maintained.
> ▸ Ventilation may be required.
> ▸ Babies who have not been vaccinated can be given prophylactic erythromycin if they develop a cough for 24 hours.

Complications Secondary bacterial bronchopneumonia, bronchiectasis, asphyxia, cerebral anoxia, convulsions and death. Subconjunctival haemorrhages can be produced by paroxysms of coughing.

TYPHOID FEVER (ENTERIC FEVER)

Science basics Due to Gram-negative bacilli *Salmonella typhi*. Paratyphoid fever is due to *S. paratyphi*. Spread by human to human transfer, especially under conditions of poor hygiene, commonly in foodstuffs. Occurs sporadically or in epidemics. Following ingestion the organisms penetrate the mucosa of the GI tract to be taken up by reticuloendothelial cells where they multiply. Incubation period up to 18 days. Septicaemic spread then occurs throughout the body. The gall bladder may act as a reservoir for ongoing infection in carriers.

Clinical features Nonspecific headache, dry cough, lethargy, constipation, pyrexia, confusion, splenomegaly, macular rose spots and relative bradycardia during the first week. If untreated the patient deteriorates with dehydration, doughy abdomen, GI bleeding and possible perforation.

Investigation • Neutropenia • Blood, urine, rose spot and stool culture • Serological tests (Widal) to both the O and H antigens of the organism have been largely superceded by ELISA.

> **Management box**
> ► Barrier nursing, rehydration, ciprofloxacin 200 mg bd iv or 750 mg bd orally is the treatment of choice except in children.
> ► Alternatives include chloramphenicol 500 mg 4-hourly, amoxicillin 500 mg 6-hourly or cotrimoxazole 960 mg 12-hourly for 2 weeks (iv initially).
> ► Carriers can be treated with ciprofloxacin 500 mg bd but may need cholecystectomy.

TUBERCULOSIS

Science basics Chronic infectious disease caused by *Mycobacterium tuberculosis* or rarely by *Mycobacterium bovis*. The disease is a major cause of both morbidity and mortality in Third World countries and although it is now less of a problem in the developed world it still occurs in some sections of society, eg alcoholics, undernourished, ethnic communities and HIV population. *M. tuberculosis* is a non-motile bacillus which is not discoloured by acid-alcohol when stained with carbolfuchsin and is therefore 'acid fast'. It is slow to grow and it may take 6 weeks for the culture result to become available. The BACTEC system allows identification of mycobacterial metabolites within 2 weeks. PCR techniques are useful in confirming the infection in difficult cases.

There are 60 known mycobacteria species, divided into 'fast growers' and 'slow growers' and they act as a potent immunogical stimulus. Tissue damage in mycobacterial disease is caused by the host immune response.

Aetiology and pathogenesis   The organisms enter the body via the skin, respiratory tract or alimentary tract. Clinical illness does not always occur and may depend on the degree of natural immunity existing, state of nourishment, age, coexisting disease (diabetes mellitus, malignancy), immunosuppression or even standard of living conditions of the affected individual. The primary infection usually occurs in the lung and a 'primary complex' is produced, which is the combination of the primary focus (Ghon focus) of infection in the lung parenchyma plus caseous involvement of the regional lymph nodes (usually mediastinal). If the initial site of infection is the tonsil or the ileum the affected nodes will be the cervical or mesenteric respectively. In the vast majority of cases the primary complex then heals and calcifies and the person remains entirely asymptomatic but becomes sensitized to tuberculoprotein. In a few cases healing may not be entirely complete and progressive pulmonary tuberculosis results. Rarely haematogenous spread may occur to produce miliary tuberculosis with widespread involvement of lungs, bone marrow, kidneys, liver, brain, bones, joints and heart. Reactivation of a partially healed primary complex can occur many years later or the person may be reinfected from an outside source with resultant postprimary tuberculosis. Blood-borne dissemination is uncommon at this stage.

Clinical features

Systemic: lassitude, weight-loss, night sweats, malaise, fever and anorexia. The disease may be asymptomatic and found incidentally.

Local:
- Lungs: cough, sputum, haemoptysis, breathlessness, hoarseness, lobar collapse, bronchopneumonia.
- Pleura: pain, breathlessness, effusion.
- Pericardium/heart: pain, arrythmias, constrictive pericarditis, cardiac failure.
- Intestine: diarrhoea, malabsorption, obstruction.
- Genitourinary tract: renal failure, haematuria, epididymitis, salpingitis, infertility.
- Skin: lupus vulgaris, erythema nodosum.

- Eyes: choroiditis, iritis, phlyctenular keratoconjunctivitis.
- Bones/joints: osteomyelitis, arthritis.
- Lymphatics: cold abscesses, lymphadenopathy, sinuses.
- Brain: meningitis, tuberculoma.
- Adrenal glands: Addison's disease.

Investigations • CXR: primary focus, lymphadenopathy, cavitation, pneumothorax, areas of calcification, pleural effusion/empyema, segmental/lobar collapse, miliary disease or secondary aspergilloma formation. Always compare with previous X-rays if possible • Chest tomography • IVU • CT scanning • Tuberculin test: Mantoux test is an intradermal injection of purified protein derivative (PPD) usually injected into the flexor aspect of the forearm and read 48–72 hours later. A positive result is an area of induration at least 5 mm in diameter with surrounding erythema. 0.1 ml of 1:10 000 dilution should be used initially, progressing to more concentrated solutions if the result is negative. Alternative tuberculin tests are available and useful for large-scale screening (Heaf and Tine tests) but they are not as accurate as the Mantoux test • Bacteriological examination: staining (Ziehl–Neelsen, fluorescent auramine), culture and BACTEC analysis of blood, sputum, pleural aspirate/biopsy, early morning urine samples (EMUs), laryngeal swabs, gastric aspirate, CSF, liver biopsy or BM aspirate to allow isolation of the organism and identification of its sensitivity profile.

Management box

▶ Prevent the disease if possible by BCG vaccination (see Table 12.5), better living standards, adequate nutrition, notification of index cases and subsequent case finding.

▶ Isolation of infected cases is rarely needed but young children should be isolated from the index case until adequate chemotherapy has had a chance to be effective.

▶ Surgery is now rarely needed.

▶ The mainstay of treatment is antibacterial chemotherapy and various drug regimens are now employed. Five drugs are commonly used in the developed world: rifampicin, isoniazid, ethambutol, pyrazinamide and streptomycin. If these drugs are used in the correct combinations for an adequate period of time they are virtually 100% effective in curing tuberculosis (Table 12.6).

▶ In developing countries less expensive drug regimens have to be used, eg streptomycin + isoniazid twice-weekly for 12 months, but standard respiratory medicine textbooks should be consulted for details on suitable treatment regimens.

▶ Anti-tuberculosis drugs:
  – Rifampicin: 10 mg/kg (400–600 mg/day) best absorbed from an empty stomach. May cause a transient rise in LFTs →

which can be ignored but the drug must be discontinued if jaundice occurs. Produces reddish discolouration of body fluids, eg urine, sweat and tears, and may irreversibly stain contact lenses. Induces liver enzymes thus making OCP less effective, and alternative forms of contraception must be used. May produce fever, vasculitis, influenza-like illness, nausea and vomiting.

- Isoniazid: 200–300 mg/day in adults. Can produce a hypersensitivity reaction (erythematous skin rash and pyrexia) and occasionally polyneuropathy (especially in slow acetylators – minimized by concurrent treatment with pyridoxine 10 mg/day). Hepatotoxicity is well recognized.
- Ethambutol: 15 mg/kg/day in adults. May cause optic neuritis. Document visual acuity before starting treatment and at regular intervals thereafter and stop the drug if visual problems occur.
- Pyrazinamide: 35 mg/kg/day up to a maximum of 2.5 g/day. May produce gout, hepatitis, arthralgia and hypersensitivity.
- Streptomycin: 0.75–1.00 mg/kg/day. Dose depends on serum level. May cause vestibular disturbance, deafness and hypersensitivity.

▶ All the drugs should be given together once-daily to ensure adequate peak serum bactericidal levels. Corticosteroids may be needed in fulminating infection, secondary Addison's disease, tuberculous pleural and pericardial effusions, lymphadenopathy, genitourinary or meningeal involvement.

Table 12.5
Current BCG recommendations

Neonates of Afro-asian origin
School children without previous BCG
Health care workers
Tuberculin-negative household contacts of respiratory TB patients
BCG is a live, attenuated vaccine and should not be given to immunocompromised individuals. It is given intradermally and confers up to 80% protection for up to 15 years.

MALARIA

Science basics Infection due to *Plasmodium falciparum, P. ovale, P. vivax* or *P. malariae*. Spread by the bite of the female anopheline mosquito and rarely by blood transfusion or transplacentally. Endemic in many tropical and sub-tropical

Table 12.6
Drug regimens in tuberculosis*

9 months' duration	Initial phase (2 months): rifampicin + isoniazid + ethambutol/streptomycin
	Continuation phase (7 months): rifampicin + isoniazid
6 months' duration	Initial phase (2 months): rifampicin + isoniazid + pyrazinamide + ethambutol/streptomycin
	Continuation phase (4 months): rifampicin + isoniazid

*Drug therapy can be modified according to bacterial sensitivity test results

countries where drug-resistance is becoming an increasing problem. Notifiable disease.

Clinical features Relapsing fever, rigors, abdominal pain, prostration, profuse perspiration, jaundice, hepatosplenomegaly, headache, vomiting, diarrhoea, increasing haemolytic anaemia. Infection with *P. ovale*, *P. vivax* and *P. malariae* tends to run a benign course but may relapse many years after the initial attack. *P. falciparum* produces a more serious illness and infection may lead to acute renal failure, hepatic failure, cerebral malaria and severe intravascular haemolysis leading to 'Blackwater fever', ARDS, DIC.

Investigations • Always consider this diagnosis in a patient with PUO especially if there is any history of foreign travel • Microscopy of thick and thin blood films looking for malarial parasites.

Management box
▶ Bed-rest, adequate hydration, paracetamol for headache.
▶ Non-falciparum: chloroquine for 3 days plus primaquine for 14 days.
▶ Falciparum: quinine 600 mg tid for 7 days plus fansidar. Mefloquine or malarone® may be used as an alternative to quinine.
▶ Transfusion may be necessary in severe anaemia.
▶ Corticosteroids help to reduce haemolysis.
▶ Unfortunately the mortality remains high in complicated cases.

Prophylaxis   This is important but is not a guarantee of protection and it is important to obtain accurate advice on drug-resistant areas before travelling abroad. Chloroquine-resistant area: chloroquine 300 mg weekly plus proguanil 100–200 mg/day, or mefloquine. Low risk of chloroquine-resistance: weekly chloroquine or daily proguanil. Repellant creams or sprays, mosquito coils and nets are also an important aspect of malaria prophylaxis.

VIRAL INFECTIONS

MEASLES

RNA paramyxovirus infection spread by droplets. Highly contagious, incubation period 7–14 days. Usually affects children. Biennial winter epidemics occur in temperate climates. One attack confers lasting immunity.

Clinical features

Catarrhal stage: fever, cough, coryza, conjunctivitis, Koplik's spots are present on the mucous membranes of the mouth (especially in the inside of the cheeks) and irritability. Most infectious during this stage.

Exanthematous stage: dark-red macular or maculopapular rash behind the ears spreading to involve the face and trunk, associated with increasing fever. The rash becomes confluent and blotchy.

Investigations • Clinical diagnosis • IgM and IgG antibodies can be measured.

> **Management box**
> ▶ Isolate from school for 10 days.
> ▶ Paracetamol for pyrexia.
> ▶ Prevention is important by active immunization of children >1 year old who have not had the disease (Table 12.1, p 261).
> ▶ Passive immunization using immunoglobulin is possible in patients with severe malnutrition.

Complications   Encephalitis, secondary bacterial otitis media, pneumonia (often with *Staph. aureus* or Gram-negative organisms in undernourished children), subacute sclerosing panencephalitis, croup, stomatitis, gastroenteritis and kwashiorkor.

RUBELLA (GERMAN MEASLES)

RNA togavirus spread by droplets. One attack confers immunity. Incubation period 18 days. Trivial disease in children but more severe in adults and may produce severe congenital abnormalities if it occurs during pregnancy (triad of blindness, deafness and cardiac defects together with hepatosplenomegaly, purpuric rash and cataracts).

Clinical features   Faint pink macular rash on face spreading to trunk and limbs. Suboccipital lymphadenopathy, fever and myalgia.

Investigations   • Viral isolation from throat swab • Rising antibody titre.

Management box
▶ None.
▶ Prevent by active immunization of girls 11–13 years who lack serum antibodies to the disease. Offer termination if the disease occurs within the first sixteen weeks of pregnancy.

MUMPS

RNA paramyxovirus spread by droplets. Low infectivity rate although some cases may be subclinical. Incubation period 18 days.

Clinical features   Fever, malaise, trismus, parotid gland swelling, orchitis in adult males, pancreatitis or oophoritis, aseptic meningitis. Rarely encephalitis.

Investigations   • Usually a clinical diagnosis. If doubt exists a rise in antibody titres or viral culture from saliva is diagnostic.

Management box
▶ Symptomatic only.

VARICELLA (CHICKEN POX)

DNA herpes virus spread by droplets or by direct contact with skin lesions. Highly infectious and usually affects children. One attack usually produces immunity but reactivation occurs and produces herpes zoster (shingles). Incubation period 14–21 days. May be disseminated in the immunocompromised host.

Clinical features   Mild fever, characteristic rash on trunk spreading to the face and limbs (initially macular, then papular, vesicular and finally pustular). The rash appears in crops.

Investigations • Clinical diagnosis • Rising antibody titre.

Complications Secondary infection, pneumonia (commoner amongst smokers and leaves calcified scars on CXR), proliferative glomerulonephritis, demyelinating encephalitis often affecting the cerebellum.

Management box

▶ Aciclovir for pneumonitis, encephalitis, severe infections and in the immunocompromised. Aciclovir may shorten course of illness if given early.
▶ If secondary skin infection occurs use topical chlorhexidine. Oral augmentin 1 tablet 8-hourly or flucloxacillin 500 mg 6-hourly may be needed for bacterial superinfection.
▶ Human anti-varicella immunoglobulin can be given to the immunocompromised.

HERPES ZOSTER (SHINGLES)

Due to invasion of posterior root ganglia by varicella virus. The virus may lie dormant for many years and reactivation is often precipitated by other infection.

Clinical features Severe pain in the distribution of the affected dorsal nerve root. The skin then becomes erythematous before the characteristic vesicular scarring rash appears. The patient may be left with intractable neuralgia for many months. Myalgia, myelitis and encephalitis may occur. Involvement of the first division of the trigeminal nerve produces ophthalmic herpes with corneal vesicles and scarring.

Investigations • Usually clinical • Confirmation by rising antibody titres.

Management box

▶ Aciclovir halts the progression of the disease if given early enough and may reduce the incidence of post-herpetic neuralgia (800 mg orally 5 times daily for 7 days, or 10 mg/kg 8-hourly for 7 days given slowly as an infusion over 1 hour in severe infections).
▶ Famciclovir is a suitable alternative to aciclovir, and better absorbed orally.
▶ Topical 5% idoxuridine 6-hourly for 7 days is useful.
▶ Pain should be treated adequately, eg regular coproxamol.
▶ Amitriptyline or carbamazepine may be useful for post-herpetic neuralgia if simple analgesics are not sufficient.

HERPES SIMPLEX (→ page 321)

INFECTIOUS MONONUCLEOSIS (GLANDULAR FEVER)

Due to infection with the Epstein-Barr virus, a herpes virus which also causes nasopharyngeal carcinoma and Burkitt's lymphoma. Mildly infectious and tends to spread by close contact, eg kissing. Tends to affect young adults. Incubation period 4–5 weeks.

Clinical features Fever, sore throat, malaise, cervical lymph-adenopathy, petechial haemorrhages on the palate, maculopapular rash (especially if ampicillin is prescribed), hepatosplenomegaly, rarely meningitis, encephalitis, haemolytic anaemia, hepatitis, thrombocytopenia and pancarditis.

Investigations • Initially a mild neutrophil leucocytosis followed by an atypical lymphocytosis (activated T lymphocytes). Similar atypical lymphocytes are seen in toxoplasmosis, CMV infection, lymphoma and leukaemia, HIV seroconversion • Heterophile antibody is present and can agglutinate sheep RBCs (Paul-Bunnell reaction). Agglutination can be prevented by prior absorption with beef RBCs, but not with guinea pig cells. The Monospot test is similar but easier and quicker to perform although not as specific • EBV antibodies titres can be measured (IgM and IgG).

> *Management box*
> ▶ Symptomatic, rest, avoid alcohol, corticosteroids are rarely needed.

FUNGAL INFECTIONS

Classification (Table 12.7)

MYCETOMA

Chronic infection of the deep soft tissues and bones. May affect the limbs, trunk or head. Due to eumycetes and actinomycetes both of which produce grains.

Clinical features Painless swelling at the site of impregnation. Sinuses, abscesses, scarring and deformity are produced.

Investigations • Microscopy and culture of pus or biopsy.

Table 12.7
Classification of fungal infections

Superficial infections:
 Dermatophytes   → Dermatology (p 323)
 Candidiasis   → Dermatology (p 323)
 Pityriasis versicolor   → Dermatology (p 324)
Subcutaneous infections:
 Mycetoma (Madura's foot)
 Chromomycosis
Systemic infections:
 Histoplasmosis
 Aspergillosis
 Coccidioidomycosis
 Cryptococcus

Management box
▸ Eumycetic infection may respond to ketoconazole.
▸ Actinomycetes may respond to penicillin, dapsone or
cotrimoxazole but amputation may be needed.

HISTOPLASMOSIS

Due to *Histoplasma capsulatum* or *duboisii*. Usually secondary to inhalation of spores.

Clinical features May be asymptomatic. Can mimic tuberculosis. Fever, anaemia, lymphadenopathy, endocarditis, hepatosplenomegaly, diarrhoea, cough and sputum.

Investigations • CXR/AXR shows calcification in lungs, liver or spleen • Tissue biopsy for microscopy and culture • Delayed hypersensitivity skin tests • Complement fixation test.

Management box
▸ Amphoteracin on alternate days for up to 1 month.
▸ Adverse reactions (fever, headache, malaise, venous thrombosis)
may be minimized by concurrent prednisolone therapy.

CRYPTOCOCCUS

Caused by *Cryptococcus neoformans*. Common in the immunocompromised, eg HIV infection.

Clinical features   Meningitis, pulmonary and gastrointestinal involvement.

Investigations • Microscopy (Indian ink dye) and culture of biopsies or CSF • Complement fixation test.

> **Management box**
> ▶ Amphoteracin plus 5-flucytosine.

ASPERGILLUS

Commonest respiratory mycosis in the UK and the cause of many diseases (Table 12.8). Aspergillus species also commonly present in the atmosphere. The demonstration of fungal hyphae in a sample of sputum is, however, always of diagnostic significance. Most cases are due to *Aspergillus fumigatus* but there are many other members of the genus (eg *A. clavatus, A. flavus* and *A. niger)*.

Asthma
Usual symptoms of allergic asthma (→ p 74). Skin hypersensitivity may be present and *A. fumigatus* may be isolated from sputum. Treatment is of the underlying asthma.

Allergic bronchopulmonary aspergillosis
A rare but important complication of asthma. May be asymptomatic and discovered on routine CXR.

Clinical features   Fever and usual symptoms of asthma may occur. Occlusion of a major bronchus by tenacious sputum may cause lobar collapse. Repeated infection can produce proximal vascular bronchiectasis.

Investigations • CXR shows various transient abnormalities (collapse/consolidation, peripheral shadows, thickened bronchial wall markings) • Peripheral blood film shows eosinophilia

---

Table 12.8
Diseases caused by Aspergillus species

Asthma
Allergic bronchopulmonary aspergillosis
Aspergilloma
Extrinsic allergic alveolitis
Invasive aspergillosis
Otomycosis

• Serum precipitating antibodies to Aspergillus species may be present, early (20 min) and late (6 hours) skin-test prick may be positive • Fungal spores/hyphae may be seen on sputum microscopy or grown on culture.

Management box
▸ Involves optimizing asthma therapy together with oral prednisolone (20–40 mg/day) reducing slowly to zero if possible.
▸ The rate of steroid reduction depends on the individual patient's response to therapy. A small proportion of patients with recurrent episodes of aspergillosis may need to be maintained on a small dose of oral prednisolone.
▸ The oral antifungal agent itraconazole may prove to be valuable in future.

Aspergilloma

Clinical features May be asymptomatic. Forms in cavities produced by previous lung diseases (eg tuberculosis, abscesses or areas of pulmonary infarction). Haemoptysis can occur and may be severe. Usually due to *A. fumigatus*. May produce secondary invasion of the lung.

Investigations • CXR (solid opacity within a cavity, often with a crescent of air between the fungal ball and the wall of the cavity) • Sputum culture may be positive, especially if the aspergilloma communicates with a bronchus.

Management box
▸ This is largely unsatisfactory although itraconazole may be useful.
▸ Surgery may be needed.
▸ Corticosteroids should be avoided if possible.

Extrinsic allergic alveolitis

Clinical features Fever, malaise, breathlessness without wheeze 6 hours after exposure to the antigen (eg *A. clavatus* in malt-worker's lung or *Micropolyspora faeni/Thermoactinomyces vulgaris* in farmer's lung), followed eventually by progressive exertional breathlessness if exposure continues.

Investigations • Microscopy and culture of sputum (24-hour specimen is most reliable), bronchial washings or transbronchial/open-lung biopsies • Immediate and delayed (6 hour) skin hypersensitivity reaction • Serum precipitins • CXR may show micronodular shadowing • Serology demonstrates precipitating antibodies, eg *Aspergillus* • Pulmonary function tests show a restrictive defect, reduced transfer factor for carbon monoxide and reduced lung volumes • ABG analysis may show type I respiratory failure • Allergen provocation tests in association with pulmonary function tests and serial temperature measurement may be needed to establish the diagnosis.

Management box
▸ Avoid the precipitating antigen if possible.
▸ Courses of prednisolone may be required during the acute illness.
▸ Established pulmonary fibrosis/respiratory failure is extremely difficult to treat.

Invasive aspergillosis

Clinical features Usually occurs in the presence of immuno-suppression and presents as a suppurative pneumonia which does not respond to conventional antibiotic regimes. It has a grave prognosis.

Investigations • CXR shows widespread parenchymal infiltration with abscess formation • Sputum microscopy and culture is required.

Management box
▸ This is with a combination of amphoteracin and flucytosine but is rarely successful unless given very early during the course of the illness.
▸ Itraconazole is a useful alternative, but may require prolonged treatment.

GASTROENTERITIS

Presents with diarrhoea, vomiting and abdominal pain following consumption of the infected food or drink.

Aetiology ($\rightarrow$ Table 12.9)

SALMONELLOSIS

This is responsible for 75% of reported cases of food poisoning in UK. Common infective sources are poultry, milk, cream, cattle and pigs. Usually due to inadequate initial cooking or rewarming partially cooked food. Outbreaks are common and may involve many people. The organism produces its effect by both invasion and by toxins. Incubation period 12–48 hours.

Table 12.9
Causes of gastroenteritis

Bacteria	*Salmonella typhimurium* and *enteritidis*
	Shigella dysenteriae, flexneri, sonnei and *boydii*
	Clostridia perfringens and *botulinum*
	Staphylococcus aureus
	Campylobacter jejuni
	Escherichia coli
	Bacillus cereus
	Yersinia enterocolitica
	Vibrio cholerae
Viruses	Rotavirus and adenovirus
	Norwalk agent
Protozoa	*Cryptosporidiosis*
	Giardia lamblia
	Entamoeba histolytica

Clinical features   Usually mild diarrhoea which lasts a few days but may produce severe diarrhoea, abdominal pain, vomiting and dehydration and in debilitated patients is occasionally fatal.

Investigations   • Epidemiological help is needed to pinpoint the source • Stool culture may remain positive for longer than 8 weeks in 30% of cases.

Management box
▶ Prevention by strict hygiene of all food handlers and adequate cooking of all foods is vital.
▶ Antibiotics (ciprofloxacin) should be limited to those few cases with systemic disease as acquired drug-resistance via plasmids is a problem.
▶ Carrier states are rarely encountered.
▶ Notifiable disease.

CAMPYLOBACTER

Due to ingestion of contaminated poultry, milk or water. Sub-clinical infection is common. Incubation period 12–48 hours.

Clinical features   Abdominal pain, diarrhoea (often bloody), rarely septicaemia, arthritis, pancreatitis and endocarditis. May mimic acute appendicitis or colitis.

Investigations   • Stool and blood cultures.

> **Management box**
> ▶ Erythromycin 500 mg 6-hourly or ciprofloxacin 750 mg bd.

SHIGELLOSIS (BACILLARY DYSENTERY)

Usually spread by faecal-oral route under conditions of poor hygiene. Commoner in tropical climates. The organism produces colonic inflammation with toxin formation which results in profuse diarrhoea.

Clinical features   These range from subclinical to severe infection. Diarrhoea (occasionally bloody), fever, colicky abdominal pain and tenderness, tenesmus, lethargy, arthralgia and iritis.

Investigations   • Stool culture.

> **Management box**
> ▶ Rehydration.
> ▶ Adequate hygiene.
> ▶ Codeine or loperamide for diarrhoea.
> ▶ Antibiotics in severe cases (ampicillin 500 mg 6-hourly or cotrimoxazole 960 mg 12-hourly or ciprofloxacin 750 mg bd), but drug-resistance can be a problem.

ESCHERICHIA COLI

Various strains exist which can produce gastroenteritis (usually in children).

Enterotoxigenic: produce heat-labile and heat-stable toxins producing watery travellers' diarrhoea with no inflammatory features.

Enteroinvasive: produce dysenteric-like illness with bloody diarrhoea.

Enteropathogenic: diarrhoea produced by unknown mechanism.

Enterohaemorrhagic: especially E0157 causing haemorrhagic colitis and is associated with haemolytic uraemic syndrome.

Clinical features   Usually acute onset diarrhoea occasionally associated with vomiting.

Investigations   • Stool culture.

> **Management box**
> ▶ Rehydration
> ▶ Codeine or loperamide.
> ▶ Antibiotics are reserved for severe cases (ciprofloxacin 750 mg bd).

YERSINIA

Due to ingestion of contaminated shellfish, water, milk or meat. Person to person spread may occur resulting in epidemics. Bowel invasion occurs.

Clinical features Abdominal pain, diarrhoea (usually watery and containing mucus but may be bloody), rashes, erythema nodosum and iritis. May mimic Crohn's disease of the terminal ileum and produce a seronegative arthropathy in individuals with HLA B27.

Investigations • Stool culture • Serology.

> **Management box**
> ▶ Antibiotics are rarely needed (chloramphenicol or tetracycline).

STAPHYLOCOCCUS AUREUS

Produces a heat-stable enterotoxin which results in an episode of acute vomiting 1-6 hours after ingestion of contaminated meat or cream cakes. Treatment is symptomatic. iv rehydration may occasionally be needed.

CLOSTRIDIUM

Clostridium perfringens: is a common cause of food poisoning especially when inadequately cooked meat is allowed to cool slowly and then reheated. Incubation period 12–24 hours. Diarrhoea is present but vomiting is uncommon.

C. botulinum: produces an enterotoxin which acts on the CNS producing paralysis and eventually death due to respiratory failure in 50% of cases. Incubation period 12–72 hours. Vomiting and diarrhoea occur. An antitoxin should be given. Artificial ventilation may be needed.

C. difficile: is associated with antibiotic-related pseudomembranous colitis. Treatment is with oral vancomycin 125 mg 6-hourly or metronidazole 400 mg tid.

BACILLUS CEREUS

Spore-bearing aerobic organism which may result in vomiting, abdominal pain and diarrhoea 1–5 hours after the ingestion of infected rice, milk and meat.

VIBRIO

Vibrio cholerae (classical and El Tor biotypes) produces cholera in man. Common in tropical and subtropical countries under conditions of poor hygiene. The organism colonizes the small intestine with production of a powerful toxin but no bowel invasion occurs.

Clinical features The disease varies from the asymptomatic carrier state to that of severe painless diarrhoea associated with vomiting and muscle cramps. Hypovolaemic shock, uraemia and hypoglycaemia may occur.

Investigations • Clinical diagnosis.

Management box
▸ Aggressive rehydration is vital using oral solutions containing sodium, glucose, potassium, chloride and bicarbonate (eg WHO solution), or iv replacement.
▸ Antibiotics are useful (tetracycline, cotrimoxazole or chloramphenicol).
▸ Cholera vaccine is of limited value and only lasts 3–6 months.

Vibrio parahaemolyticus can contaminate shellfish and produce profuse watery diarrhoea. Treatment is by rehydration and antibiotics (tetracycline or chloramphenicol).

VIRAL DIARRHOEA

Rotaviruses, adenoviruses and the Norwalk agent can all produce diarrhoea especially in children. They act by destroying gut villi. Management is by rehydration. Vaccines are being developed.

GIARDIASIS

Infection due to the flagellated protozoan *Giardia intestinalis* (*Giardia lamblia*), common in tropical areas and North America. May be entirely asymptomatic or produce severe malabsorption.

Clinical features Acute diarrhoea, abdominal pain and distension, flatulence, lethargy, nausea and weight-loss.

Investigations • Demonstration of cysts on microscopy of fresh stool or trophozoites in jejunal aspirate.

> **Management box**
> ▶ Metronidazole 400 mg tid for 14 days (avoid alcohol because of antabuse effect), or tinidazole 0.5–2.0 g as a single dose repeated after 1 week if necessary.

AMOEBIASIS

Due to infection with *Entamoeba histolytica*. Spread occurs by the ingestion of food contaminated by cysts. Trophozoites form in the colon with invasion of the bowel wall producing amoebic dysentery. Haematogenous spread may occur resulting in amoebic liver abscesses. Incubation period from 2 weeks to many years.

Clinical features

Amoebic dysentery: abdominal discomfort, episodes of diarrhoea alternating with constipation, blood-stained mucus is often passed PR, rarely bowel perforation may occur or a localized amoebic granuloma ('amoeboma') may be mistaken for a colonic carcinoma.

Hepatic amoebiasis: lethargy, swinging pyrexia, sweating and tender hepatomegaly with referred shoulder-tip pain. The liver abscess may rupture catastrophically into the pleural, pericardial or peritoneal cavities.

Investigations • Identification of trophozoites by microscopy of fresh stool • Sigmoidoscopy and biopsy reveals colonic ulceration • Hepatic amoebiasis can be diagnosed by US, radioisotope or CT scanning, and confirmed by serological tests (immunofluorescent antibody test).

> **Management box**
> ▶ Amoebic dysentery: metronidazole 800 mg tid for 5 days or tinidazole 2 g daily for 3 days. Both should be followed by diloxanide furoate 500 mg tid for 10 days to eliminate any luminal cysts.
> ▶ Hepatic amoebiasis: treatment as above but aspiration may be needed if the abscess is large. Secondary bacterial infection may occur and should be treated with appropriate broad spectrum antibiotics. Cure is not always complete.

ACQUIRED IMMUNODEFICIENCY SYNDROME

Science basics HIV infects cells bearing the CD4 molecular binding site. Once the virus is bound it is released into the cell cytoplasm and travels to the cell nucleus where integration into the host's DNA occurs. Transcription and translation of viral

Table 12.10
Classification of HIV infection

Stage 1	Seroconversion (CD4 > 800×10^6/l)
Stage 2	Asymptomatic disease (CD4 $350–800 \times 10^6$/l)
	Persistent generalized lymphadenopathy is common, skin diseases, eg herpes zoster, seborrhoeic dermatitis and pruritic folliculitis.
Stage 3	Infection (CD4 $200–350 \times 10^6$/l)
	Complications begin, typically with organisms that are common in the immunocompetent but infections are more severe and frequent, eg TB, pneumonia, oral candidiasis, vaginal candidiasis, weight-loss and constitutional disease (intermittent diarrhoea, fever, fatigue and myalgia)
Stage 4	Opportunistic infections and malignancies (CD4 < 200×10^6/l)
	PCP, Kaposi's sarcoma, cerebral toxoplasmosis, diarrhoea (cryptosporidium, CMV)
Stage 5	Multiple opportunistic infections (CD4 < 50×10^6/l)
	Systemic fungal /CMV/candidiasis, AIDS dementia complex (ADC), high-grade B cell non-Hodgkin's lymphoma

Table 12.11
Modes of transmissions of AIDS

Sexual intercourse	Anal and vaginal
Contaminated needles	Intravenous drug abuse, needle-stick injuries (very rare)
Contaminated blood and blood products	Transfusion
Contaminated organ and tissue donation	Bone marrow, organ transplant
Vertical mother to child	In utero, at birth, breast milk

RNA occurs with ongoing viral replication. A number of viral proteins are toxic to cells and it is probable that the reduction in CD4 population is due to a combination of viral-mediated cell killing and clearance of virally infected cells by the host's immune system. As the CD4 count falls, progressive immunological deficiency results and the patient is then left vulnerable to malignancies and opportunistic infections. The normal CD4 count is $>800 \times 10^6/l$. For classification and transmission see Tables 12.10 and 12.11.

Table 12.12
Organ involvement in AIDS

Lungs	*Pneumocystis carinii* pneumonia Tuberculosis – typical and avium-intracellulare Cytomegalovirus Bacterial pneumonia – *Strep. pneumoniae*, *Staph. aureus*, *H. influenzae* Fungi – invasive candidosis Lymphocytic interstitial pneumonitis Pulmonary Kaposi's sarcoma
GI tract	Oropharynx – candidosis, HSV, leucoplakia, Kaposi's sarcoma Stomach – tuberculosis, Kaposi's sarcoma, cryptosporidium Small intestine – cryptosporidium, giardia, salmonella, campylobacter, CMV, microsporidia, lymphoma Large intestine – HSV, cryptosporidium, CMV, Kaposi's sarcoma, lymphoma
Liver/biliary tract	Atypical mycobacteria, HSV, histoplasmosis, toxoplasmosis, cryptosporidium, CMV
Skin	Kaposi's sarcoma, non-Hodgkin's lymphoma, atypical mycobacteria, folliculitis, seborrhoeic dermatitis, herpes zoster, HSV, molluscum contagiosum, bacillary angiomatosis
Nervous system	Encephalopathy, transverse myelitis, peripheral neuropathy, myelopathy, dementia, depression, demyelination encephalitis, retinitis, focal intracranial lesion (toxoplasmosis, lymphoma), abscess (cryptococcus, asperigillus, mycobacteria, candida) Progressive multifocal leucoencephalopathy

Clinical features (Table 12.12). The initial infection is usually asymptomatic but as progression occurs there is increasing evidence of immunodeficiency with recurrent common infections, increasing constitutional symptoms and finally opportunistic infections and the occurrence of unusual tumours. These lead to an early death.

Seroconversion (Stage 1): occurs 1–6 weeks after infection and may be asymptomatic. A mononucleosis-like illness may occur with fever, diarrhoea, myalgia, arthralgia, headache, nausea, sore throat, rash, transient lymphadenopathy and rarely meningo-encephalitis. A period of asymptomatic infection then follows and this may last from a few months to many years.

Persistent generalized lymphadenopathy (Stage 2) nodes >1 cm diameter in two extrainguinal sites for >3 months. There is usually no evidence of any other symptoms or signs of disease at this time, other than skin diseases.

AIDS-related complex (Stage 3): symptomatic disease with evidence of constitutional upset and minor opportunistic infections (Table 12.13). This stage is one short of fully developed AIDS.

AIDS (Stages 4 and 5): severe immunodeficiency due to HIV infection. There is evidence of life-threatening opportunistic infections and/or unusual tumours (pneumocystis pneumonia,

Table 12.13
Features of AIDS-related complex*

Symptoms	Lethargy, malaise, fever, night sweats, weight-loss > 10%, diarrhoea > 1 month
Signs	Oral candidiasis/leucoplakia, tinea, dermatitis/folliculitis, pityriasis versicolor, impetigo, molluscum contagiosum/warts, herpes simplex, herpes zoster, hepatosplenomegaly, PUO > 2 months, persistent generalized lymphadenopathy
Investigations	HIV isolation, HIV antibody positive, lymphocytopenia, thrombocytopenia, anaemia, raised ESR, anergy to three common antigens ↓ CD4 lymphocyte count

*To qualify for a diagnosis of AIDS-related complex (ARC) the patient must have two symptoms, two signs and two positive investigations

cerebral toxoplasmosis, CMV, cryptosporidiosis, cerebral lymphoma, non-Hodgkin's lymphoma, mycobacterial infection, Kaposi's sarcoma). Neurological problems (encephalopathy, myelopathy, neuropathy, encephalitis, demyelination, retinitis and dementia are all common and may be present in up to 50% of cases.

Investigations • Detection of virus/viral antigen allowing the viral load to be assessed (HIV RNA copies/ml) • Detection of antibody (HIV antibody test): seroconversion usually occurs about 2 months after exposure to the virus. Techniques include ELISA assays and Western blot • Lymphocytopenia $< 1.5 \times 10^9$/l • Reduced T4(CD4) lymphocyte (helper/inducer) cell count $<0.4 \times 10^9$/l • Thrombocytopenia $<150 \times 10^9$/l • Anaemia • Raised ESR • Polyclonal rise in Igs (IgA in homosexuals; IgM in children) • Anergy to three recall antigens • Decreased HIV p24 antibody level • Increased HIV p24 antigen level.

Management box

▶ The optimal time to start antiretroviral therapy has not been fully established but is generally based on clinical symptoms and a CD4 count $< 500 \times 10^6$/l and/or HIV RNA viral load > 10000–20000 copies/ml.

▶ As with TB treatment triple combination therapy is superior to mono or dual drug therapy.

▶ There are three groups of antiretroviral drugs:
  – Nucleoside reverse transcriptase inhibitors (NRTIs): zidovudine, stavudine, didanosine.
  – Non-nucleoside reverse transcriptase inhibitors (NNRTIs): nevirapine.
  – Protease inhibitors (PIs): indinavir, nelfinavir, ritonavir and saquinavir.

▶ Various combinations of these three drug groups are used. The preferred option is a combination of two NRTIs and a PI. This is known as highly active antiretroviral therapy (HAART).

▶ Zidovudine (AZT) is an analogue of the nucleic acid thymidine. Acts by interrupting the transcription of viral RNA to DNA by inhibiting viral DNA polymerases. Half-life 1 hour and is able to penetrate the CNS. Metabolized in the liver. Adverse reactions include nausea, vomiting, bone marrow suppression and myalgia.

▶ Stavudine and zalcitabine should not be used together because of an increased risk of peripheral neuropathy.

▶ Two protease inhibitors may be used for viral treatment in those intolerant of nucleoside analogue.

▶ The choice of drugs depends on previous drug exposure, development of resistance, tolerability, concomitant medication and compliance.

▸ The aim is to reduce viral load by 10-fold within 8–12 weeks.
▸ An effective HIV vaccine is also being sought.
▸ The most important aspect of HIV control is the avoidance of possible risk-factors and education with the adoption of 'safer sex' techniques (Table 12.14).
▸ Further information and updates on HIV treatment can be found at http://www.hivatis.org

---

Table 12.14
Safer sex guidelines

Avoid casual sexual contact with multiple partners
Avoid unprotected sexual intercourse with casual partners (use a condom)
Avoid high-risk activities – anal sex, sex acts which draw blood
Regular venereological screening for high-risk groups, eg prostitutes

KAPOSI'S SARCOMA

Commonest tumour in AIDS and is present in 25% of cases although almost exclusively in homosexual men. May affect any organ although CNS involvement is rare. Usually multifocal at presentation and is locally invasive.

Clinical features Commonly affects the skin and presents as a firm, non-tender, non-pruritic, purple coloured lesion in the skin or subcutaneous tissue. May be initially mistaken for a bruise.

Investigations • Biopsy reveals spindle-shaped cells, intracellular clefts and extravasated RBCs.

Management box
▸ Unsatisfactory. Local radiotherapy is useful.
▸ Chemotherapy: a-interferon or vinblastine and bleomycin may be needed in rapidly advancing cases but this may provoke development of opportunistic infections.

PNEUMOCYSTIS CARINII PNEUMONIA

Commonest life-threatening opportunistic infection in AIDS and is the presenting feature in 50% of cases. Due to a protozoan. It is still the commonest AIDS-defining illness.

Clinical features   Gradually increasing breathlessness (may be over months), fever, lethargy, retrosternal chest discomfort, cough (worse on inspiration), night sweats, tachycardia, tachypnoea, occasionally cyanosis. Chest auscultation may reveal scanty crackles.

Investigations   • CXR may be normal, but typically shows bilateral, diffuse perihilar interstitial shadowing with relative sparing of the peripheral lung fields until late in the disease, may show pneumothorax • ABG reveals hypoxaemia and often hypocapnia. Hypoxaemia is most marked following exercise (using finger oximetry) • Decreased KCO and abnormalities on gallium scanning are early features • Immunofluorescent antibody test on induced sputum • Bronchoscopy with bronchoalveolar lavage and transbronchial biopsies may be needed to confirm the diagnosis and exclude other opportunistic infections.

Management box

▶ High-dose contrimoxazole 120 mg/kg qid is the treatment of choice. The drug should be given iv initially followed by the oral preparation. Adverse reactions are common and include rashes, fever and BM suppression (use folinic acid supplements).

▶ Corticosteroids (prednisolone 60 mg/day) may be given to severely ill patients with pO_2 < 10 kPa on supplemental oxygen.

▶ Alternatively pentamidine 4 mg/kg/day can be used (slow intravenous infusion or via nebulizer) but this drug often produces hypoglycaemia and hypotension.

▶ If neither drug can be tolerated trimethoprim plus dapsone or clindamycin plus primaquine may be effective.

▶ Prophylaxis against further infections should be undertaken using cotrimoxazole 960 mg twice weekly or using nebulized pentamidine 300 mg once per month (via a Mizer type system) or dapsone 100 mg/day. Bronchospasm may be minimized by using nebulized salbutamol before pentamidine.

CRYPTOSPORIDIUM

Protozoan which may produce diarrhoea, malabsorption, weight-loss, fever and abdominal pain.

Investigations   • Stool culture (oocytes) • Small-bowel biopsy which can also exclude other causes of diarrhoea (*Salmonella*, mycobacteria, *Giardia*, *Microsporidia*, *Campylobacter*).

Management box

▶ Spiramycin 1 g 6-hourly or paromomycin in combination with anti-diarrhoeal agents (codeine, loperamide).

▶ Adequate hydration.

NON-SPECIFIC URETHRITIS

Science basics Also known as non-gonococcal urethritis. Commonest sexually transmitted disease in the UK. Incubation period 7–21 days. Due to *Chlamydia trachomatis* in most cases but may be caused by *Ureaplasma urealyticum*, *Trichomonas vaginalis*, HSV and *Candidia*. May be promoted by stress, alcohol or frequent change of sexual partner.

Clinical features Insidious onset and produces only mild discomfort (rather than the abrupt onset dysuria with gonococcal urethritis).

Investigations • By exclusion of gonococcal infection • Endocervical and urethral swabs for *Chlamydia* culture • *Chlamydia* serology • Microscopy of wet mount from vaginal fornices for *Trichomonas*.

> **Management box**
> ▶ Tetracycline 500 mg qid for 5 days or erythromycin 500 mg bd for 7 days for each sexual partner.

SYPHILIS

Science basics Systemic infection due to the spirochaete *Treponema pallidum*. Incubation period 10–90 days. The time interval dividing early from late syphilis is 2 years. For classification see Table 12.15.

Clinical features

Primary: small papule which erodes to form a small painless ulcer at the site of infection (chancre). Serous exudate from this ulcer is highly infectious. Painless, rubbery regional lymphadenopathy occurs.

Table 12.15
Classification of syphilis infection

Congenital		
Acquired	Early	Primary
		Secondary
		Latent
	Late	Latent
		Tertiary
		Quaternary

Secondary: begins 1–4 months after healing of the primary chancre. Generalized, non-pruritic macular rash (may involve palms and soles), flat papular condylomata lata develop in moist areas (eg perianally), generalized painless lymphadenopathy, superficial ulceration on mucous membranes ('snail-track' ulcers), fever, arthritis, anterior uveitis, hepatosplenomegaly and meningitis may occur. The disease can then enter a latent stage which may last many years.

Tertiary: chronic infection which may appear 30 years after the primary stage and involves gumma formation in bones, skin and subcutaneous tissues. The disease may finally progress to the quaternary stage.

Quaternary stage: the main systems involved are cardiovascular and nervous systems (aortic dilatation, aortic valve incompetence, tabes dorsalis, Argyll Robertson pupils – small, irregular, unequal, do not react to light but respond to convergence and show an impaired response to mydriatics – general paralysis of the insane and meningovascular syphilis). The features of neurosyphilis are due to either endarteritis obliterans or to the formation of localized gummatae.

Congenital syphilis may result in spontaneous abortion, still-birth or fetal abnormalities, failure to thrive, rash, iritis, bone and teeth involvement, VIII nerve deafness, tabes, paralysis and early death.

Differential diagnosis HSV, traumatic genital ulceration, drug eruption, lichen planus, viral warts, HSV, IM, AIDS, *condyloma acuminata* and yaws.

Investigations • *T. pallidum* can be identified by dark ground microscopy of serum from primary chancre or secondary mucous patches • Serological tests are positive 1 month after infection. VDRL is a non-specific test and may be falsely positive in IM, SLE, malaria and leprosy. It may also be negative in tertiary and quaternary cases. TPHA or FTA are more sensitive and specific. These tests can be carried out on blood or CSF. An antitreponemal IgG ELISA test is available and is both sensitive and specific, titres <0.9 are negative, 0.9–1.1 are equivocal and values >1.1 are positive • The CSF in neurosyphilis shows increased protein (gamma globulin fraction), lymphocytosis and positive serology.

Management box
▶ Penicillin (long-acting im procaine benzlpenicillin (procaine penicillin) 600 mg/day for 10–12 days in primary, 14–15 days in secondary, tertiary and latent cases and 21 days in quarternary).
▶ The Jarisch-Herxheimer reaction 6–12 hours after the first penicillin injection may occur and is a febrile episode due to release of endotoxin from dead spirochaetes.
▶ In cases of penicillin allergy tetracycline 500 mg/day for up to 28 days can be used.
▶ Contact tracing should also be undertaken.

GONORRHOEA

Science basics Due to Gram-negative intracellular diplococcus Neisseria gonorrhoeae. Incubation period 2–10 days.

Clinical features Urethritis with dysuria and mucopurulent discharge (may be asymptomatic in 50% females), prostatitis, salpingitis, pelvic inflammatory disease, pustular/erythematous rash on limbs, arthritis, rarely endocarditis and meningitis. In male homosexuals pharyngitis or proctitis may be produced.

Differential diagnosis *Chlamydia trachomatis*, *Ureaplasma urealyticum*, Reiter's disease, or candidiasis.

Investigations • Gram stain and culture of discharge, blood culture or joint aspirate.

Management box
▶ Ampicillin 2 g plus probenecid 1 g orally or ciprofloxacin 250 mg if allergic to penicillin.
▶ Erythromycin 500 mg qid for 7 days in pregnant women.
▶ Pharyngeal infection should be treated with ciprofloxacin 250 mg bd or ampicillin 250 mg qid for 5 days.

13

Dermatology

DEFINITIONS

Abscess: collection of pus in a cavity >1.0 cm in diameter.

Angioedema: diffuse oedema which extends to the subcutaneous tissues.

Annular: ring-like.

Arcuate: curved.

Atrophy: thinning due to diminution of all the layers of the skin and subcutaneous fat.

Bulla: circumscribed elevation of skin >0.5 cm diameter and containing fluid (Fig. 13.1).

Circinate: circular.

Comedo: plug of keratin and sebum wedged in a dilated pilosebaceous orifice. Open comedones are blackheads.

Crust: flake composed of dried blood or tissue-fluid.

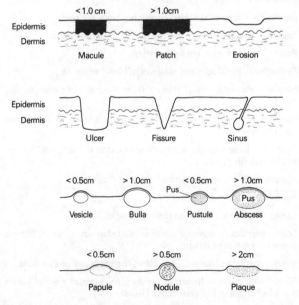

Fig. 13.1 Skin lesions.

Cyst: epithelial lined cavity containing fluid or semi-solid material.

Discoid: disc-like.

Erosion: area of skin denuded by a complete or partial loss of the epidermis.

Erythema: area of reddened skin which blanches on pressure.

Excoriation: an ulcer or erosion produced by scratching.

Fissure: slit in the skin.

Gyrate: wave-like.

Haematoma: swelling from gross bleeding in dermis or deeper structures.

Koebner phenomenon: the occurrence of skin lesions (eg psoriasis) at the site of skin trauma.

Lichenification: thickened skin with exaggerated skin lines.

Macule: small flat area of altered colour or texture <1.0 cm.

Nodule: solid palpable mass in the skin >0.5 cm in diameter.

Nummular: round or coin-like.

Papilloma: nipple-like mass projecting from the skin.

Papule: small solid elevation of skin <0.5 cm diameter.

Patch: macule >1.0 cm in diameter.

Petechiae: pinhead-sized macules of blood in the skin.

Plaque: elevated area of skin >2.0 cm diameter but without any depth.

Poikiloderma: combination of atrophy, reticulate pigmentation and telangiectasia.

Purpura: large macule or papule of blood in the skin which does not blanch on pressure

Pustule: visible accumulation of pus in the skin.

Retiform and reticulate: net-like.

Scale: a flake arising from the horny layer.

Scar: permanent replacement of normal skin structures by fibrous tissue as a result of healing.

Sinus: cavity or channel that allows the escape of pus or fluid.

Stria: a streak-like, linear, atrophic, pink, purple or white lesion due to changes in the connective tissue.

Telangiectasia: visible dilatation of cutaneous blood vessels.

Tumour: enlargement of the tissues by normal or pathological material or cells that form a mass usually >1.0 cm in diameter.

Ulcer: area of skin from which the whole of the epidermis and at least the upper part of the dermis has been lost.

Vesicle: circumscribed elevation of skin <0.5 cm in diameter and containing fluid.

Weal: elevated white compressible evanescent area produced by dermal oedema usually surrounded by a red axon-mediated flare.

PSORIASIS

Science basics A chronic relapsing and remitting papulo-squamous skin disease which affects both sexes equally, may appear at any age and involve any part of the skin. The incidence is approximately 1–2% in the Caucasian population and 30% of patients have a first-degree relative with the disease.

Clinical features Erythematous, scaly lesions commonly involving the extensor aspects of the knees, elbows and scalp. Each lesion is elevated, palpable and topped by greyish-white scales. If the lesions are rubbed pinpoint bleeding occurs from dilated superficial capillaries (Auspitz's sign).

Variants

Guttate: commoner in children, multiple small lesions mainly on the trunk.

Seborrhoeic: classical scalp lesions associated with lesions in the groins, axillae and inframammary regions.

Erythrodermic: extensive erythema leading to loss of thermo-regulation and high-output cardiac failure.

Pustular: sterile pustules at the advancing edge of psoriatic lesions.

May be asymptomatic or pruritic. Usually runs a chronic course. Nail involvement is common – pits, ridges, onycholysis, sub-ungual hyperkeratosis and discolouration. Mutilating sero-negative psoriatic arthropathy may be present and involves the distal interphalangeal and sacroiliac joints. A higher incidence of arthropathy is seen in patients with nail changes. Scalp hair may be thin.

Differential diagnosis Reiter's disease, lichen planus, pityriasis rosea, seborrhoeic dermatitis and pityriasis rubra pilaris.

Investigations • Clinical diagnosis • If in doubt perform a skin biopsy.

Management box

▶ *Topical*: coal tar preparations (1–20% ointment, paste or lotion) as antimitotic agent +/– salicylic acid as a keratolytic agent. These preparations are grey or black and tend to stain clothes and bedding and are unsuitable for use on the face and scalp. Alternatively anthralin or dithranol can be used as they are cosmetically more acceptable than tar. Scalp lesions are commonly treated with salicylic acid preparations (2–20%), light oils (olive oil) or tar shampoos. Vitamin D analogues such as calcipotriol may be effective.

▶ *Ultraviolet light*: commonly in association with systemic psoralens (PUVA) is now established for widespread disease but concern still exists over possible long-term adverse reactions (eg skin malignancy).

▶ *Cytotoxic drugs*: methotrexate or ciclosporin may be indicated in a small proportion of severely affected patients attending dermatology clinics.

▶ *Topical steroids*: use is controversial with often only a short-lived response and more unstable disease when discontinued. Possible pituitary-adrenal axis suppression is also a draw-back. The management of both nail changes and psoriatic arthropathy is largely unsatisfactory.

▶ *Retinoids*: Analogues of vitamin A such as etretinate are currently showing much promise in severe cases but adverse reactions can prove troublesome, eg hypercholesterolaemia, LFT abnormalities, ossification of the paraspinal ligaments, DISH syndrome (disseminated interstitial skeletal hyperostosis) and teratogenicity. Refinement of these agents, perhaps in combined modality therapy (eg with PUVA) may be successful.

LICHEN PLANUS

Science basics A condition of unknown aetiology characterized by intensely pruritic flat-topped papules most commonly seen on the inner aspect of the wrists and elbows. The mucous membranes are usually affected and spontaneous resolution often occurs.

Clinical features Intensely itchy shiny red or purple papules on the skin. The lesions inside the mouth or on the genitalia may be asymptomatic. With time the skin lesions become violaceous and develop a fine white network on their surface (Wickham's striae). As in psoriasis, new lesions appearing at sites of trauma (Koebner's phenomenon) is a feature of the active disease.

Differential diagnosis Usually clearcut. Psoriasis, contact dermatitis or drug-induced eruption.

Investigation • Clinical diagnosis • Occasionally a biopsy is required.

> **Management box**
> ▶ Systemic antihistamines, 1–2% menthol in calamine lotion, weak coal tar preparations or topical steroids may be required to combat the intense itch.
> ▶ Etretinate or systemic steroids may be needed in severe cases.
> ▶ Vitamin A (retinoic acid) or the newer synthetic retinoids may also be useful.

PITYRIASIS ROSEA

Science basics A self-limiting disorder characterized by the development of asymptomatic erythematous macules on the trunk. Increased incidence in spring and autumn possibly due to viral infection.

Clinical features Herald patch: an isolated erythematous area on the trunk with a peripheral collar of fine scales followed by oval macules on the trunk ('Christmas-tree' distribution), thighs and arms. Purpuric lesions are rare. Usually remits spontaneously in 4–8 weeks.

Differential diagnosis Drug eruptions, pityriasis versicolor, secondary syphilis, guttate psoriasis.

Investigations • Usually clinical • Rarely a biopsy is needed.

> **Management box**
> ▶ Reassurance as the disease is self-limiting.
> ▶ Topical antipruritic (eg 1–2% menthol in calamine or aqueous cream).
> ▶ Neither topical or systemic corticosteroids are usually indicated.

ECZEMA (DERMATITIS)

Science basics A chronic remitting pruritic cutaneous disorder which may be caused by a variety of genetic and environmental factors.

Exogenous: irritant, allergic contact and photodermatitis.

Endogenous: (constitutional) atopic, seborrhoeic, discoid (nummular), pompholyx, gravitational (stasis).

Unclassified: asteatotic, neurodermatitis, juvenile plantar dermatosis.

Clinical features   May be divided into acute, subacute and chronic phases. All three phases may coexist simultaneously.

Acute: redness and swelling, usually with an ill-defined border. Papules, vesicles, large blisters, crusting, white dermatographism and scaling may be present.

Subacute: erythema and crusting are present without the extreme oedema and exudation of acute reactions.

Chronic: less vesicular and exudative, more scaly, pigmented and thickened. More likely to be lichenified and have fissures. Asthma and rhinitis are often associated with the atopic form.

Differential diagnosis   Psoriasis, fungal infections, scabies, lichen planus, angio-oedema, pityriasis rosea, drug reactions, head lice.

Investigations   • Usually clinical diagnosis. • *Atopic*: patch testing, serum IgE levels, specific antigen detection (Radio Allergo Sorbent Test = RAST) • *Contact*: search for any possible sensitizing antigen (patch test important) • Biopsy may be required • Exclude fungal infections by culture of scrapings.

Management box

▶ *Acute*: apply wet dressing impregnated with 1% ichthamol in calamine lotion or 1:8000 solution of potassium permanganate to weeping sites. Each soaking followed by a smear of corticosteroid cream or lotion. Preparations containing tar or ichthamol applied on top of the steroid reduce the quantity of steroid required. Systematic antihistamines can be used to control itch. Secondary infection by Staphylococcus may occur, and should be treated with a 5-day course of flucloxacillin.
▶ *Subacute*: steroid creams or lotions (dose depends on the severity of the attack).
▶ *Chronic*: steroids in an ointment base, or ichthammol and zinc cream. Treat the associated dry skin with emollients (eg oilatum). Avoid perfumed soaps. Bacterial superinfection can often be controlled by the incorporation of antibiotics or antiseptics (eg vioform) into the steroid formulation. A short course of systemic corticosteroids may be needed in severe attacks. Avoid precipitating antigen if possible.

Complications   Higher incidence of warts and fungal infections in the atopic form. Occasionally widespread viral infections (eg herpes simplex or vaccina Kaposi's varicelliform eruption). Time may be lost from work or alternative employment may be necessary.

ACNE VULGARIS

Science basics   A disorder characterized by comedones, papules, and pustules centered on the pilosebaceous follicles. Affects most teenagers, usual age of onset is 12–14 years. Androgens stimulate sebum secretion. Genetic factors may be important. The role of *Proprionibacterium acnes* is uncertain.

Clinical features Comedomes, papules and pustules on the forehead, nose, chin, upper chest and back. In severe cases the whole face may be involved and the lesions may heal with scarring. The skin is usually greasy.

Variants

Tropical: affects young Caucasians in hot humid environments.

Steroid: patients on systemic steroids.

Chemical: due to contact with cutting oils or chlorinated hydrocarbons.

Infantile: rare, exclude androgen-secreting tumour.

Differential diagnosis Drug eruptions (eg anti-epileptics and anti-tuberculous medication), rosacea and pyogenic folliculitis.

Investigation • Clinical diagnosis.

Management box
▶ *Local*: regular cleansing with soap and water or anti-bacterial cleansers (eg chlorhexidine), benzoyl peroxide (begin with 2.5% solution), abrasive pastes, topical antibiotics (eg tetracycline, clindamycin), sulphur preparations, alcoholic solutions of aluminium chloride, cosmetic camouflage.
▶ *Systemic*: antibiotics (eg tetracycline 250 mg qid for at least 4 months, may be needed for a year or two) but avoid in pregnancy. Tetracycline may produce stained teeth and dental hypoplasia in children. Hormonal treatment with a combined antiandrogen/oestrogen pill (2 mg cyproterone acetate and 0.035 mg ethinylestradiol) may be useful in women only. Retinoids (eg 13-cis-retinoic acid) inhibit sebum excretion, the growth of *P. acnes* and acute inflammatory processes but are reserved for severe or resistant cases. There is little evidence to suggest that the avoidance of certain foods (eg chocolate) helps.
▶ *Physical*: local exision of cysts, intralesional injections of steroids, dermabrasion or collagen injections.

ROSACEA

Science basics The association of facial erythema, flushing, and acneform features in adults.

Clinical features Cheeks, nose, centre of forehead and chin are commonly affected with sparing of the periorbital and perioral areas. Intermittent flushing is followed by fixed erythema and telangiectasia. Papules, pustules and nodules but no comedones or seborrhoea occur. Rhinophyma and lymphoedema may be present. Ocular complications can occur (eg blepharitis, conjunctivitis, keratitis, corneal ulceration).

Investigation • Clinical diagnosis.

Management box
▶ Systemic antibiotics (eg tetracycline 250 mg bd for 3–6 months) are the mainstay, topical agents are of doubtful help (eg 2% sulphur or 2% ichthamol), topical steroids should be avoided as rebound flare-ups occur.
▶ Topical agents such as tetracycline or metronidazole may be useful.
▶ Sunscreens are useful.
▶ Severe rhinophyma may need surgery.

PEMPHIGUS

Science basics A group of conditions characterized by the formation of blisters in the epidermis. An antibody is directed against the intercellular substance of the epidermis. Acantholysis occurs in which individual keratinocytes lose their normal intercellular bridges and they may be seen floating freely in the resultant blister.

Varieties: vulgaris, foliaceus, vegetans and erythematosus.

Clinical features Painful mouth and genital ulcers followed by fragile skin blisters. Clinically normal skin may demonstrate the Nikolsky's sign – if lateral pressure is put on the skin surface with the thumb the epidermis appears to slide over the underlying dermis.

Investigations • Skin biopsy (immunoflurescent – IgG and C3 binding in intercellular area of epidermis) • Circulating IgG intercellular antibodies.

Management box
▶ Systemic steroids (may need 60–100 mg/day initially reducing slowly to a probable lifelong maintenance dose).
▶ Steroid-sparing immunosuppressives (eg azathioprine or cyclophosphamide) or plasmapheresis may be useful.
▶ Topical treatment is symptomatic to protect raw skin and prevent infection (eg ripple beds).

BULLOUS PEMPHIGOID

Science basics A chronic blistering disorder characterized by large tense blisters on an erythematous base. Commoner than pemphigus in the UK, may be associated with malignancy. Seen especially in the elderly, the blister is subepidermal and as such is relatively resilient and may remain intact for days.

Clinical features Itchy blisters with an urticated base on the arms and thighs. Oral lesions are less common than in pemphigus.

Investigations • Skin biopsy, (immunofluorescent – linear band of IgG and C3 along the basement zone between the epidermis and the dermis) • Circulating IgG antibodies.

> **Management box**
> ▶ Systemic steroids (begin with 30–60 mg/day but the dose can usually be reduced slowly and eventually stopped).
> ▶ Dapsone can also be a very useful single or adjuvant therapy.
> ▶ Azathioprine has a useful steroid-sparing effect.

DERMATITIS HERPETIFORMIS

Science basics An intensely itchy blistering condition associated with a gluten-sensitive enteropathy. M>F. Blisters are subepithelial but smaller than pemphigoid. Aggregations of leucocytes are present at the tips of dermal papillae ('microabscesses'). No circulating antibody to skin has yet been discovered.

Clinical features Intense burning itch on the affected sites (eg knees, scalp, scapula, buttocks and elbows). Small blisters are quickly excoriated leaving raw lesions. Most patients have no evidence of malabsorption but a jejunal biopsy should be performed and reveals villous atrophy.

Investigations • Skin biopsy of surrounding uninvolved skin (immunofluorescent – granular deposits of IgA and C3 in the dermal papillae and superficial dermis) • Jejunal biopsy • Antibodies to muscle endomysium.

> **Management box**
> ▶ Gluten-free diet, dapsone or sulfapyridine (can both cause rashes, haemolytic anaemia, leucopenia, methaemoglobinaemia and peripheral neuropathy).

ERYTHEMA MULTIFORME

Science basics An erythematous disorder characterized by annular target lesions which may develop into blisters. Often of unknown aetiology (50%) but may be secondary to viral (eg herpes simplex or orf), fungal, parasitic or bacterial infection (eg mycoplasmal pneumonia), drugs, pregnancy, malignancy, or connective tissue disease.

Clinical features Symptoms of an URTI followed by annular lesions on the palms, soles, legs and forearms. Lesions enlarge but clear centrally to form 'targets'. Blisters may occur. The Stevens-Johnson variant is the association of erythema multiforme with fever and mucous membrane involvement. Severe lesions in the tracheobronchi may produce asphyxia, or corneal ulceration may lead to blindness. The lesions appear in crops.

Differential diagnosis Urticaria, pemphigus, pemphigoid, dermatitis herpetiformis.

Investigations • Clinical diagnosis • Skin biopsy • Search for a cause: Tzanck smears, viral culture from scrapings, CXR, atypical pneumonia titres, autoantibodies and drug history.

> **Management box**
> ▶ Identify and remove the cause if possible.
> ▶ Antihistamines; systemic steroids may be needed in Stevens-Johnson syndrome.
> ▶ Prevent secondary infection and dehydration.
> ▶ Aciclovir 200 mg 5 times daily orally for 5 days or 5–10 mg/kg 8-hourly iv for 10 days if herpes simplex infection is present.

SKIN TUMOURS

Science basics An important factor in the aetiology of skin tumours is excessive exposure to sunlight (especially ultraviolet light in the UVB 280–320 nm part of the spectrum). The risk is higher in fair-skinned Caucasians. Genetic factors may be important.

PREMALIGNANT CONDITIONS

Actinic keratoses (senile keratoses)
Multifocal scaly, hyperpigmented or ulcerated lesions. Use sunscreens, eg 4% mexenone (Uvistat) prophylaxis. Cryotherapy, local exision or topical cytotoxic preparations (eg 5-fluorouracil) for established lesions.

Kerato-acanthoma
Grows rapidly as a papule which develops into a nodule and may rarely transform into a squamous carcinoma. Histological differentiation between kerato-acanthoma and well differentiated squamous carcinoma is extremely difficult and not possible without special cytokeratin stains. Excise or curette and cauterize.

Intra-epithelial carcinoma (Bowen's disease)
Slowly expanding pink, scaly plaque with a sharply defined border. May develop into an invasive squamous carcinoma. Treat by excision or cryotherapy.

BENIGN CONDITIONS

Viral warts
Caused by human papilloma virus (HPV), typical appearance, treat with wart paint containing salicylic acid. If unsuccessful after 8–12 weeks try paint containing formaldehyde or glutaraldehyde. Cryotherapy or excision may be needed.

Squamous cell papilloma
Arises from keratinocytes and may form a horn-like excrudescence – excise or curette with cautery and check histology.

Seborrhoeic keratosis (basal cell papilloma or seborrhoeic wart)
Flat, raised, or pedunculated yellow or dark brown 'stuck-on' lesions, usually multiple. Leave alone or treat by excision, cryotherapy, or curettage.

Skin tags
Excise if cosmetically unacceptable.

Melanotic naevi
Unknown cause, may be congenital or acquired (junctional, compound, intradermal, Spitz or blue). May swell and become painful, depigment but rarely become malignant. Signs of possible malignant transformation: enlargement, itch, increased or decreased pigmentation, irregularity of edge or surface, asymmetry, ulceration, inflammation or bleeding. Excise and examine histologically if in any doubt.

MALIGNANT CONDITIONS

Basal cell carcinoma
Commonest skin cancer, usually of middle-aged or elderly,

invade locally but rarely if ever metastasize. Develop on sun-damaged skin on the face or in scar tissue. Initially a red nodule which expands leaving a characteristic rolled edge with central ulceration: 'rodent ulcer'. Treat by surgery or radiotherapy. Excellent prognosis.

Squamous cell carcinoma

Derived from keratinocytes, often on sun-exposed skin. Dangerous sites for metastases include ears and lips. Hyperkeratotic, ulcerated, rapidly expanding nodule. Metastatic spread to the local draining lymph nodes and beyond may occur. Excision or radiotherapy is required.

Cutaneous malignant melanoma

Derived from melanocytes, increased sun exposure is important in the aetiology. Risk is highest in those with dysplastic naevi or congenital melanocytic naevi. A pre-existing naevus is seen histologically in 30%. F:M = 2:1.

Signs suggestive of malignancy: • asymmetry • border irregularity • increasing size • diameter >6 mm • colour irregularity.

Varieties: • lentigo maligna • superficial spreading and • nodular. Treat by excision and skin grafting. Histological analysis of the tumour allows microstaging – Breslow's method assesses the height from the granular cell layer to the deepest part of the tumour. Clark's method assesses the degree of penetration. The 5-year survival is 90% with shallow tumours (<1.0 mm) but worsens with increasing penetration. Regional node clearance may be required in thicker tumours (2.0–3.5 mm). Adjuvant chemotherapy may be required in advanced tumours but is rarely curative. Campaigns to educate both doctors and patients to recognize melanoma at an early curable stage are vital.

Paget's disease of the nipple

Well-defined red and scaly plaque over and around the nipple due to invasion of the epidermis by cells from an underlying intraductal breast carcinoma. Biopsy to confirm the diagnosis, mastectomy may be required.

Cutaneous lymphoma

Most originate from T cells (unlike other forms of lymphoma), eg mycosis fungoides which occurs in middle age as a pruritic cutaneous plaque which may form a nodule or ulcerate. Biopsy reveals T cell lymphoid infiltration. May progress to involve local lymph nodes or metastasize. Treat with topical steroids, ultraviolet light, PUVA or radiotherapy. Responds poorly to systemic chemotherapy and treatment is aimed at controlling the disease rather than curing it.

URTICARIA

Science basics Recurrent transient cutaneous swellings and erythema due to fluid transfer from the vasculature to the dermis. Wide spectrum exists from trivial forms to life-threatening angio-oedema with laryngeal involvement. Sometimes caused by an allergy but is often mediated by non-allergic methods.

- *Allergens*: may be contacted in a number of ways – ingestion, inhalation, instillation, insertion, injection, insect bites, infestations and infections.
- *Physical*: cold, solar, heat, cholinergic, dermatographism, delayed pressure.
- *Inherited*: hereditary angio-oedema, hypersensitivity.
- *Pharmacological*: due to histamine release by various agents, eg drugs, food, bites, inhalants, pollens, insect venoms, animal dander.
- *Miscellaneous*: connective tissue disorders, hyperthyroidism, diabetes, pregnancy, intestinal parasites, neoplasia.
- *Contact and idiopathic.*

Clinical features Sudden appearance of pink, annular, itchy weals which usually disappear over a few hours. In the acute form weals may cover most of the skin surface but in the chronic form only a few weals may develop each day. Angio-oedema affects the subcutaneous tissues and may produce swelling of the tongue, laryngeal mucosa, airways, periorbital, perioral and genital mucosa.

Differential diagnosis Erythema multiforme, urticarial vasculitis, dermatitis herpetiformis, pemphigoid, erysipelas.

Investigations • History is vital (including all drugs) • FBC • Urinalysis • LFTs • CXR • Sinus X-rays • MSU • Stool examination • ANF, complement and C1 esterase inhibitor level • Autoantibodies.

Management box
▶ Eliminate the cause if possible.
▶ Antihistamines (eg terfenadine 60 mg bd).
▶ Systemic steroids should only be used in acute cases.
▶ Topical agents (eg menthol 1–2% in calamine lotion) are useful in relieving itch.
▶ Subcutaneous adrenaline and maintenance of the airway may be life-saving in acute cases.
▶ Methylprednisolone, trasylol, danazol, stanozolol and fresh plasma may all be needed in hereditary angio-oedema.
▶ Salicylates, benzoates and azo-dyes (widely used as food additives) should also be avoided as they are well recognized histamine-releasing agents.

ICHTHYOSIS

Science basics A disorder of keratinization characterized by excessive dry and scaly skin.

Varieties: vulgaris (autosomal), nigricans (sex-linked), lamellar, Refsum's syndrome, epidermolytic hyperkeratosis, acquired (secondary to Hodgkin's disease, lymphoma, leprosy, malabsorption, poor diet or sarcoidosis).

Clinical features Excessively dry scaly skin, accentuated skin creases. Appears in the first few years of life in the inherited forms and persists throughout life. Can be severely handicapping.

Investigations Usually none are required.

> **Management box**
> ▸ Regular use of emollients (eg emulsifying ointment, soft white paraffin, E45 or unguentum merck), avoid excessive use of soap.
> ▸ Long-term use of retinoids can perhaps be justified in severe cases as they may produce a marked improvement but hyperostosis is an inevitable adverse reaction.

DISORDERS OF SKIN PIGMENTATION

ALBINISM

A condition characterized by a lack of melanin production by melanocytes in the epidermis, the eye and hair bulb. Autosomal recessive in inheritance.

Clinical features Lack of normal pigmentation, poor tolerance of sunlight, photophobia and rotatory nystagmus.

> **Management box**
> ▸ Avoid sun exposure, use sun-barrier creams, watch for the development of skin tumours.

VITILIGO

Islands of skin depigmentation secondary to loss of normal melanocyte function. Possible genetic association (link with autoimmune disorders, eg thyroid disease, Addison's disease, diabetes mellitus and pernicious anaemia).

Clinical features Sharply demarcated patches with relative lack of skin pigmentation commonly affecting the dorsum of the hands, wrists, knees, neck and around body orifices. Koebner's phenomenon is present. May improve spontaneously.

Investigations • Usually obvious but exclude fungal infection • Leprosy should be excluded by biopsy if considered relevant.

Management box
▶ Artificial tanning creams, cosmetic masking creams or PUVA in selected patients.
▶ Avoid sunburn.

CHLOASMA

Hormonally stimulated increase in pigmentation mainly affecting the face in pregnancy or when taking the OCP.

Clinical features Increased pigmentation.

Management box
▶ Self-limiting condition.
▶ Use cosmetic masking creams.

HAIR DISORDERS

Science basics The scalp contains approximately 100 000 hairs, we shed 100 hairs each day and each hair grows for about 1000 days.

ALOPECIA

Localized hair-loss can be divided into two types:

Non scarring: alopecia areata, androgen, hair-pulling habit, scalp ringworm, traction alopecia.

Scarring: radiodermatitis, aplasia cutis, carbuncle, sarcoid, basal cell carcinoma, SLE, lichen planus.

Aetiology (→ Table 13.1)

Alopecia areata
Characterized by either localized or generalized sudden loss of hair from the scalp or other body sites. May be a genetic link. Commoner in Down's syndrome. Two subgroups exist: • atopic tendency • associated autoimmune disease eg vitiligo, diabetes. No scarring occurs. Hairs plucked from the margin of the

Table 13.1
Causes of diffuse hair-loss

Androgenic (male pattern baldness)
Telogen effluvium (post partum, fever, 'stress')
Syphilis
Endocrine (eg hypo/hyperthyroidism)
Nutritional (eg iron deficiency)
SLE
Drug-induced (eg cytotoxics, anticoagulants, ethionamide
    carbimazole, excess vitamin A)
Alopecia areata
Trichotillomania
Hair-shaft defects (eg pilo torti, monilethrix)

affected area are often broken leaving behind remnants that resemble 'exclamation marks' which are diagnostic. The nails are often pitted and ridged. Exclude fungal infection by scraping and the use of Wood's light. Most cases are self-limiting but occasionally UVB light, intralesional steroids, topical minoxidil or wigs are useful.

HIRSUTISM → Chapter 16, page 413

Investigations • Exclude an underlying remediable cause • Check menstrual history • Perform tests of endocrine function as indicated (eg diurnal cortisol levels, ACTH, dexamethasone suppression test, testosterone, glucose tolerance test with GH measurement, abdominal US, LH, FSH).

Management box
▶ Treat any remediable cause as indicated.
▶ Remove excess hair by shaving, bleaching, depilatory cream or waxing.
▶ Antiandrogen drugs (ie cyproterone) may be helpful.

NAIL DISORDERS

Beau's lines
Transverse ridges due to temporary interference with nail growth, eg following severe illness. Usually self-limiting.

Koilonychia
Loss of the normal nail contour resulting in a flat or depressed

surface. Nails are brittle. Reputed to be associated with iron deficiency anaemia.

Paronychia

Inflammation of the nail fold, may be bacterial (Staphylococcal, *Pseudomonas* or *Proteus*), or fungal (*Candida*). Exacerbated by immersion in water. Treat with appropriate antibiotic (eg flucloxacillin, nystatin or amphoteracin).

LEG ULCERATION

VENOUS

Accounts for 70–80% of lower limb ulceration. Due to incompetence of valves resulting in an increase in capillary pressure, capillary damage, fibrosis and a poorly nourished skin which is easily damaged by even minor trauma.

Clinical features Often affects obese women with a history of varicose veins and DVTs. Ulcer forms over the medial malleolus, is usually pain-free and the surrounding skin is discoloured due to extravasated blood.

Differential diagnosis Exclude diabetes, sickle cell disease, RA, malignancy, syphilis.

> *Management box*
> ▸ Weight reduction.
> ▸ Supportive elastic stockings, protective dressings, multiple-layer bandaging, leg elevation, clean the ulcer and dress with paraffin tulle (plain or impregnated with 0.5% chlorhexidine) or apply an absorbant dressing (eg granuflex or seaweed based).
> ▸ If infected apply a dressing containing eg potassium permanganate (1:10 000).
> ▸ Use diuretics if cardiac failure exists.
> ▸ Systemic antibiotics are reserved for spreading infections and the choice depends on swab results.
> ▸ Analgesia as required.
> ▸ Avoid systemic steroids.

ARTERIAL

Usually painful, M>F, often in association with poor peripheral circulation. Punched out in appearance and may be associated with diabetes, atherosclerosis, RA, Buerger's disease and connective tissue diseases. Varicose veins are usually absent.

> *Management box*
> ▶ Symptomatic, topical therapy as for venous ulceration, rest and warmth, sympathectomy.
> ▶ Systemic vasodilators are of limited use.

LYMPHOEDEMA

Science basics Swelling of the limbs which is firm, pits poorly and is often longstanding.

Aetiology (→ Table 13.2)

Clinical features Swelling of one or more limb which may not appear until puberty or adulthood.

> *Management box*
> ▶ Elevation, compression bandages, diuretics and antibiotics if infection is present.
> ▶ Surgery is occasionally needed.

VASCULITIS

Science basics A pathological inflammatory process based primarily on blood vessel walls (mainly small and medium-sized vessels) resulting in nodules, purpura and ulceration. The different types are listed in Table 13.3.

ERYTHEMA NODOSUM

A lymphocytic vasculitis predominantly affecting the lower limbs. F:M = 5:1.

Table 13.2
Causes of lymphoedema

Primary
Due to a developmental defect in the lymphatic system

Secondary	
Recurrent lymphangitis	Erysipelas
Lymphatic obstruction	Filariasis, tumour, tuberculosis
Lymphatic destruction	Tumour, radiation therapy, surgery
Unknown aetiology	Yellow nail syndrome, rosacea

Table 13.3
Types of vasculitis

Predominant cell type in infiltrate	Clinical condition
Lymphocyte	Lupus pernio
	Chillblains
	SLE
	Erythema nodosum
Polymorph	Henoch-Schönlein purpura
	Polyarteritis nodosa
Granuloma formation	Pyoderma gangrenosum
	Temporal arteritis
	Churg-Strauss syndrome
	Erythema induratum
	Wegener's granulomatosis

Clinical features   Painful, palpable, dusky blue-red lesions on the calves, shins and forearms, malaise, fever and arthralgia.

Aetiology   Streptococcal infections, drugs (eg sulphonamides, OCP), sarcoidosis, viral and chlamydial infections, tuberculosis, ulcerative colitis, Crohn's disease, Behçet's disease, *yersinia*, mycoplasma, *Rickettsia*, fungi (eg coccidioidomycosis), leprosy.

Differential diagnosis   Trauma, cellulitis, abscess, phlebitis.

Investigations   • FBC • ESR • CXR • Throat swab • ASO • Mantoux test • Kveim test • Acute and convalescent viral titres.

> **Management box**
> ▶ Mainly symptomatic as the disease is usually self-limiting.
> ▶ Antibiotics if due to a bacterial infection, bed-rest, NSAIDs for analgesia.
> ▶ Systemic steroids are not usually needed.

POLYARTERITIS NODOSA

A rare, severe, generalized disease characterized by necrotizing polymorph arteritis.

Clinical features   Febrile, malaise, weight-loss, abdominal pain, chest pain, skin ulceration, subcutaneous nodules, purpura, gangrene, splinter haemorrhages, livido reticularis, myalgia, neuropathy, hypertension and signs of renal failure.

Differential diagnosis   • Panniculitis • Wegener's granulomatosis • SLE • RA, tissue infarction.

Investigations • FBC • ESR • Gammaglobulins • RF, cryoglobulins, HBsAg may be positive • Biopsy of involved organs (eg skin or kidneys). These investigations often yield non-specific results.

> **Management box**
> ▶ Systemic steroids and steroid-sparing immunosuppressives (eg azathioprine or cyclophosphamide) but the mortality remains high.

PYODERMA GANGRENOSUM

Clinical features   Characterized by large and rapidly spreading ulcers with a blue, indurated, undermined or pustular margin. Due to underlying thrombosis and vasculitis. Associated with RA, ulcerative colitis, Crohn's disease, monoclonal gammopathy or myeloma.

Investigations   Look for the underlying disease.

> **Management box**
> ▶ Systemic corticosteroids (eg prednisolone 60–100 mg/day reducing slowly to zero).
> ▶ Dress with sofratulle.

TEMPORAL ARTERITIS (giant cell arteritis)

Affects large vessels of head and neck, most commonly in elderly people and is associated with polymyalgia rheumatica.

Clinical features   Tender, pulseless temporal arteries in association with severe headaches. Necrotic ulcers may appear on the scalp and blindness may occur due to involvement of the retinal arteries.

Investigations   • Elevated ESR • C-reactive protein in active disease.

> **Management box**
> ▶ Systemic corticosteroids without delay (prednisolone 30–60 mg/day).

WEGENER'S GRANULOMATOSIS

Granulomatous vasculitis of unknown aetiology.

Clinical features Fever, malaise, weight-loss, nasorespiratory symptoms (eg hearing-loss, rhinitis, haemoptysis, sinusitis), skin lesions (ulcers or papules). Arthralgia, haematuria, eye, heart, lung and nerve involvement.

Investigations • Antineutrophil cytoplasmic antibody • Elevated KCO • CXR • Biopsy of nasal mucosa, lung or kidney.

Management box
▶ Cyclophosphamide alone or with corticosteroids.

CHURG–STRAUSS SYNDROME

A granulomatous condition characterized by eosinophilia ($>1.5 \times 10^9$/l), and vasculitis commonly affecting the lungs, the skin, and the peripheral nerves. Most patients have a past history of asthma or rhinitis.

Clinical features Worsening asthma, dyspnoea, haemoptysis, fever, nerve involvement, subcutaneous nodules, purpuric lesions.

Investigations • CXR shows patchy pneumonia-like shadows • Antineutrophil cytoplasmic antibody • Tissue biopsy.

Management box
▶ Systemic corticosteroids with cyclophosphamide.

HENOCH–SCHÖNLEIN PURPURA

Vasculitis which may be an allergic reaction to ingested drugs or bacteria and is associated with fever, lethargy, renal and gastro-intestinal disease.

Clinical features Multiple purpuric lesions on the limbs and buttocks, fever, malaise, arthralgia, abdominal pain and haematuria. May be a preceding streptococcal sore throat.

Investigations • Normal platelet count • Exclude connective tissue diseases and other forms of vasculitis • May need renal biopsy • Urinalysis.

Management box
▶ Usually symptomatic as the disease is self-limiting.
▶ Steroids for severe systemic disease.

BACTERIAL INFECTIONS

IMPETIGO

A superficial infection caused by either streptococci or staphylococci. Highly contagious, especially under conditions of poor hygiene.

Clinical features Thin-walled blisters which burst rapidly leaving areas of exudation and yellowish crusting, usually on the face.

Investigations • Swab lesions and send for culture.

Management box
▶ Remove crusts, apply topical antibiotics (eg fucidin), systemic antibiotics for severe cases (eg erythromycin, flucloxacillin, penicillin V).
▶ May complicate eczema or acne and may rarely lead to glomerulonephritis.

ERYSIPELAS

Cutaneous streptococcal infection with a sharply demarcated edge, commonly on the face.

Clinical features Fever, malaise, shivering followed by the development of a red skin eruption with a well defined advancing edge. Infecting organism gains entry through a small abrasion.

Investigations • Swab but do not delay treatment.

Management box
▶ Penicillin V or erythromycin.

CELLULITIS

Inflammation of the skin involving deeper tissues than erysipelas.

Clinical features Raised, hot, tender area of skin with a less well demarcated margin than erysipelas. Organism enters through an abrasion. Fever and rigors may occur.

Investigations • FBC • Multiple blood cultures • Swab lesions

---

Management box
▶ Systemic antibiotics (eg penicillin V, erythromycin and flucloxacillin).

CUTANEOUS TUBERCULOSIS

Lupus vulgaris

Firm skin nodule occurring after primary infection in people with a high degree of natural immunity. F>M.

Clinical features Discrete reddish-brown nodule which may invade deeper tissues and scar. Malignant change may occur.

Investigations • Diascopy (pressure with a slide) shows characteristic 'apple jelly' appearance • Biopsy reveals tuberculoid granulomata.

Scrofuloderma

Cutaneous tuberculosis with involvement of the lymphatic system.

Clinical features Fistulae, abscesses and scars most commonly occurring in the neck.

Investigations • Biopsy and culture.
Erythema nodosum (→ Vasculitis p 314–315).

Erythema induratum (Bazin's disease)

Cutaneous tuberculosis with deep ulcerating nodules on the calves.

Tuberculides

Recurring crops of firm dusky ulcerating papules usually at the knees or elbows.

> *Management box*
> (→ Table 12.6, p 271).

LEPROSY

Infection due to *Mycobacterium leprae*.

Clinical features Depend on the degree of immune response of the patient. If high resistance exists the tuberculoid form occurs, if low resistance exists the lepromatous form occurs. The borderline form lies between the two ends of the spectrum.

Tuberculoid

Organisms hard to find, non-infectious, localized lesions and positive lepromin test. Well formed granulomata invade the dermis from within the nerve trunks. Anaesthetic depigmented plaque or macule. Palpable enlarged nerves.

Lepromatous

Many organisms, infectious, generalized lesions and negative lepromin test. Macules, papules, nodules and ulceration occurring at sites where tissue temperature is low (eg nostrils and nasal septum leading to collapse of the nasal bones).

Borderline

Some organisms, slightly infectious, scattered lesions and intermediate resistance.

Investigations • Biopsy • Ziehl-Neelsen stain and culture of skin or sensory nerve • The lepromin test is of no use in diagnosing the condition but is useful in determining the form of disease which is present (eg negative in lepromatous and positive in tuberculoid).

Management box
▸ Combination of dapsone, rifampicin and clofazimine. Drugs may have to be continued for life in the lepromatous form.
▸ Two forms of lepra reactions may occur during treatment:
  – Type I (in tuberculoid and borderline) lesions become increasingly inflamed and painful and paralysis may occur.
  – Type II (in lepromatous) immune complex-mediated vasculitis, eg erythema nodosum.

VIRAL INFECTIONS

WARTS

Benign cutaneous tumours due to the human wart virus (human papilloma virus – HPV). Transmitted by direct contact.

Varieties: common wart (verruca vulgaris), plantar wart (verruca plantaris), anogenital, mosaic and planar.

Clinical features Raised, multiple, hyperkeratotic nodules which may develop into clusters. Demonstrate Koebner's phenomenon and may be resistant to treatment. May enlarge rapidly during pregnancy or may be large and persistent if malignancy (eg leukaemia) coexists. Some forms of genital warts may predispose to cervical carcinoma.

Differential diagnosis Plantar corns, granuloma annulare, amelanotic melanoma • molluscum contagiosum, condyloma lata, periungual fibromata of tuberose sclerosis.

Investigations • Usually clinical • Can be identified by electron microscopy • If in doubt always biopsy.

> *Management box*
> ▸ Usually improve spontaneously.
> ▸ Salicylic acid paint (12–20%) for 3 months, cryotherapy with liquid nitrogen or carbon dioxide, paint containing glutaraldehyde or formaldehyde.
> ▸ Podophyllin in soft paraffin may be useful in genital warts (not in pregnancy).

VARICELLA (CHICKEN POX) → p 273

HERPES ZOSTER (SHINGLES)

Cutaneous infection caused by herpes varicellae (→ also Chapter 12, p 274).

Clinical features   Usually reactivation of virus which has remained dormant in a dorsal root ganglion since an earlier episode of chickenpox. Pain in a dermatome followed by malaise, pyrexia and a linear erythematous blistering band along this dermatome. Postherpetic neuralgia may develop. Ramsay-Hunt syndrome is involvement of the geniculate ganglion with blistering of the external auditory meatus. The ophthalmic division of the trigeminal nerve with subsequent damage to the eye may occur. Zoster may become disseminated in the immunocompromised and may prove fatal.

Investigations   • Usually clinical • If in doubt send blister fluid for culture and electron microscopy.

> *Management box*
> ▸ Symptomatic for mild cases, systemic aciclovir for early severe infections.
> ▸ The management of postherpetic neuralgia is unsatisfactory but carbamazepine may be helpful.

HERPES SIMPLEX

Cutaneous infection due to herpes virus hominis. Two types have been isolated: Type 1 causes 'cold sores', Type 2 causes genital lesions.

Clinical features

Type 1: febrile illness with painful ulcerated blistering perioral lesions and cervical lymphadenopathy which last for up to a week and resolve spontaneously. The eye may also be involved.

Type 2: produces painful genital lesions.

Investigations • Usually clinical • If in doubt take a thick smear and send for culture and electron microscopy • Check acute and convalescent antibody titres.

Management box
▶ Symptomatic, topical aciclovir or 5-idoxuridine applied 5–6 times daily. Systemic acyclovir can be used in severe infections. Antibiotics for secondary infections.

MOLLUSCUM CONTAGIOSUM

Cutaneous lesion caused by the pox virus.

Clinical features Elevated, smooth red papules seen on the face, neck and trunk. The lesions have a characteristic central punctum.

Investigations • Usually clinical • Examine debris expressed from the lesions under microscopy and identify large swollen epidermal cells.

Management box
▶ Destructive measures which induce an inflammatory reaction, eg squeezing, piercing or curetting the lesions or applying liquid nitrogen or carbon dioxide, although may lead to scarring. If left alone may clear spontaneously without scarring.

ORF

A rapidly growing cutaneous lesion due to a pox virus. Usually secondary to contact with sheep.

Clinical features Red papule which develops rapidly 1 week after infection and commonly affects the finger. The lesion may grow to 10 mm in diameter and may ulcerate. Fever, lymph-adenopathy and erythema multiforme may occur.

Management box
Spontaneous recovery occurs and confers immunity but if secondary infection occurs systemic antibiotics are required.

FUNGAL INFECTIONS

Science basics Two main groups of fungi affect man: dermatophyte (ring-worm), candida (thrush, candidiasis).

DERMATOPHYTE INFECTIONS

Produce athlete's foot, tinea corporis, nail infections and scalp ringworm. Invade keratin only and do not penetrate living tissue, the resulting inflammation is due to metabolic products produced by the fungus or to delayed hypersensitivity. Three genera exist:

- Microsporum – nail and skin infections
- Trichophyton – nail, skin and hair infections
- Epidermophyton – skin and nail infections

Clinical features

Athlete's foot (tinea pedis):   usually affects toe webs with soggy scaling. Itching may be prominent.

Ringworm (tinea corporis):   itchy erythematous rash on the axillae or groin with a raised advancing edge.

Tinea infection of the nails: produces yellow discolouration with crumbling and subungual hyperkeratosis.

Scalp infections: can produce boggy swelling, pustules, kerion and scarring alopecia. Epidemics may occur in schools, public baths and swimming pools.

Investigations • Microscopic examination of skin or nail scrapings • Culture and examination under UV Wood's light revealing green fluorescence.

> **Management box**
> ▸ *Local*: topical antifungal agents, eg miconazole or clotrimazole.
> ▸ *Systemic*: used for tinea infections of the scalp and nails or for skin infections which have failed to respond to topical therapy, eg griseofulvin (500 mg daily for up to 18 months), but adverse reactions such as nausea, vomiting, rashes and headache may occur and it should be avoided in pregnancy, porphyria and liver disease.

CANDIDA

Normal commensal of the gastrointestinal tract but may become pathological in the immunocompromised or diabetic.

Clinical features   Napkin dermatitis in infants and intertrigo affecting the submammary folds, groins and axillae in the elderly, present as shiny red areas and are characterized by satellite lesions with occasional fissures. Commonly seen on hands chronically immersed in water. May also affect mucous membranes producing raised white patches which leave raw bleeding areas if scraped

Itchy balanitis or vulvovaginitis associated with a white vaginal discharge may occur. Chronic paronychia may affect the nails. If candidiasis is generalized immunosuppression should be suspected (eg AIDS).

Investigation • Swab affected areas and send for microscopy, and culture • Exclude diabetes mellitus.

> **Management box**
> ▶ Eliminate predisposing factors, eg poorly fitting dentures, keep hands dry, topical amphoteracin or nystatin (eg mouth-washes, pessaries or lozenges).

PITYRIASIS VERSICOLOR

A fungal infection of the skin due to *Malassezia furfur* which is usually asymptomatic.

Clinical features Fawn-coloured or depigmented areas with brawny scaling. Usually affects the upper trunk. Reinfection may occur.

Investigations • Usually clinical but microscopic examination of scrapings is useful • Pale yellow fluorescence under Wood's light.

> **Management box**
> ▶ Topical application of 2.5% selenium sulphide applied for 12 hours at weekly intervals for 3 weeks.

CUTANEOUS INFESTATIONS

SCABIES

A persistent and intensely itchy skin eruption due to the mite *Sarcoptes scabei*.

Clinical features Severe itch especially after bathing and at night. Classically affects the finger webs, fingers, wrists, elbows, areolae, genital area and periumbilical skin. Papules, linear burrows and pustules.

Investigations • Extract the acarus from its burrow.

Management box
▶ Malathion or permethnin. The entire family has to be treated.
▶ Crotamiton cream controls the itch.
▶ Launder all clothes and sheets.

CUTANEOUS MANIFESTATIONS OF SYSTEMIC DISEASES

Science basics Many diseases have a cutaneous component and these are listed in Table 13.4.

Table 13.4
Cutaneous manifestations of systemic diseases

Diabetes mellitus	Necrobiosis lipoidica, granuloma annulare, candida infections, staphylococcal infections, diabetic dermopathy, vitiligo, pruritus, eruptive xanthomas, neuropathic ulcers, tight waxy skin on fingers, atherosclerosis
Addison's disease	Buccal pigmentation
Acromegaly	Seborrhoea, soft tissue hypertrophy
Hypothyroidism	Alopecia, coarse broken hair, xeroderma, oedema, pruritus
Hyperthyroidism	Alopecia, pruritus, pretibial myxoedema, exophthalmos
Cushing's syndrome	Obesity, buffalo hump, acne, striae, oedema, moon face
Sarcoidosis	Erythema nodosum, lupus pernio, plaques, nodules, papules, scars, granulomata
Renal disease	Dry skin, pruritus, yellow pigmentation, 'half-and-half' nails
Porphyria	Photosensitivity, blisters, skin fragility, pigmentation, hypertrichosis, hirsutism
Hyperlipidaemias	Xanthelasmata, xanthomata-tendinous, tuberous, planar, eruptive
Scurvy (vitamin C deficiency)	Bleeding gums, purpura, poor wound healing
Pellagra (nicotinic acid deficiency)	'3 Ds': diarrhoea, dermatitis, dementia, erythema after sunlight
Tuberous sclerosis	Shagreen patch, adenoma sebaceum, periungual fibromata
Neurofibromatosis	Cutaneous neurofibromata, axillary freckling, cafe-au-lait spots

Table 13.4
Cutaneous manifestations of systemic diseases (*Cont'd*)

Graft-v-host disease	Acute: morbilliform rash, skin desquamation, toxic epidermal necrolysis
	Chronic: pigmentation, vesicles
Malignancy	Acne, flushing, jaundice, acanthosis nigricans, erythema gyratum repens, necrolytic migratory erythema, dermatomyositis, generalized pruritus, superficial thrombophlebitis
Liver disease	Spider naevi, bruising, palmar erythema, pigmentation in PBC, xanthelasma, scratch marks, jaundice, oedema, finger clubbing, leukonychia, 'paper-money skin'

DRUG ERUPTIONS

Always be aware of the possibility of a drug-related aetiology with any rash (consider all the medications that a patient is taking including over the counter preparations) (Table 13.5).

Management box
▶ Withdraw the offending drug.
▶ In severe anaphylactoid reactions emergency administration of subcutaneous adrenaline (epinephrine) (0.5 ml of 11 000 solution) given slowly may be life-saving.
▶ Systemic antihistamines (eg 10 mg of chlorphenamine (chlorpheniramine) iv), systemic corticosteroids (100–200 mg of hydrocortisone iv followed by oral prednisolone 40–60 mg/day). The steroids can be reduced slowly to zero over 7–10 days.
▶ Nebulized salbutamol (5 mg) is needed if wheeze is present.
▶ Soothing topical therapy, eg calamine lotion or 1–2% menthol in calamine cream, may be helpful.
▶ Report possible drug eruptions to the Committee for Safety in Medicine (CSM).

Table 13.5
Drug reactions

Reaction	Likely drug
Urticaria	Salicylates
Toxic erythema	Sulphonamides
	Ampicillin
Acne, gingival hyperplasia	Phenytoin
Erythema multiforme	Sulphonamides
Erythema nodosum	OCP, sulphonamides
Vasculitis, purpura	NSAIDs, heparin
	Phenytoin
Psoriasis	Lithium, β-blockers
Toxic epidermal necrolysis	Phenylbutazone
	Allopurinol
	Phenytoin
	Carbamazepine
	Penicillins
Photosensitivity	Phenothiazines
	Tetracycline
Alopecia	Cytotoxics
	Warfarin
SLE-like syndrome	Antibiotics
	Hydralazine
Exfoliative dermatitis	Gold, isoniazid
Blistering disorder	Barbiturates
	Penicillamine
Pustules	Bromide

14
Oncology

Science basics Cancer is second only to cardiovascular disease as a leading cause of death in Western society. It is the end result of a variety of mutations in specific genes. These mutations may lead to either underactivity or overactivity of gene function, producing irreversible and unregulated cellular proliferation.

There is interaction between genetic and environmental factors (eg smoking, exposure to ionizing radiation, drugs, alcohol, viruses, occupation) in the genesis of the majority of cancers. DNA sequences are generated by tumour-producing oncogenes (onc) and they may act by overexpressing proteins important in the regulation of cell proliferation and programmed cell death (apoptosis). Tumour suppressor genes have also been identified and may be important in balancing the tendency of oncogenes to drive the production of cancer cells.

In order for a cancer to grow and spread, new blood vessels are needed to serve the tumour's metabolic requirements. This process is called angiogenesis and may be influenced by the production of peptides from the cancer cells. The cancer cells must also break free from neighbouring cells to allow dissemination via lymphatics and the bloodstream.

ASSESSMENT

It is important to fully assess the degree of spread of the cancer to allow some prediction regarding prognosis to be made. A variety of anatomical tumour-staging systems have been developed (eg TNM – tumour, node, metastasis) but it is also important to assess the patient's functional performance status before deciding which treatment option is most appropriate (eg Karnowsky Performance Status, Table 14.1)

Table 14.1
Karnowsky Performance Status

Status	Description
100	Normal, no restriction on activity, asymptomatic
90	Able to continue with normal activity but has minor symptoms
80	Normal activity with effort
70	Self-caring but unable to carry out normal activities or work
60	Needing occasional assistance
50	Needing considerable assistance
40	Disabled
30	Severely disabled, often hospitalized
20	Very sick, needing active support
10	Moribund

Response to treatment can be assessed in terms of tumour shrinkage as well as overall, 1, 2 or 5-year survival. Accurate pre-treatment staging involves a variety of radiological (plain X-ray, ultrasound, CT, NMR) and biochemical measurements (LFTs, calcium, albumin, FBC, tumour markers) which are important in determining the response.

TREATMENT

Various treatment options are available to the multidisciplinary team caring for the patient (Table 14.2).

RADIOTHERAPY

A dose of ionizing radiation is delivered to the tumour to either kill all cancer cells (if possible – curative) or palliate symptoms. The total energy dose (measured in units of Gray (Gy)) is given in a number of fractions over a number of days, in order to reduce toxicity.

Indications • Haemoptysis • Dysphagia • SVC obstruction • Painful bony metastases • Brain metastases • Spinal cord/nerve root compression.

Table 14.2
Treatment options in oncology

Surgery	Curative v debulking
Chemotherapy	Curative
	Palliative
	Adjuvant
Radiotherapy	Radical
	Palliative
Combination:	
Adjuvant	Any additional treatment given after initial treatment for a primary tumour, designed to target occult micrometastases (eg tamoxifen after breast cancer surgery)
Neoadjuvant	Administration of adjuvant therapy before the primary treatment (eg chemotherapy before surgery)
Endocrine	Some cancers express sex hormones receptors which can be blocked (eg LHRH analogues in breast cancer – oophorectomy, tamoxifen)

Side-effects • Oesophagitis • Nausea/vomiting • Alopecia • Diarrhoea • Skin discomfort/desquamation.

Most side-effects are localized to the irradiated site and short-lived (<3 months) but occasional late sequelae can occur (bowel, ureteric strictures, pulmonary alveolitis/fibrosis, development of secondary malignancies).

CHEMOTHERAPY

A variety of drugs can be used in an attempt to cure/palliate cancer. These drugs damage DNA or prevent tumour-cell reproduction by a variety of mechanisms (Table 14.3).

Chemotherapy is a systemic treatment and may be used as the sole treatment in cancer or in combination with other treatment modalities (eg surgery, radiotherapy). Some extremely chemo-sensitive tumours (eg teratoma, seminoma, high-grade lymphoma) may be cured, but most tumours relapse at some stage following initial response. Treatment is usually given with multiple drugs simultaneously (as part of a clinical trial if possible) at intervals of 3–4 weeks for 4–6 cycles, with restaging to gauge clinical

Table 14.3
Chemotherapeutic agents

Drug class	Example	Mode of action
Antimetabolites	Methotrexate 5-Fluorouracil	Inhibit enzymes involved in DNA synthesis or incorporate themselves into DNA/RNA
Ankylating agents	Cyclophosphamide Chlorambucil Busulfan	Form covalent bonds with DNA to prevent cell division
Antitumour antibiotics	Bleomycin Doxorubicin	Incorporate into DNA or generate oxygen free radicals
Plant-derived antitumour agents	Vinca alkaloids Etoposide	Inhibit microtubular function
Heavy metals	Cisplatin Carboplatin	Form covalent bonds with DNA interfering with function
Tubulin-binding drugs	Taxanes	Inhibit microtubular function

response. The 'pulsed' nature of this treatment allows normal tissue repair (Table 14.4) and regrowth to occur while maximizing cancer-cell death.

Table 14.4
Common side-effects of chemotherapy

Side-effect	Possible drug involved
Haematological	Alkylating Agents
– Neutropenia	
– Anaemia	
– Thrombocytopenia	
Diarrhoea	Methotrexate
Nausea/vomiting	Most types
Peripheral neuropathy	Vinca alkaloids
Renal failure	Cisplatin
Haemorrhagic cystitis	Cyclophosphamide
Pulmonary fibrosis	Bleomycin
Cardiomyopathy	Doxorubicin

PALLIATIVE CARE

This describes the active care of the patient whose disease has not responded to curative treatment. It involves a multidisciplinary team approach and includes the coordinated help of doctors, nurses, physiotherapists, occupational therapists, family members, clergy and the patient to allow a caring and dignified death.

Physical symptoms (eg pain, breathlessness, nausea, vomiting and constipation) as well as emotional, social and spiritual concerns can be addressed in a holistic approach to patient care.

15

Psychiatric disorders and clinical medicine

INTRODUCTION

All medical students and doctors will be exposed to patients with psychiatric disorders and it is essential that these are recognized. It should be remembered, however, that mental disorders cannot be separated from general health and often the mind reflects physiological disturbances and vice versa. In this chapter the psychiatric disorders that are of most relevance to physicians will be considered. For a more complete list see Table 15.1.

DELIRIUM

Science basics Delirium or acute organic reactions have an abrupt onset with disturbance of several aspects of psychological functioning. For causes see Table 15.2.

Table 15.1
Classification of mental and behavioural disorders*

1. Organic mental disorders including Alzheimer's disease and vascular dementia, organic amnesic syndrome, delirium (non-alcohol related), mental, personality and behavioural disorders due to brain damage
2. Mental and behavioural disorders due to psychoactive substances
3. Schizophrenia, schizotypal and delusional disorders
4. Mood (affective) disorders including mania, bipolar affective disorders, depression
5. Neurotic, stress-related and somatoform disorders including phobias, anxiety, obsessive-compulsive and dissociative disorders and stress-adjustment disorders
6. Behavioural syndromes associated with physiological disturbances and physical factors including eating and non-organic sleep disorders, non-organic sexual dysfunction and abuse of non-dependence-producing substances
7. Disorders of adult personality and behaviour including personality, impulse and gender identity disorders and disorders of sexual preference
8. Mental retardation
9. Disorders of psychological development including speech, language and reading disorders and autism
10. Behavioural and emotional disorders with onset usually occurring in childhood and adolescence including hyperkinetic conduct and tic disorders
11. Unspecified mental disorder

---

*From ICD-10 Classification of mental and behavioural disorders

Table 15.2
Causes of delirium

Toxic, eg alcohol or drugs, either intoxication or withdrawal
Infection, eg pneumonia, meningitis, AIDS
Brain disease, eg cerebral vascular accident, subdural
  haematoma
Electrolyte imbalance, eg hypercalcaemia, hyponatraemia
Metabolic disease, eg hepatic failure
Intracranial tumour either primary or secondary
Cerebral hypoxia, eg respiratory or cardiac failure
Epilepsy, eg psychomotor seizure or post-ictal state

Clinical features These are characterized by a distinctive pattern of impairment of several cognitive functions including: clouding of consciousness which, if mild, can be readily overlooked; memory impairment, particularly of new information; perceptual disturbances, most commonly visual; thought processes slowed, disorganized and incoherent; mood changes, most often perplexity, anxiety; and psychomotor changes which may vary from agitation with repetitive purposeless movements to diminished motor behaviour with the patient lying immobile in bed.

Investigations • Temperature • FBC, U&E, LFT, Ca^{2+} and thyroid function • CXR • Urine examination • EEG, CT, LP and CSF examination • HIV serology.

> **Management box**
> ▶ This is the treatment of the underlying cause, such as antibiotics for infection and correction of electrolyte disturbances.
> ▶ Skilled nursing care is important and patients should be nursed in a well-lit room and sedative medication avoided unless the patient is distressed and/or a risk to himself or others.
> ▶ Drugs most commonly used are neuroleptics including haloperidol.
> ▶ These, however, should be avoided in patients with *delirium tremens* or other conditions associated with convulsions, because of the risk of epilepsy. Benzodiazepines such as chlordiazepoxide or diazepam are the drugs of choice in these patients.

DEMENTIA

Science basics This is a chronic organic reaction involving wide cerebral disturbance. Dementia can be defined as an acquired global impairment of intellect, memory and personality, but without

Table 15.3
Aetiology of dementia

Primary degeneration, eg Alzheimer's disease, Pick's disease,
  Huntington's chorea
Vascular, eg cerebral vascular disease
Normal-pressure hydrocephalus
Neoplasia
Trauma, eg punch-drunkenness
Metabolic, eg hypothyroidism, hepatic failure
Infections, eg syphilis, AIDS
Toxic, eg alcohol
Vitamin deficiency, eg vitamin B_{12}
Hypoxia

impairment of consciousness. It is important to realize that the condition is not necessarily irreversible.

Aetiology → Table 15.3.

Clinical features Predominantly but not exclusively a disorder of the elderly, characterized by a general decline in intellectual function with slowing of thought and poor concentration. There is usually poverty of speech, reduction in spontaneity and reduction in vocabulary. Global impairment of memory is characteristic and often an early feature. Its severity varies widely. Social behaviour progressively deteriorates and there may often be emotional lability and caricaturing or loss of personality traits.

Investigations • These should seek to identify the underlying cause as well as confirm the diagnosis and its severity and should include FBC, U&E, LFT and thyroid function • CXR • CT brain scan • Syphilis and HIV serology • Folate and vitamin B_{12} • EEG. Psychometric tests eg Wechsler adult intelligence scale (WAIS) are useful in determining the severity and response to treatment. Presenile dementia is usually differentiated from senile dementia (occurring before the age of 60). The latter is rarely investigated thoroughly while the former usually is. Approximately 5% of cases are wholly/significantly reversible.

Management box

▸ Correcting any underlying cause, if present, otherwise social and family support.
▸ Drug therapy should be used sparingly and should only treat episodes of confusion or agitation, eg thioridazine.
▸ A number of newer drugs are being developed to improve mental functioning but at present these are largely experimental.

WERNICKE'S ENCEPHALOPATHY AND KORSAKOFF'S SYNDROME

Science basics Wernicke's encephalopathy, due to a deficiency of dietary thiamine most often in alcoholics, is characterized by confusion, disorientation and memory impairment. Other features such as ophthalmoplegia, nystagmus, ataxia and peripheral neuropathy may be present. Once diagnosed urgent treatment with intravenous thiamine (50 mg) is essential as substantial improvement may occur. Failure of recognition leads to the chronic state of Korsakoff's syndrome characterized by profound memory impairment, particularly of recent events and near total inability to acquire new information. Confabulation is a common feature.

SCHIZOPHRENIA

Science basics Schizophrenic disorders are characterized by fundamental distortions of thinking and perception with inappropriate affect. Clear consciousness and intellectual capacity are maintained. Difficulty thinking or a sense of losing control of one's thoughts are key features. Other symptoms include auditory hallucinations, persistent delusions, mood changes, eg incongruous or blunted emotions, apathy and social withdrawal. The severity of the disorder may vary considerably and diagnosis is essential as specific psychiatric treatment is important.

MOOD DISORDERS

Science basics These are characterized by fundamental disturbance in mood, usually depression or elation (mania), accompanied by changes in thinking, outlook and behaviour. The mood changes may be unipolar with either mania or depression, or bipolar alternating between the two. The severity of the disorder varies widely and in the more severe forms accompanying psychotic symptoms with delusions and hallucinations may be present. The condition is important to recognize and specific psychiatric care should be sought.

ACUTE STRESS REACTIONS

Science basics These represent transient disorders which subside within hours or days in response to exceptional, physical or mental stress. There is great variation in an individual's vulnerability and capacity to cope following acute stress and a typical reaction is the initial state of 'daze', narrowing of attention, inability to comprehend stimuli and disorientation. This may be followed by withdrawal, agitation and over-activity.

Sympathetic autonomic features such as tachycardia and sweating may be present. It is different from post-traumatic stress disorder which arises as a delayed response to an exceptionally threatening and stressful event. Clinical symptoms of the latter include 'flashbacks' or dreams and a background of emotional numbing, social detachment, avoidance of situations likely to revive memories of the trauma and features of hyperarousal.

ADJUSTMENT DISORDERS

Science basics These are states of subjective distress and emotional disturbance following a significant life change or stressful life event. Again there is considerable inter-individual vulnerability and symptoms include depressed mood, anxiety and feelings of inability to cope, either at present or in the future. Markedly dramatic behaviour is recognized but is uncommon. In children regressive phenomena such as bed-wetting and thumb-sucking are common. The onset is usually within 4 weeks of the stressful event and lasts not usually more than 6 months.

EATING DISORDERS

Science basics These comprise two clear-cut syndromes: anorexia nervosa and bulimia nervosa.

ANOREXIA NERVOSA

Anorexia nervosa is characterized by deliberate weight-loss induced by the patient and most commonly arises in adolescent girls and young women, but not exclusively. Although the cause remains unknown cultural factors are undoubtedly important.

The disorder is associated with malnutrition of varying severity and secondary endocrine and metabolic changes and disturbances of bodily function. Diagnostic criteria which have to be fulfilled include a voluntary weight reduction to at least 15% below that expected and which is induced by avoidance of 'fattening' foods. Self-induced vomiting or self-induced purging, use of appetite suppressants or diuretics and excessive exercise may be features. These is a distortion of body image with a dread of fatness which persists as an over-valued idea with the patient imposing a low weight threshold for themselves. There may be secretive behaviour. Patients not uncommonly present with physical complications such as secondary amenorrhoea, unexplained weight-loss, abdominal pain, with abnormal eating habits denied!

BULIMIA NERVOSA

Bulimia nervosa is characterized by repeated bouts of over-eating with an excessive preoccupation to control the body weight and the adoption of measures to mitigate the effects of the ingested food. It is closely related to anorexia nervosa with the difference that the weight is ± 15% of normal. The effects of repeated vomiting may give rise to profound disturbances of electrolytes with complications including cardiac arrhythmias, tetany, epilepsy and weakness.

PERSONALITY DISORDERS

Science basics Personality disorders entail a severe disturbance in the constitution and behaviour of individuals, usually associated with considerable personal and social disruption. These usually appear in late childhood or adolescence and continue into adult life. A number of well recognized patterns are seen including paranoid personality disorder, with excessive sensitivity, tendency to bear grudges, suspiciousness and a tendency to experience excessive self-importance; schizoid personality disorder, with emotional coolness, detachment, apparent indifference to criticism or praise, preference for solitary activity, lack of close friends; dysocial personality disorder, characterized by callous unconcern for others' feelings, gross irresponsibility, poor tolerance of frustration, discharge and aggression and marked proneness to blame others; and histrionic personality disorder characterized by self-dramatization, suggestibility, shallow and labile affect, over-concern with physical attractiveness and continual seeking for excitement.

DRUG AND ALCOHOL MISUSE

ALCOHOL

Approximately 25% of male patients in general medical hospital wards have present or past alcohol problems.

Alcoholism is a term used to describe harmful (to patient or family) drinking. Alcohol dependence includes features such as drinking taking undue priority in life, tolerance to the effects of alcohol, withdrawal symptoms and relief of these with alcohol intake. Psychological problems caused by alcohol include: depression and morbid jealousy. Withdrawal symptoms include shaking, anxiety, confusion, seizures (most hospitals will have detoxification protocols which should be followed), Wernicke's encephalopathy or Korsakoff's psychosis.

DRUGS

Drug abuse is particularly common in young people. 2% of the population regularly take benzodiazepines in the UK and there are up to 100 000 opiate addicts. It is important to enquire about drug misuse in appropriate circumstances. Drug abuse varies in effect and can produce physical and psychological dependence. The most important drugs abused, from a clinical perspective, are benzodiazepines and opiates.

Benzodiazepine dependence occurs usually after use for several months and results in withdrawal symptoms on abrupt cessation of the drug, which include anxiety, fits and psychosis.

Cannabis Use may produce psychological dependence, but rarely tolerance. Heavy consumption may precipitate a toxic confusional state or acute psychosis. Long-term use may lead to 'amotivational syndrome' with apathy.

Opiates May cause physical dependence within weeks of use causing dose escalation. Withdrawal symptoms include craving, lacrimation, diarrhoea and vomiting, and abdominal pain.

Amphetamines Chronic ingestion may present like paranoid schizophrenia. Depression, anxiety or fatigue are common.

Ecstasy A synthetic amphetamine which has hallucinogenic properties. It has few addictive properties but may cause cardiac arrhythmias, DIC, liver and renal failure and cerebral haemorrhage.

Cocaine Use may cause a toxic psychosis with tactile hallucinations.

Section 3:
Problem solving and medical emergencies

16

Clinical problem solving

346

WEIGHT-LOSS

Causes ($\rightarrow$ Table 16.1) The commoner causes of weight-loss will be somewhat different in the older as compared to the younger subject. Thus, in an older patient, malignancy would be more prominent as a cause of weight-loss but AIDS less so. Social and geographical factors are also important. Assessing patients' weight in relation to their height is often useful: this can be calculated as the body mass index (BMI):

BMI = Weight (kilos)/Height (meters)^2

The normal range for BMI is 20–25 for a male, 19–24 for a female.

History • Thirst and polyuria • Mood (the patient with anorexia nervosa typically says that everything is fine and, in particular, does not complain of weight-loss) • Heat or cold intolerance • Symptoms of organ-specific disease, eg cough, sputum, breathlessness, pain • Dysphagia, vomiting, diarrhoea and steatorrhoea.

Examination • Anaemia • Clubbing • Lymphadenopathy • Skin rashes • Signs of thyrotoxicosis • Abdominal mass, especially the liver or spleen • Signs of endocarditis in any susceptible patient • Signs of iv drug abuse.

It is important to do a dipstick urine test for glucose.

Table 16.1
Causes of weight-loss

Common	Uncommon
Diabetes mellitus	Tuberculosis
Malignancy	Adrenal insufficiency
Thyrotoxicosis	Oesophageal stricture
Depression	
Anorexia nervosa	
AIDS	
Malabsorption:	
Coeliac disease	
Pancreatic insufficiency	
Blind loop syndrome	
Chronic disease with muscle wasting, eg	
rheumatoid arthritis, neurological disorders	
Chronic ill health leading to depression of	
appetite, eg uraemia, chronic obstructive pulmonary disease	

Investigations • Full blood count (FBC) and film, ESR or plasma viscosity • Biochemical profile, including liver function tests (LFTs) • Blood glucose • Thyroid function tests • CXR • Blood cultures in patients with a pyrexia:

Patients who might have AIDS must be nursed as if HIV-positive until the results of serology are known ($\rightarrow$ p 288).

FEVER

Causes Fever is commonly (but not invariably) caused by infection and infection, if present, may be bacterial, viral, protozoal, fungal, etc. Therefore the golden rules for dealing with a febrile patient are:

- Do attempt to find out the cause of the fever by means of a proper history and examination.
- Do take proper samples for culture and for serology and make sure they are properly stored.
- Do not give a febrile patient antibiotics without a diagnosis unless he/she is seriously ill.
- Do not, in adults, give an antipyretic unless the patient is extremely uncomfortable because of the fever. You will simply confuse the issue.

Remember that a low-grade pyrexia (less than 38°C) is often normal in patients who are receiving a blood transfusion or in the first 24 hours after an operation; there is no need to do anything in such cases unless the patient is unwell.

History • Ask about symptoms related to the common fevers, ie sore throat, cough, sputum, dysuria, pain in any site, diarrhoea, purulent discharge. • If history of pancreatic or biliary disease, he/she may be at risk of cholangitis • Consider a drug-induced fever • Ask about weight-loss, night sweats (a feature of lymphomas and tuberculosis), foreign travel (including aircraft stopovers), contact with infectious disease or animals, recent medication, any appearance of a rash.

Examination • How ill the patient looks, check for the presence of a rash and note other general pointers such as lymphadenopathy, clubbing, splinter haemorrhages • Check any iv infusion sites to make sure that the patient does not have phlebitis or cellulitis • Examine the mouth and throat • Examine the heart (checking especially for signs of heart failure and for new murmurs) • Examine the lungs • Check any sites of pain • Check the abdomen for masses and for tenderness in the right upper quadrant • Check for signs of deep vein thrombosis (DVT) if the patient has been bed-bound.

Investigations For significant fever (sustained temperature above 38°C): • Perform a full blood count and ESR or PV

• Take blood for LFTs and blood cultures • Do a dipstick test on the urine to check for protein and blood • Depending on history and examination, send off samples of urine, sputum, stool, throat swab, etc, for culture • Arrange a CXR • If myocardial infarction (MI) or pulmonary embolism (PE) is suspected, do an ECG • Take blood for viral and bacterial serology • Consider arterial blood gas measurements or a perfusion lung scan if the patient is at risk of pulmonary embolism • Consider requesting an abdominal ultrasound examination • Consider tests for collagen/vascular diseases, eg ANA, c-ANCA (Wegener's granulomatosis) • If there is a history of foreign travel, take blood for thick and thin film examination for malaria and consider other common tropical fevers such as typhoid, amoebic liver abscess and dengue (Table 16.2) • If the patient is known or suspected to be HIV-positive, consider unusual infections (Table 16.3).

Immunocompromised patients In neutropenic patients (white cell count less than $2 \times 10^9/l$) infections can progress rapidly and be extremely serious or even fatal; the same is true in patients with advanced chronic renal failure or (to a lesser extent) diabetes. Episodes of fever should be assessed as a matter of urgency and treated aggressively. If an immunocompromised patient becomes febrile, you should go through the routine described above but, in addition, take blood for culture from any central venous lines or Hickman lines. Make sure you inform a more senior member of your team if an immunocompromised patient becomes febrile. (Table 16.3)

Table 16.2
Causes of fever in people recently returned from abroad

Pneumonia (including Legionnaire's disease)
Dysentery (bacterial or amoebic)
Typhoid
Brucellosis
Hepatitis A or B
Malaria (central and south America, west and central Africa, India, south-east Asia)
Urinary tract infection
Dengue fever (Asia, south America, Africa)
Amoebic liver abscess
Viral haemorrhagic fevers (yellow fever, Lassa, Marburg or Ebola fever) (South America, central and west Africa)
HIV
Other viral infections

Table 16.3
Causes of fever in HIV-positive people

Pneumocystis carinii pneumonia
Bacterial pneumonia, including *Haemophilus influenzae* and
  Pseudomonas
Tuberculosis
Atypical mycobacteria
Cryptococcal pneumonia or meningitis
Toxoplasmosis (intracranial mass lesion)
Cytomegalovirus infection, eg GI tract
Cryptosporidiosis (leading to diarrhoea)
Herpes simplex infection
Hepatitis
Tumours, eg non-Hodgkin's lymphoma

Management box
▶ If the patient is well and the fever is only mild (less than 38ºC)
   it is wise not to treat until a firm diagnosis has been made. If
   the patient is poorly or the temperature is higher than 38ºC,
   treatment should be based on the most likely clinical
   diagnosis. The British National Formulary (BNF) gives
   guidance on the use of antibiotics in specific circumstances;
   a summary of the recommendations is given on p 577. You
   should also check with your local hospital formulary, which
   might make slightly different recommendations from those in
   the BNF.

JAUNDICE AND ABNORMAL LIVER FUNCTION TESTS

Jaundice can be conveniently divided into haemolytic, hepatic or
obstructive causes, based largely on LFTs (Fig. 16.1). Mild
abnormalities of LFTs (without jaundice) are very common
(Table 16.4).

Causes   The common causes of jaundice in adults are: • Viral
hepatitis (A, B, C, etc) • Alcoholic hepatitis • Other viral
infections (Epstein-Barr or CMV) • Biliary obstruction, due
either to gallstones or to malignancy • Drug-induced jaundice
(either hepatitic or cholestatic) • Multiple hepatic metastases
• Cirrhosis (late stage).

Very sick patients, especially those with septicaemia, may also
become jaundiced, as may patients with congestive heart failure
(rarely). Jaundice in a patient who is otherwise reasonably well
should make you think of inherited conditions such as Gilbert's
and Crigler-Najjar's syndrome.

Table 16.4
Common causes of asymptomatic abnormal LFTs

Bilirubin	ALT	Gamma GT
Gilbert's syndrome (bilirubin alone elevated; worse with fasting)	Obesity	Isolated elevation: drugs, alcohol
Haemolysis	Diabetes	Elevated with ↑ alkaline phosphatase: biliary disease
	Drugs	
	Chronic viral hepatitis	

History • First symptom to appear before the jaundice: 'flu-like illness will often precede viral hepatitis; biliary colic suggests a stone in the cystic or common bile duct; rigors suggest biliary obstruction; itching suggests biliary obstruction or cholestasis; several months of malaise and anorexia suggest a carcinoma of the pancreas • Duration of the jaundice • Have there been pale stools or dark urine • Alcohol history in detail (including previous drinking) • Contact with infectious disease in family and friends • Foreign travel • Tattoos • Drug history, especially phenytoin, rifampicin, methyldopa, oral testosterone • Abdominal pain • Weight-loss • Recent blood transfusion • Homosexual behaviour in men (a cause of hepatitis B) • Drug abuse, especially by injection.

Physical examination • Signs of chronic liver disease: spider naevi, clubbing, Dupuytren's contracture, testicular atrophy, palmar erythema • Evidence of hepatomegaly: nodularity of the liver, pain and tenderness in the abdomen, splenomegaly, ascites.

Contrary to traditional teaching, the liver can be enlarged in a patient with cirrhosis, especially if there is associated alcoholic hepatitis or fatty infiltration. Another clinical myth is that painless jaundice is always due to malignancy. It is quite possible for obstruction secondary to gallstones to produce painless jaundice.

Also look for signs which will help to assess the degree of liver dysfunction, eg extent of any spontaneous bruising. Hepatic encephalopathy should be tested for by checking for the presence of a flapping tremor; another useful test is to ask the patient to copy a five-pointed star.

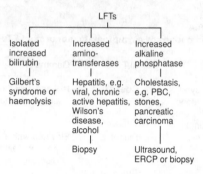

Fig. 16.1 Scheme for the differential diagnosis of jaundice

Investigations • Urinary urobilinogen (haemolysis) and bilirubin (hepatitis and obstruction) • LFTs (Fig. 16.1) • Viral hepatitis serology • Glandular fever screening test • FBC • Coagulation screen • If there is a possibility of obstruction, cirrhosis or metastases, ask for an ultrasound scan of the liver • If there is a possibility of autoimmune disease or chronic liver disease, send blood for anti-nuclear factor and antibodies against smooth muscle and mitochondria • If you are considering haemolysis, ask for haptoglobin, a blood film and a Coombs' test.

Patients with jaundice should *always* be assumed to represent a high risk for transmission of hepatitis and all specimens from these patients should be labelled as 'high risk'.

Management box

▶ Will depend on the cause. Carefully observe for evidence of hepatic decompensation and encephalopathy (Grades of hepatic coma → page 443). Regular checks on clotting status and blood count. If evidence of decompensation, treatment should include:
  – a high-carbohydrate, low-protein, very low-salt diet
  – large doses of thiamine
  – intravenous vitamin K if there is a clotting abnormality
  – regular cultures of blood, urine, etc, and aggressive treatment of any infection
  – oral lactulose and neomycin
  – avoidance of sedatives.

See Hepatology (Chapter 6) for management of specific conditions.

CHEST PAIN

Chest pain is a common symptom, the cause of which may be serious. The most important features of the pain, so far as making a diagnosis is concerned, are:

- What type of pain is it? Patients are not always good at describing pain so it is worth offering the patient a list of choices, eg burning, stabbing, crushing, pulling
- Where is the pain and is it localized or more diffuse?
- Does the pain radiate to a distant site?
- Is the pain affected by breathing or movement?
- Are there any associated symptoms such as shortness of breath, nausea or faintness?

Beware of the patient who says he/she has a 'sharp-pain'. Patients often describe a pain as 'sharp' when they mean that it is severe.

Serious causes

The commonest serious causes of chest pain are angina, MI, PE, pericarditis, pleurisy, pneumothorax, aortic dissection and malignant infiltration. Acute pancreatitis and cholecystitis should also be considered.

Angina

History: • Usually a heavy or crushing pain in the centre of the chest radiating to one or both arms (especially the left), the neck or the jaw • It is sometimes described as sharp and is usually brought on by exertion or emotion; pain which occurs irrespective of exercise is less likely to be angina • Left-sided pain alone, especially if localized to a small area under the left breast (without radiation), is usually not angina • Relief by glyceryl trinitrate (GTN) supports a diagnosis of angina but may also occur if the pain is due to oesophageal spasm • Relief by antacids, unfortunately, does not exclude a cardiac cause for the pain.

Myocardial infarction (MI)

History: • This pain is like that of angina but is said to be more severe and is often accompanied by sweating, faintness, shortness of breath or nausea • Occasionally patients feel that death is imminent • Cardiac pain lasting for more than 15 minutes is likely to be due to infarction rather than angina; in practice, however, the distinction is often impossible.

Examination: This may be normal but look especially for: • pallor, sweating, degree of distress • tachycardia • hypotension • chest wall tenderness (usually mild if it is cardiac pain) • gallop rhythm • signs of pulmonary oedema • pericardial friction rub (occasionally).

Investigations: • ECG, indeed, you must request an ECG in anyone who might have ischaemic cardiac pain even if you think other diagnoses are more likely • ECG done during pain is particularly helpful (Figs 17.3–17.11 (→ pp 422–423, 426–431)) • FBC • U&E • Glucose and cardiac enzymes • Cardiac enzymes at 12 and 24 hours after the onset of the chest pain.

Remember in the early stages of an MI the ECG may be normal.

Management box

▸ If you think that an MI is very probable or strongly possible, you should arrange urgent transfer to a coronary care unit (CCU).

▸ Give analgesia (usually diamorphine, 5 mg iv with pro-chlorperazine 12.5 mg), oxygen and (if breathless) intravenous furosemide (frusemide) (40 mg) before transfer and make sure that intravenous cannula is in place before leaving. If no bed is available on the CCU, arrange bedside cardiac monitor and ask the nursing staff to check pulse and blood pressure (BP) every half hour. Treatment with a thrombolytic agent or with inotropic drugs (dobutamine, adrenaline (epinephrine)) may need to be considered: for this and other reasons you should inform the duty medical registrar (→ p 419). If the diagnosis of MI is definite or highly probable, thrombolysis should be given as soon as possible.

If a patient complains of angina-type pain which has been coming on more frequently, lasting longer and provoked by lesser degrees of exertion, but the initial ECG is normal, the diagnosis may be unstable angina; this can be diagnosed more confidently in someone with a long history of stable angina (months or years). The treatment for unstable angina consists of:

- bed rest with cardiac monitoring
- β-blockade (unless contraindicated)
- aspirin (unless contraindicated)
- nitrates (buccal or intravenous)
- sc low molecular weight heparin (eg enoxaparin 1 mg/kg every 12 hours) or intravenous heparin.

Serial ECGs (at 2, 24 and 48 hours) and cardiac enzymes tests (at admission and at 12 and 24 hours after the onset of pain) should be requested to exclude an MI.

Unstable angina carries a high risk of progression to MI. If the pain cannot be controlled easily with simple treatment or in a patient who fails to settle quickly and who might be a candidate for coronary artery surgery or angioplasty, you should discuss the management with a cardiologist.

Pulmonary embolism (PE)

→ Chapter 4, p 93–94, Chapter 17, p 437. If a patient with a suspected PE is hypotensive or shocked, you are faced with a grave emergency → p 467; contact your SHO or registrar immediately.

Pericarditis

Clinical features: • The pain resembles angina but is more definitely made worse by breathing and may be affected by change of position, eg sitting forward • There is often a tachycardia and there may also be a pericardial friction rub.

Examination: • ECG may show sinus tachycardia and widespread ST segment elevation.

> **Management box**
> ▶ Treatment is with analgesics. Non-steroidal anti-inflammatory drugs (NSAIDs) such as naproxen or indometacin are often effective. Ask the nursing staff to carry out regular observations of pulse and BP. Some patients with pericarditis will develop a pericardial effusion or tamponade.

Pleurisy

Clinical features: • This is rare nowadays as an isolated phenomenon, but often accompanies lobar pneumonia • There is usually a history of several hours to several days of malaise, cough, fever, shortness of breath and pleuritic-type chest pain (ie localized and markedly exacerbated by deep breathing or coughing) • The onset may be surprisingly sudden (mimicking a PE) • Ask about recent foreign travel: Legionnaire's disease is common in some favourite holiday spots and can cause lobar pneumonia.

Examination: • Physical examination may reveal fever, reduced chest movement on the affected side, tachycardia and an area of dullness with crackles or a pleural friction rub • CXR typically shows an area of dense, uniform opacification corresponding to one or more lobes.

> **Management box**
> ▶ Treatment consists of antibiotics, analgesia, rehydration and oxygen and physiotherapy as required.

Pneumothorax

Clinical features: • This occurs in two major groups of patients: firstly the young, fit, asthenic person and secondly the middle-aged or elderly person with chronic obstructive pulmonary disease, chiefly emphysema • Pneumothorax may also complicate acute asthma • The pain usually begins very abruptly and may be felt over an area of the chest wall or over the shoulder • The patient may say that 'something seemed to snap and then the pain and shortness of breath suddenly began' • The pain is usually pleuritic • Dyspnoea can vary from mild to very severe depending on the size of the pneumothorax and whether there is tension within it or not • Physical signs are often absent but if the pneumothorax is large there may be hyperresonance on the affected side, together with reduced breath sounds • In the case of a tension pneumothorax the patient is often very breathless, pale and cyanosed and the trachea may be displaced to the opposite side; in such a case more senior help should be sought urgently.

Investigations: • CXRs taken in inspiration (the standard view) and expiration (to show evidence of a small pneumothorax) • Blood gas analysis is helpful if the patient is very symptomatic.

Management box
→ Chapter 17, p 435 and Chapter 18, p 490.

Aortic dissection This condition is uncommon but, when it occurs, has a high mortality. The pain may mimic that of MI or it may begin in, or radiate to, the interscapular area. Patients often describe the pain as tearing or pulling in nature and say that it gets relentlessly worse over an hour or two after its onset. Physical signs are often absent but you should look for inequality of brachial and radial pulses between the two sides, inequality of BP readings between the two arms and evidence of an aortic diastolic murmur.

Investigations: • ECG may be normal or may show changes suggesting acute MI • Most helpful routine investigation is CXR, which typically shows widening of the mediastinal shadow • If CXR is unhelpful, next investigation of choice is an urgent CT scan of the chest or transoesophageal echocardiogram.

Management box
▸ Should begin with a phone call to your SHO or registrar. The patient should be given adequate analgesia (usually diamorphine) and oxygen. BP must be lowered to minimize the risk of extension of the dissection and agitated patients should be given sedation. BP should be lowered to a level below 120 mmHg systolic using intravenous labetalol, hydralazine or nitroprusside, if necessary. Urgent investigation is needed to

confirm the diagnosis and to assess the extent of the dissection: CT scanning of the chest and/or transoesophageal echo-cardiography are the investigations of choice. If a dissection is suspected, your SHO or registrar should ring the on-call team at the nearest cardiac surgical unit. Anticoagulants and thrombo-lytic agents are absolutely contraindicated.

Malignant infiltration of the chest wall and ribs

Clinical features: • Pain from this cause is usually of longer duration • Often has a boring or deep aching quality, keeps the patient awake at night and is affected to a varying degree by respiration • Most likely malignancies to produce this disorder are carcinomas of the bronchus, breast or prostate, myeloma and mesothelioma.

Examination: • May reveal local chest-wall tenderness or signs of a pleural effusion • May also be evidence of disease elsewhere such as clubbing, lymphadenopathy or an enlarged liver • Remember to examine the breasts in women.

Investigations: • Will vary according to the probable under-lying cause but likely to include blood count • ESR • LFTs • Rib X-rays • Bone scan • Aspiration of any associated pleural effusion.

Acute pancreatitis

Clinical features: • Pain of pancreatitis is typically felt in the epigastrium or upper abdomen but it may radiate to the inter-scapular area • Nausea and vomiting are usually present.

Examination: • There is usually abdominal tenderness • Guarding and/or rigidity of the abdomen may be present • Patient may be shocked.

Investigations: • Serum amylase and/or lipase the key investi-gations • Although amylase may be raised in a variety of other disorders such as perforated peptic ulcer or cholecystitis, a value more than 4 times the upper limit of the reference range (ie above 400 iu/l) is virtually diagnostic of acute pancreatitis • FBC • U&E • Glucose • Serum calcium (remember hypocalcaemia is a complication of acute pancreatitis) • LFTs • Clotting screen and 'group and save' • Plain X-rays of the abdomen may be needed to exclude other causes of the patient's symptoms • US of the abdomen will also be required at some stage and CT or MRI scanning may also be used.

Management box
▶ The patient should be nil by mouth and should receive iv fluids, usually saline and a plasma expander such as Haemaccel. Nasogastric suction may be needed. Adequate analgesia (using pethidine or buprenorphine, not morphine) should be given. Peritoneal lavage and protease inhibitors are, in general, NOT necessary.

Cholecystitis

Clinical features: • Pain is typically felt in the right upper quadrant but may radiate to the right shoulder or to other parts of the chest.

Examination: • There is often guarding and/or rigidity in the right upper quadrant • Acute tenderness in the right subcostal area on inspiration (Murphy's sign) may be present.

Management box
▶ Ask for a surgical opinion. iv fluids may be necessary. It is best, if at all possible, to withhold analgesics until the surgical team have seen the patient but you may give anti-emetics if needed.

Less serious causes

Less serious causes of chest pain include reflux oesophagitis or gastritis, oesophageal spasm, benign chest-wall pain and herpes zoster.

Reflux oesophagitis or gastritis

Clinical features: • Pain does not usually radiate to the arms (though it may to the back) • Bears no relation to exercise and typically has a burning or squeezing quality • There may be a history of previous indigestion • The pain may, in the past, have been brought on by bending, stooping or lying flat.

Examination: • This is usually negative though there may be some tenderness in the epigastrium.

Management box
▶ Treatment is with antacids, H_2 receptor antagonists or proton pump inhibitors (omeprazole, lanzoprazole, etc) and reassurance.

Oesophageal spasm

Clinical features: • This can sound very like angina but does not radiate to the arms and is not exercise-related • May be relieved by nitrates or calcium antagonists • Differentiation from cardiac pain can sometimes be made by considering other risk-factors (age, family history, smoking history, gender) • In some cases it requires an exercise test or other cardiac investigations.

Management box
▶ Treatment is by reassurance and the use of nitrates, calcium antagonists, H_2-receptor antagonists or motility agents such as metoclopramide.

Benign chest-wall pain

Clinical features: • May result from musculoskeletal strain and typically gives rise to pain following exertion which is localized to a small area of the chest and is accompanied by chest-wall tenderness • Tietze's syndrome is a particular form of chest-wall pain in which the patient feels sudden, intense pain in a very small area of the chest wall which remits after 2–3 seconds. The cause is unknown.

Herpes zoster → Chapter 13, p 321

HAEMOPTYSIS

Causes (→ Table 16.5)

History • First make sure that the patient is actually describing haemoptysis and not haematemesis: try to see a specimen of sputum if possible • Haemoptysis is usually bright red and may be frothy, whereas haematemesis is more likely to be granular

---

Table 16.5
Causes of haemoptysis (in order of frequency)

Small haemoptysis
   PE
   Pneumonia
   Carcinoma of the lung
   Pulmonary oedema
   ENT causes (nose or pharynx)
Large haemoptysis
   Bronchial carcinoma
   PE
   Bronchiectasis
   TB
   Severe thrombocytopaenia
   Lung cavity (eg abscess, mycetoma)

and reddish-brown • Ask about chest pain, breathlessness, purulent sputum, weight-loss, past history of chest disease and heart disease.

Examination • Look at the patient generally for evidence of anaemia, finger clubbing, lymphadenopathy and cachexia • Examine the heart and chest fully, looking for asymmetry of chest movement, deviation of the trachea, cardiac murmurs, signs of pulmonary oedema and signs of lobar consolidation. Listen for a pleural friction rub • Examine the abdomen for hepatomegaly (carcinoma or TB) • Examine the legs for signs of a DVT.

Investigations • Key investigation is a CXR (postero-anterior and lateral) • Sputum culture (1 specimen), cytology (3 specimens) and, where appropriate, tubercle bacilli • Consider an FBC, LFTs and ECG • The patient is likely to need a bronchoscopy at some stage.

> *Management box*
> ▶ According to the underlying cause.

BREATHLESSNESS

It is useful to subdivide causes of breathlessness into acute (coming on within minutes or hours) and subacute or chronic (coming on over days or weeks) (→ Tables 16.6 and 16.7).

First steps • If you are telephoned by a ward to tell you that a patient is breathless, try to find out: • Over what length

Table 16.6
Causes of acute dyspnoea (in order of frequency)

Pulmonary oedema
   Left ventricular failure
   Mitral valve disease
Bronchopneumonia (including exacerbations of chronic
   bronchitis)
Asthma
Pulmonary embolism
Lobar pneumonia (especially pneumococcal)
Pneumothorax
Anaphylaxis
Inhalation of foreign body
Extrinsic allergic alveolitis
Psychogenic

Table 16.7
Causes of subacute dyspnoea (in order of frequency)

Chronic bronchitis
Pulmonary oedema
    Left ventricular failure
    Mitral valve disease
Asthma
Bronchopneumonia
Anaemia
Lobar pneumonia
Pleural effusion
Carcinoma of the lung
Recurrent pulmonary embolism
Pericardial effusion
Fibrosing alveolitis

of time the dyspnoea has come on • How ill the patient is (eg is there any clouding of consciousness?) • Bedside observations, ie pulse, BP, temperature and respiratory rate • Associated symptoms such as chest pain, cough, sputum, wheezing, haemoptysis.

History • How severe the dyspnoea is, ie whether it occurs at rest as well as on exertion • Time-scale • Whether the problem is worse at night (as with asthma) • Associated symptoms as above • Any previous history of chest disease (and what was the patient's exercise-tolerance when well) • Any risk factors for pulmonary embolism ($\rightarrow$ Chapter 4, p 93) • In audible wheeze, ask about a past history of asthma, whether there are pets at home, any history of occupational exposure to allergens, review the drug history with particular reference to β-blockers and NSAIDs • In lobar pneumonia, if the patient has a fever and localized, pleuritic chest pain, ask about foreign travel and contact with infectious disease.

Examination • Perform a full cardiovascular and respiratory examination, including pulse rate, respiratory rate and BP • Important points to remember: • A person can be hypoxic without being cyanosed • Tachypnoea is an important physical sign, especially in the elderly, where it may be the first sign of bronchopneumonia (before there is any fever) • In a patient with asthma: pallor, exhaustion, tachycardia (greater than 120 beats/min), inability to speak more than one or two words, quiet breath sounds are all signs of *severe asthma* ($\rightarrow$ p 434) • In cases of PE, a pleural rub is the exception rather than the rule; it is more useful to check for a raised JVP and a gallop rhythm • Many cases of PE have no physical signs.

Investigations

Acute dyspnoea: • Hb and white cell count • CXR (if you suspect a pneumothorax, ask for both an inspiratory and an expiratory film) • ECG (for suspected MI, PE or heart failure).

More than mild dyspnoea: • Check ABG • an arterial PO_2 of less than 8 kPa (60 mmHg) indicates severe hypoxaemia • Consult your SHO or registrar.

Febrile patients: • Blood and sputum cultures should be performed.

Suspected PE: • Check D-dimers: a positive result carries no diagnostic value but a negative result makes a PE unlikely • Check arterial blood gases: there may be mild hypoxaemia with relatively normal oxygen saturation • Arrange ventilation/perfusion lung scan as soon as possible • Alternatives would be a spiral CT scan, MRI scan or a pulmonary angiogram.

Subacute dyspnoea • Hb and white cell count • CXR • ECG • Sputum culture • Sputum for cytology (if a carcinoma is suspected) • ABG at rest and after exercise • In suspected asthma, measurements of peak expiratory flow rate (PEFR) 8-hourly, usually before and after bronchodilators.

Asthma: • Consider an eosinophil count, IgE and radio allergosorbent test (RAST) to look for specific allergens.

Suspected extrinsic allergic alveolitis: • Send blood for avian precipitins and precipitins against aspergillus and other fungi.

Consider requesting spirometry or fuller lung function tests, with transfer factor.

Management box

Acute dyspnoea

Pulmonary oedema: → Chapter 17 p 432.

Bronchopneumonia (eg exacerbation of chronic bronchitis):

▶ Nebulized salbutamol, 2.5–5 mg every 4 to 6 hours, depending on the severity of the condition.

▶ Oxygen 24% (2 l/min) if there is a previous history of chronic obstructive airways disease, otherwise 40% (10 l/min). Aim to keep the patient's oxygen saturation (by pulse oximeter) above 90% but **do regular measurements of arterial blood gases** to check for CO_2 retention.

▶ Having taken blood and sputum cultures, give antibiotic in the form of amoxicillin, 500 mg every 8 hours. If the patient is allergic to penicillin, give trimethoprim, 200 mg every 12 hours or clarithromycin (oral dose: 250 mg every 12 hours; iv dose: 500 mg every 12 hours, given into a large vein).

→

▶ If the patient has a lot of tenacious sputum, arrange chest physiotherapy.
▶ If the patient is very breathless despite nebulized salbutamol, add nebulized ipratropium bromide (Atrovent), 250–500 µg four times daily.
▶ Consider an oral theophylline or, if the patient is very breathless despite nebulized bronchodilators, aminophylline by iv infusion: first give 5 mg per kg as an iv injection over *20 minutes*. Dilute aminophylline 500 mg in 500 ml of 5% glucose or 0.9% saline. The rate of infusion will depend on whether the patient has been taking an oral theophylline before admission or not, on co-existing medical conditions and on his/her size. *If the patient is relatively well otherwise and has not been taking an oral theophylline at home*, give iv aminophylline as follows:

Small patient   600–1000 ml/24 hours
Medium-sized patient   900–1500 ml/24 hours
Large patient   1100–2000 ml/24 hours

If the patient has been taking an oral theophylline at home, take blood for measurement of theophylline level, then give iv aminophylline at the above rate but without the initial loading dose. If the patient is over 55, has heart failure or liver disease or is taking drugs which potentiate the actions of aminophylline such as erythromycin, ciprofloxacin or oral contraceptives, the rate of aminophylline infusion should be half that given above.
▶ If the patient can swallow, start oral prednisolone, 40–60 mg once daily in the morning. If he/she cannot swallow, give hydro-cortisone, 100 mg iv followed by a second dose 6 hours later.

Pulmonary embolism (PE): → Chapter 17, p 437.

Asthma: The management of asthma is discussed more fully on pages 434–435. As a general rule, patients who are ill enough to need admission for their asthma should be treated aggressively with nebulized or iv bronchodilators and with steroids.

Lobar pneumonia: In early pneumococcal pneumonia, the most useful investigation for identifying the organism is blood culture.
▶ Give antibiotics in the form of benzylpenicillin 1.2 g 6 hourly iv or clarithromycin, 500 mg 12 hourly iv given into a large vein; give clarithromycin if the patient is penicillin-allergic. If the pneumonia is severe give clarithromycin as above, plus cefuroxime, 750 mg-1.5 g iv 6-hourly or cefotaxime, 2 g iv 12-hourly. If an 'atypical' pneumonia (*Mycoplasma* or *Legionella*) is possible, take blood for viral studies (which usually includes these organisms) or for specific *Mycoplasma* and *Legionella* serology and check urinary *Legionella* antigen, then start the clarithromycin.
▶ If the patient is known to have AIDS or if this is a strong possibility, the pneumonia could be due to *Pneumocystis carinii*. →

This will require treatment with high-dose cotrimoxazole, possibly combined with dapsone. Another possible cause would be tuberculosis or opportunistic pathogens: induced sputum or bronchoscopy may be required. Consult your SHO or registrar.

▶ Give analgesia as required if there is pleuritic pain. Do not be afraid to use opiates if these appear necessary.

▶ If the PaO_2 is less than 10 kPa (75 mmHg) give oxygen, 40% (10 l/min) unless there is a previous history of chronic obstructive airways disease, in which case you should give 24% (2 l/min).

Pneumothorax: If the pneumothorax is small (just a rim of air around the lung) and the patient is not significantly breathless, no treatment is required other than analgesia and observation. If the pneumothorax is larger or the patient is very breathless then aspiration or formal drainage will be needed (→ p 488).

If you think the patient has a tension pneumothorax (indicated by severe dyspnoea and an obvious shift of the mediastinum to one side), ask your SHO or registrar for urgent help: a large-bore (18-gauge) needle should be inserted into the second intercostal space in the mid-clavicular line. If your SHO/registrar cannot come immediately you should put the needle in yourself. Once the tension has been relieved the patient will need a chest drain.

Psychogenic dyspnoea: Be wary of making this diagnosis unless the patient is known to be hysterical or very neurotic or there is a past history of a similar episode. In severe cases the patient will breathe deeply and rapidly and may complain of peri-oral tingling or paraesthesiae in the hands. As the condition progresses there may be carpopedal spasm or even loss of consciousness. Treatment is by encouraging patients to re-breathe their own expired air using a large paper bag. Once the acute attack is over a psychiatric assessment and/or sedative drugs may be indicated.

Management box

Subacute or chronic dyspnoea

▶ **Chronic bronchitis**: In mild cases the patient may require nothing more than a bronchodilator inhaler for intermittent use. Most older people, however, are not very good at using a traditional metered-dose inhaler and do better with a breath-actuated inhaler (Ventolin Easi-Breathe, Aerolin Auto-haler) or a dry powder inhaler (Ventolin Rotahaler or Bricanyl Turbo-haler). In more severe cases, especially where reversible airways obstruction can be demonstrated on spirometry, the patient may benefit from a steroid inhaler such as Aero-Bec, Becotide Rota-haler, Pulmicort Turbo-haler or (if the patient prefers) Becotide or Becloforte inhaler. An oral theophylline (eg Uniphyllin, →

Phyllocontin Continus, Slo-Phyllin, etc.) is often useful, particularly where nocturnal breathlessness is a problem.

Treatment of patients taking oral theophyllines should be monitored by measurements of plasma theophylline concentrations. The level should be maintained at 10–20 mg/l (55–110 µmol/l).

▶ **Left ventricular failure (LVF)** Once the acute episode is over the patient may be adequately treated with a small dose of diuretic, eg furosemide (frusemide), 40 mg once or twice daily; this is often combined with a potassium-sparing diuretic in a compound tablet such as Frumil, Frusene or Burinex A. If, however, the dose of diuretic required is more than 80 mg of furosemide (frusemide) per day (2 mg bumetanide per day) it is often appropriate to treat the patient with an ACE inhibitor (→ p 536). After starting an ACE inhibitor the patient's U&E should be checked every second or third day. Because ACE inhibitors cause potassium retention there is usually no need to give a potassium-sparing diuretic: furosemide (frusemide) (or bumetanide) alone should be used.

▶ **Asthma** (→ also p 363): Once the patient is recovering to a point where he/she is almost ready to come off nebulized bronchodilators (usually the peak flow rate will be above 300 l/min), start inhaled steroids and an inhaled β_2-adrenergic agonist. Check that the patient is able to use his/her inhalers properly. Talk to the patient about how to reduce/stop oral steroids and about measuring his/her own peak flow rates at home. Some patients may require long-acting β_2 agonists (eg salmeterol) or an oral theophylline.

▶ **Pleural effusion**: Symptomatic relief can often be achieved by aspirating a pleural effusion. You should observe the procedure on one or two occasions before doing it yourself and should be supervised during your first few attempts (→ p 488).

▶ **Pericardial effusion**: If moderately large or very large this may require aspiration, which must be done by a senior person, so consult your SHO or registrar.

ABDOMINAL PAIN

Those patients who are admitted as an emergency because of abdominal pain will usually come under the care of a surgical team. However, you should be aware of the problem of abdominal pain in 'medical' patients, either as an accompaniment to the admission diagnosis or occurring during a stay on a medical ward.

Causes (→ Tables 16.8, 16.9 and 16.10) • A word of caution: a patient with a 'medical' condition and abdominal pain

Table 16.8
Common causes of abdominal pain accompanying an acute medical diagnosis

Gastroenteritis
Food poisoning
Peptic ulcer
Pancreatitis (in a patient admitted with a fever of unknown cause or with jaundice)
Inflammatory bowel disease (IBD) (especially Crohn's disease)
Myocardial infarction
Basal pneumonia (may simulate gallbladder disease)
Mesenteric embolism (especially in a patient with AF, a recent MI or severe heart failure)
Hepatitis or hepatic congestion
Ketoacidosis
Addison's disease
Acute intermittent prophyria
Lead poisoning

Table 16.9
Causes of abdominal pain arising de novo in medical in-patients

Surgical acute abdomen (Table 16.10)
Reflux oesophagitis
Gastritis
Constipation
Urinary tract infection (UTI)
Irritable bowel syndrome (IBS)

Table 16.10
Surgical causes of acute abdominal pain

Cholecystitis
Biliary colic
Perforated viscus
Intestinal obstruction
Appendicitis
Ruptured aortic aneurysm
Mesenteric infarction
Diverticulitis
Pancreatitis
Ectopic pregnancy

is quite entitled to have more than one diagnosis, so do not be too ready to attribute the pain to the medical disorder.

Clinical assessment • You will obviously need to take a proper history and carry out an appropriate examination. Try to answer the following questions specifically: • Is the patient shocked? • Is there any evidence of peritonism? • If you are considering urinary tract infection (UTI), make sure that the urine is dip-stick tested as soon as possible, then send a midstream specimen of urine (MSSU) to the laboratory.

Investigations • If the cause of the pain appears potentially serious, ask for an FBC and U&E • If there is a possibility of pancreatitis, ask for a serum amylase – a value greater than 4 times the upper limit of the reference range (ie above 400 iu/l) is virtually diagnostic of acute pancreatitis • If the patient has known heart disease or the pain might be due to cardiac causes

---

Management box

This will depend on the cause, but certain general principles apply.

▶ Keep the patient nil by mouth.
▶ Ask the nurses to perform half-hourly pulse and BP.
▶ If the patient is shocked, take blood for a coagulation screen and for 'group and save' and resuscitate with iv fluids (usually a colloid such as Haemaccel or Gelofusin).
▶ If the patient is systemically ill, is shocked or has signs of peritonism, involve your SHO or registrar at an early stage. You may also need an urgent surgical opinion.
▶ If the patient has pancreatitis he/she should be nil by mouth and should receive iv fluids, usually saline and a plasm expander such as Haemaccel. Nasogastric suction may be needed. Adequate analgesia (using pethidine or buprenorphine, not morphine) should be given. Peritoneal lavage and protease inhibitors such as Trasylol are, in general, NOT necessary. In all but the mildest cases, be sure to inform your SHO or registrar (Pancreatitis → p 441).
▶ Less serious causes of abdominal pain can be managed symptomatically. The patient who has gastritis or a peptic ulcer which is associated with *Helicobacter pylori* infection should be treated with a 'triple therapy' eradication regime for 7 days; this consists of omeprazole 40 mg daily plus 2 antibiotics, eg clarithromycin, 250 mg bd plus metronidazole 400 mg bd or amoxicillin 1 mg bd plus clarithromycin 500 mg bd or amoxicillin 500 mg tid plus metronidazole 400 mg tid. Note that the antibiotic doses used vary according to the combinations in which they are included.

or the patient might have to go to theatre or the patient is shocked, arrange an urgent ECG • If the patient is shocked or has evidence of peritonism, your SHO or registrar needs to be informed immediately • In such a case, arrange an X-ray of the chest (erect) and of the abdomen (erect and supine).

SWALLOWING DIFFICULTIES

Difficulty in swallowing is commonly associated with a sore throat due to an upper respiratory tract infection. If dysphagia rather than sore throat is the main symptom, however, it needs to be taken seriously as many of the causes are malignant. If the complaint is of a lump in the throat not associated with eating then the most likely cause is either a goitre or globus hystericus.

Causes (Table 16.11)

History As well as the dysphagia itself, you should ask about other associated symptoms such as weight-loss, dyspepsia and/or reflux, hoarseness. More specifically: • If the dysphagia is worse for solids than for liquids a mechanical obstruction is likely. If, however, the problem is as bad or worse with liquids as with solids, a motility disorder is more likely (eg achalasia, diabetic neuropathy) • If it is difficult to perform the swallowing movement (and especially if the patient coughs on swallowing), bulbar or pseudobulbar palsy should come high on your list • If the dysphagia is constant you are probably dealing with a malignant

---

Table 16.11
Causes of dysphagia (in order of frequency)

Reflux oesophagitis
Local oropharyngeal problems e.g. poorly fitting dentures, candidiasis
Cerebrovascular disease (bulbar or pseudobulbar palsy)
Peptic stricture secondary to long-standing reflux
Carcinoma of the oesophagus, stomach or larynx
Extrinsic compression (carcinoma of bronchus, lymphadenopathy, retrosternal goitre, etc)
Psychiatric (globus hystericus)
Neuromuscular disorders, eg Guillain-Barré syndrome, Parkinson's disease, diabetic neuropathy, multiple sclerosis, myasthenia gravis, motor neurone disease, chronic alcoholism, achalasia, Huntington's chorea

stricture, a progressive neurological disorder or a CVA, especially one involving the brain stem.

Examination This is often normal but it is nevertheless useful to check for the following: • Evidence of wasting • Stridor • Hoarseness of the voice (eg Ca larynx, recurrent laryngeal nerve palsy with Ca bronchus) • Posture when eating/drinking • Physical stimulation of the swallow reflex • 'Wet' voice: food debris or liquid from the mouth falling into an unprotected airway will do this because it will remain on the vocal cords • Nature of the cough ('bovine', etc) • Lymphadenopathy • Goitre or other mass in the neck • Asymmetrical chest movement • Other evidence of malignancy such as an enlarged liver or a mass in the epigastrium.

Investigations • Routine blood tests (FBC, U&E and LFTs) • Plain CXR is often helpful (for example, in showing a large shadow behind the heart in someone with a hiatus hernia) • More specific investigations would consist of a barium swallow and/or upper GI endoscopy with biopsy • In a few cases oesophageal manometry (motility disorders), video-fluoroscopy, 24-hour pH monitoring (reflux) or radionuclide gastric emptying studies (motility or neuromuscular disorders) will be needed • In cases of difficult dysphagia, especially those due to neuromuscular disorders, advice from, and involvement of, a speech therapist is often invaluable • Close liaison with a dietitian regarding nutrition is also important, as is full cooperation from the patient's carers.

Management box

This will obviously depend on the diagnosis:

▶ **Benign peptic strictures** These can usually be treated by endoscopic dilatation. If there is associated oesophagitis this is treated with a proton pump inhibitor (omeprazole, lanzoprazole, etc), together with advice about losing weight, raising the head of the bed, etc.

▶ **Extrinsic compression** This requires surgical treatment or, if the lesion is inoperable, radiotherapy.

▶ **Carcinoma of the oesophagus or stomach** These should be treated by surgical excision if this is possible. Very often, however, excision is not possible but useful palliation can be achieved either by passing a tube through the lesion or by burning away part of the tumour by means of an endoscopic laser.

▶ **Neuromuscular disorders** These require a variety of approaches, including long-term intragastric tube feeding (see below).

→

▶ **Muscular incoordination or a peripheral neuropathy** Alteration of food textures is often useful. A motility agent such as domperidone may be effective.
▶ **Bulbar or pseudobulbar palsy** The patient should be assessed by a doctor experienced in rehabilitation and by a speech therapist.
▶ **Total inability to swallow** It may be necessary to introduce a fine-bore nasogastric tube so as to provide water and nutrients. Remember that rehabilitation of the swallow can take place while nasogastric feeding is being carried out. In cases of persistent, severe dysphagia or aphagia a feeding tube can be introduced into the stomach through a small abdominal incision under endoscopic control, a so-called percutaneous endoscopic gastrostomy (PEG).

VOMITING

Causes • There are many possible causes of vomiting, most of which are quite common, so keep an open mind (Table 16.12).

History • Take a careful history, including associated symptoms such as diarrhoea, abdominal pain, weight-loss, headache • Ask about drugs and alcohol • In young women, ask about the date of the last menstrual period.

Table 16.12
Causes of vomiting

Gastrointestinal
  Hiatus hernia, oesophageal stricture, oesophageal carcinoma, oesophageal compression, gastritis, gastroenteritis, food poisoning, dietary indiscretion (including alcohol), gastric ulcer, pyloric stenosis, gastric volvulus, duodenal ulcer, cholecystitis, pancreatitis, intestinal obstruction, appendicitis, strangulated hernia, severe constipation*
Central nervous system (CNS) disease
  Raised intracranial pressure (ICP), meningitis, brain-stem stroke, Ménière's, disease*, labyrinthitis*
Metabolic/chemical
  Drugs (especially antibiotics, opiates, chemotherapy, digoxin, oestrogens), pregnancy, diabetic ketoacidosis, Addison's disease, uraemia, hypercalaemia*
Reflex/constitutional
  MI, any severe infection, glaucoma*

Rare

Examination This needs to include an assessment of the patient's state of hydration and a careful review of the abdomen. Do not forget the hernial orifices.

Investigations • Baseline tests will usually include an FBC and U&E • If there is abdominal pain, ask for a serum amylase • If there is a significant chance of a 'surgical' cause, discuss the case with your SHO or registrar; you may need to consider a plain X-ray of the abdomen (erect and supine) • In young women, consider a pregnancy test.

Management box

This will depend largely on the cause.

▶ It is usually possible to give an anti-emetic im or iv, such as prochlorperazine or metoclopramide.

▶ If the nausea is secondary to chemotherapy, ondansetron may be more effective.

▶ If the patient is dehydrated, rehydrate with iv, normal saline and 5% glucose ($\rightarrow$ p 517).

▶ If a 'surgical' cause is likely, keep the patient nil by mouth until seen by the surgeons.

▶ If vomiting is profuse, ask the nursing staff to pass a nasogastric tube.

HAEMATEMESIS OR MELAENA

First a few basic points about haematemesis and melaena:

- Altered food in the vomitus can resemble altered blood. Do not ask the patient a leading question such as: 'Did it look like coffee grounds?' Try to be neutral when asking about the colour of vomitus and stools.
- Patients' estimates of the volume of blood lost by haematemesis are notoriously inaccurate: try to obtain more information from a witness.
- Blood mixed with the stool can arise from bleeding in *any part* of the GI tract. Similarly, melaena may occur with both upper and lower GI tract bleeding. A history of blood per rectum (PR) is only of value for localization if the blood is bright red and liquid and there is no melaena mixed in with the blood *and* no haematemesis.
- If the patient is taking oral iron, the stools will be dark grey but they are usually firmer than melaena and have a different odour.

Causes $\rightarrow$ Tables 16.13, 16.14 and 16.15.

Table 16.13
Causes of haematemesis

Mallory-Weiss tear
Oesophagitis
Gastritis (including alcoholic)
Gastric erosions or ulcers
Duodenitis
Duodenal ulcer
Oesophageal varices
Angiodysplasia
Gastric carcinoma
Additional contributory factors:
    Steroids, NSAIDs, coagulation disorders, over-anticoagulation
    (warfarin, heparin, streptokinase)

Table 16.14
Causes of melaena

All of the conditions in Table 16.13, especially:
    Duodenal ulcer
    Gastric ulcer
    Oesophageal varices
Right-sided colonic lesions, eg angiodysplasia, carcinoma

Table 16.15
Causes of bleeding per rectum

All of the conditions in Table 16.13 and 16.14
Inflammatory bowel disease
Carcinoma
Polyps
Diverticular disease
Ischaemic colitis
Infective colitis
Fissure-in-ano
Haemorrhoids

Initial approach to the patient with GI bleeding
• Has there been a significant bleed? If the patient has lost more
  than 100 ml of blood or there has been definite haematemesis
  or definite melaena then the bleeding is significant.

Patients whose initial Hb concentration is < 10 gm/dl are also likely to require transfusion at an early stage.

- Is the patient shocked? There may be obvious signs such as pallor, cold, clammy skin, tachycardia (> 100/min) or hypotension (systolic BP < 100 mmHg): if present, these indicate major volume depletion (several litres). If there are no obvious signs of shock you should check for postural hypotension (BP lying versus sitting upright): if the systolic BP falls by more than 10 mmHg or drops to below 100 mmHg then the patient is volume-depleted.
- If there is evidence of shock or volume depletion then resuscitation must be carried out immediately: detailed history and examination can be carried out during or after resuscitation.

Resuscitation in volume-depleted patients

1. Take blood for FBC, U&E, LFTs, cross-match (whole blood, not packed red cells; order at least 4 units initially) and clotting screen.
2. Insert the largest iv cannula possible.
3. Give one or two units of plasma expander (Haemaccel or Gelofusin) as rapidly as possible, then give blood as soon as it is available.
4. Inform your SHO or registrar of the patient's existence and for assessment. He/she should inform the surgical team on call and the on-call endoscopist. A CVP line may be needed to monitor fluid replacement.
5. Arrange admission of the patient to a high-dependency area. This is especially important if the patient is aged over 60.
6. Keep the patient nil by mouth and ask the nurses to do quarter-hourly pulse and BP.
7. If the patient is aged over 40, obtain an ECG.
8. If liver disease is present, avoid sedation. Clear the bowel with magnesium sulphate mixture, 10 ml 3 times a day or an enema.
9. *Do not* give intravenous ranitidine: there are obvious theoretical attractions, but clinical trials have failed to show any benefit from such treatment in acute GI bleeding.

Further assessment

History • Try to find out as much as you can about the circumstances of the acute bleed and about associated symptoms such as nausea, vomiting, diarrhoea or abdominal pain • Ask about previous history of peptic ulcer or GI haemorrhage • Ask about previous liver disease, heart, lung or renal diseases and about alcohol intake • Review the drug history, especially in relation to steroids and NSAIDs.

Examination • If the patient is elderly or infirm or if there is a relevant history, check the cardiovascular and respiratory systems for evidence of disease • Examine the abdomen carefully • Perform a rectal examination.

> **Management box**
> Detailed → Chapter 17 p 438.

DIARRHOEA

Diarrhoea is defined as the passage of loose, semisolid or liquid stools, which are passed at a frequency greater than is usual for the patient.

Causes • (→ Table 16.16) In subjects who have recently been abroad, consider tropical diseases such as amoebiasis, cholera, shigella.

History • Ask about the timing of the diarrhoea (both onset and frequency) and about details of the stool character, ie whether it is completely liquid or semi-formed, the colour, whether the stool is greasy and offensive (as in malabsorption), presence of blood or mucus in the stool • Ask about the health of family and friends, recent eating of unusual foods, occupation, contact with known infectious disease and foreign travel • Ask about associated symptoms such as weight-loss, abdominal pain, nausea and vomiting.

Examination • Assess state of hydration (eyes, skin turgor, fall in BP from lying to standing) • Note whether the patient is

---

**Table 16.16
Causes of diarrhoea in the UK**

Food poisoning/infections
  Staphylococcus aureus, Salmonella, viruses (Norwalk, Rotavirus),
  Campylobacter, Escherichia coli, Clostridium perfringens
Inflammatory
  Ulcerative colitis, Crohn's disease, pseudomembranous colitis,
  (patients who have been on antibiotics for several days)
Drugs
  Antibiotics, laxatives, antacids, methyldopa, digoxin,
  colchicine
Miscellaneous
  Diverticular disease, malabsorption, ischaemic colitis, colonic
  neoplasm, thyrotoxicosis, faecal impaction with overflow,
  irritable bowel syndrome

febrile • Examine the abdomen and do a rectal examination • In the elderly a rectal examination must be performed to exclude faecal impaction.

Clinical syndromes

- Antibiotic-induced: usually begins 2 or 3 days into a course of antibiotics. There may be associated nausea and vomiting but abdominal pain is rare.
- Pseudomembranous colitis, characterized by cramping abdominal pain and diarrhoea with mucus and sometimes blood in the stool, begins between 4 days and 6 weeks after the start of a course of antibiotics.
- Acute food poisoning: vomiting and diarrhoea usually begin within 24 hours of ingesting contaminated food; incubation period may be up to 5 days in the case of *Campylobacter*, while in staphylococcal food poisoning it may be as little as a couple of hours.
- Acute watery diarrhoea: caused by enterotoxin-producing or invasive organisms transmitted by contaminated water or food. May be caused either by viruses (Rotavirus, Norwalk) or bacteria (*E. coli, Salmonella, Vibrio cholerae*).
- Diarrhoea due to a carcinoma of colon: may be subacute and intermittent. Should be thought of especially in older patients or if there is blood or a lot of mucus in the stool.
- Bloody diarrhoea: blood mixed with the stool suggests a serious intestinal infection (including *pseudomembranous colitis*) or the presence of *inflammatory bowel disease*.
- If the stool consists entirely of fairly fresh blood, check for haemorrhoids; a bloody stool associated with abdominal pain suggests ischaemic colitis.
- Chronic diarrhoea alternating with constipation in a patient who is relatively well and has not lost weight suggests irritable bowel syndrome.
- Chronic diarrhoea with pale stools, weight-loss and chronic abdominal pain suggests malabsorption secondary to chronic pancreatitis.

Investigations

Blood tests • These should be performed in all but mild cases; they include FBC, U&E, blood cultures (if febrile or if *Salmonella* infection is suspected), blood glucose and thyroid function tests where appropriate • If you think the patient might have a flare-up of Crohn's disease, check ESR or plasma viscosity (PV), CRP and orosomucoid.

Stool examination: • Send samples for culture and sensitivity (including *Clostridium difficile* where appropriate) • If there has been foreign travel or contact with infectious disease, send a sample for ova, cysts and parasites • If the patient is ill, dehydrated or has a high fever, immediate microscopy of a direct stool smear is indicated: the presence of polymorphs indicates that the diarrhoea is probably due to *E. coli*, *Campylobacter*, *Shigella* or (occasionally) *Clostridium difficile*; if there are no polymorphs, *Salmonella*, *E. coli* or *Clostridium difficile* are likely.

X-rays: • If inflammatory bowel disease is suspected, the patient must have a plain X-ray of the abdomen to look for toxic dilatation of the colon; this may need to be repeated daily • A water-soluble contrast enema is sometimes necessary in patients with diarrhoea. Consult a more senior colleague.

Other tests: • Sigmoidoscopy (without prior bowel preparation) should be carried out within the first 24 hours if IBD is suspected

---

Management box

▸ **Isolation** Any patient suspected of having an infectious cause for diarrhoea should be isolated in a single room and barrier-nursed. Involve the control of infection nurse and his/her team.

▸ **Rehydration** This may be carried out orally in milder cases. You will need to give about 50 ml/kg initially, ie 2.5–3.5 litres in the first 12 hours, followed by a similar volume in each 24 hours. If the patient is anorexic, vomiting or more severely ill, rehydration should be by intravenous infusion using roughly equal parts of 0.9% saline and 5% glucose, with at least 40 mmol of potassium per litre. 4–6 litres of fluid per day may be required, depending on the severity of the diarrhoea (→ p 517–18).

In patients needing iv rehydration because of diarrhoea, U&E measurements must be carried out at least once per day.

▸ **Anti-diarrhoeal drugs** These should be avoided in all but mild cases since, if infection is present, they will prolong it. If symptomatic anti-diarrhoeal treatment is required, use loperamide or codeine phosphate.

▸ **Antibiotic** These are not required in most cases of infective diarrhoea. If a positive stool culture is obtained or if diarrhoea persists for more than 5 days, consult your local micro-biologist. As a general rule, the antibiotic agents used in infective diarrhoea are those listed in Table 16.17.

▸ **Steroids and other drugs for inflammatory bowel disease** Any patient with IBD who is ill enough to need hospital admission will usually require systemic steroids, such as prednisolone 40 mg per day or hydrocortisone 100 mg iv 6-hourly. Other treatments such as rectal steroids, a 5-ASA derivative (sulfasalazine, mesalazine) or parenteral nutrition may be required: consult your SHO or registrar.

Table 16.17
Antibiotic agents used in infective diarrhoea

Organism	Antibiotic
Salmonella	Ampicillin, co-trimoxazole, chloramphenicol
Campylobacter	Erythromycin, ciprofloxacin, tetracycline
Clostridium difficile	Vancomycin, metronidazole
Yersinia	Tetracycline

• US or CT scanning of the abdomen may be indicated if a pancreatic cause is suspected • Rarely, a faecal fat collection will be required in patients suspected of having malabsorption.

PRURITUS

Pruritus may be a symptom of local skin conditions, but can also be a manifestation of systemic disease without obvious skin lesions. Localized itch, such as pruritus ani, indicates local disease while generalized pruritus has a wide differential diagnosis. Many factors have been implicated in the pathogenesis of itch such as proteases, histamine, prostaglandins, kinins and bile acids, but the underlying mechanism in many disorders remains unclear, as is the relief obtained by scratching.

Local skin conditions • Scabies • Atopic eczema • Candidiasis • Urticaria • Insect bites.

Systemic disorders • Chronic cholestasis (eg PBC) • Chronic renal failure • Polycythaemia rubra vera • Pregnancy • Hyper- and hypothyroidism • Myeloproliferative diseases (Hodgkin's disease, leukaemia, myeloma) • Carcinoid syndrome • Iron deficiency • Drug hypersensitivity • Mastocytosis • Diabetes mellitus • Brain tumour (especially fourth ventricle).

OEDEMA

Oedema is said to exist when soft-tissue swelling occurs due to the collection of interstitial fluid. Such fluid collects either when increased formation or impaired reabsorption exists.

Generalized oedema • This occurs when greater than 3 l of interstitial fluid collects and is always associated with renal retention of sodium • The predominant site of collection varies with the underlying disorder; pulmonary and ankle oedema are typical of cardiac failure, periorbital oedema in renal failure and ascites in cirrhosis • The mechanisms involved also vary with the disease.

Cardiac failure: • reduced cardiac output • increased venous pressure • reduced renal blood flow • secondary aldosteronism, all result in sodium retention.

Cirrhosis: • portal venous hypertension • secondary aldosteronism • intra-renal vascular shunting • hypoproteinaemia, are all believed important.

Renal failure: • impaired renal sodium excretion results in oedema if the sodium intake is not regulated.

Nephrotic syndrome: • hypoalbuminaemia and reduced plasma volume are important.

Other causes: • pregnancy • idiopathic oedema • angioneurotic oedema • steroid therapy • hypothyroidism • starvation (especially on refeeding) • localized oedema, the commonest example is unilateral lower limb oedema complicating a DVT • blockage of large veins elsewhere may produce oedema such as in SVC, IVC or subclavian vein obstruction • lymphoedema, due to lymphatic obstruction, may be acquired or congenital (eg Milroy's disease) • a paralysed limb may also become oedematous • localized inflammation may result in localized fluid collection in adjacent potential spaces, eg pleural effusion or ascites.

History and examination • Enquire and look for evidence of underlying cardiac, renal or liver disease • Enquire about the duration of the oedema.

Investigations • FBC, LFTs, albumin, TFTs • Urinalysis and 24-hour urine collection for proteinuria and creatinine clearance if indicated • CXR and echocardiogram if indicated • US of abdomen • Doppler or venogram of leg veins.

Management box

▶ Depends upon the underlying cause.
▶ In generalized oedema sodium restriction is generally necessary and diuretics are advocated in most cases.
▶ Since in many instances the plasma volume is reduced, overvigorous diuresis should be avoided.
▶ Intravenous diuretic administration may be necessary when intestinal oedema results in diuretic resistance.

ACUTE PAIN IN THE LEG

This section is concerned with pain which affects the whole of the calf or the whole leg, not pain confined to a single joint or a pair of joints.

Causes (→ Table 16.18)

History • Ask about: • Duration of the pain • Nature of the pain • Whether it came on gradually or suddenly • Whether it affects the whole leg or a part • Whether it is worse when walking or when the patient moves to stand up • Any risk factors for DVT (Table 16.19).

Examination • Inspect the leg for: • Skin colour • Temperature (use the back of your hand) • Swelling • Distended veins

---

Table 16.18
Causes of acute pain in the leg

Mechanical: trauma, sprain, etc
Thrombophlebitis
DVT
Cellulitis
Bursitis
Ruptured knee joint/ruptured Baker's cyst
Embolism to the femoral artery or its branches
Neuropathic pain, eg diabetes

Table 16.19
Factors predisposing to a DVT

Elderly
Previous history of proven DVT or PE
Immobilization
Recent trauma, especially to leg
Major abdominal or pelvic surgery
Recent surgery to hip, leg or knee
Pregnancy or puerperium
Myocardial infarction
Disabling heart failure or COPD
Malignant disease, especially abdominal or pelvic, metastatic
  disease or recent chemotherapy
Recent stroke or spinal cord injury
HRT or oral contraceptives

• Breaks in skin, blisters, ulcers, etc • If you think the leg is swollen, measure the circumference with a tape measure. For the calf, identify the tibial tuberosity on each side, then measure 10 cm down from this on the anterior surface. Mark the skin with a pen and measure the circumference just below the mark. A difference of 1.5 cm or more between the two sides is significant. For the thigh, measure 25 cm from the anterior superior iliac spine and mark the leg with a pen. A difference of 1.5 cm or more between the two sides is significant • Check for the presence of femoral, popliteal and foot pulses • If you think the pain might be neuropathic, check light-touch, pinprick and vibration sense (joint position sense is not helpful in this situation) and examine the knee and ankle reflexes.

Clinical syndromes

Deep vein thrombosis (DVT): • the history is usually of a fairly rapid (but not abrupt) onset of pain, over a period of hours. The patient may say that he or she has been immobile for some time prior to the event (eg a long coach or plane journey) or there may be other risk factors present (Table 16.19) • pain may get acutely worse if the patient puts the foot to the ground to stand up • on examination the affected leg is swollen, warm and pink and there may be visible distended veins • the calf may be acutely tender posteriorly • venous thrombosis is relatively rare in rheumatoid arthritis • if a patient with known rheumatoid arthritis develops a painful, swollen calf it is more likely to be a ruptured knee joint (below) than a DVT.

Cellulitis: • there may be a history of recent bite or trauma to the leg • on examination, the affected area is hot, swollen and red (the redness is usually much more marked than in DVT) • the affected area of the leg may have an irregular boundary which does not follow obvious anatomical landmarks.

Ruptured knee joint/Baker's cyst: • there may be a history of arthritis (either osteo or rheumatoid) in the relevant knee • on examination the leg is swollen and may be very red and tender over the posterior and lateral calf.

Arterial thromboembolism: • the pain comes on very abruptly and is often intense • there may be a history of atherosclerotic vascular disease, valvular heart disease or atrial fibrillation • the leg is often very pale, sometimes with peripheral purplish or bluish discoloration, and feels cold • the acutely ischaemic leg is a surgical emergency: contact your SHO or a member of the on-call vascular surgical team immediately (see below).

Neuropathic pain: • this is characteristically sharp and stabbing or burning in nature, or the patient may say that it feels like walking on sharp pebbles • on examination there is usually impairment of at least one sensory modality and absence of the ankle jerks.

Investigations • If there are any broken areas of skin or ulcers, take swabs from these for culture • If the patient is febrile or you suspect cellulitis, take blood cultures • If you suspect a DVT, even if you are not sure, the patient must have a Doppler ultrasound scan of the leg or a venogram as the diagnosis can be extremely difficult to make clinically • If the initial Doppler ultrasound is negative but the clinical suspicion of DVT is strong, it is wise to anticoagulate the patient with sc low-molecular-weight heparin (→ below and p 569) and repeat the scan after 48 hours • Another approach which is gaining popularity is to measure the level of D-dimers (breakdown products of fibrin) in the blood: if the initial Doppler scan is negative and the level of D-dimer, measured by a reliable assay, is normal, then a DVT is very unlikely • If there is going to be any delay in obtaining a scan/venogram the patient should be given analgesics and sc low-molecular-weight heparin • If you suspect a ruptured knee joint the investigation of choice will be an arthrogram; it is wise to discuss the case with your SHO or registrar before ordering this.

Management box

▶ **Deep venous thrombosis (DVT)** • The patient should be given analgesia and commenced on a low-molecular-weight (LMW) heparin, eg tinzaparin, 175 µ/kg by once-daily sc injection (Table 19.7). Once the diagnosis of DVT is confirmed, start treatment with warfarin, 10 mg in the early evening; adjust the dose as indicated in Table 19.5 • Once the patient has had LMW heparin for 5 days and the INR is within the therapeutic range, the heparin can be stopped • Warfarin will need to be continued for 6 weeks if the DVT has an obvious precipitant such as an operation, 3–6 months if the cause is unknown (each consultant will have a particular preference) • Should be fitted with an elastic, graduated compression stocking (TED stocking) and early mobilization encouraged • If the patient has had a large ilio-femoral thrombosis and there is a lot of tension in the tissues, there is a risk of venous gangrene and streptokinase may be needed: consult your SHO or registrar.

▶ If a patient presents with a DVT **without any apparent cause**, an underlying malignancy should be considered • Likely primary tumours include carcinomas of the pancreas and liver and brain tumours • There is also an association with cancers of the prostate, ovary and uterus, also non-Hodgkin's lymphoma and leukaemia • Alternatively, the patient may →

▶ **Cellulitis** • Give analgesics and antibiotics in the form of benzylpenicillin, 600 mg–1.2 g 6-hourly iv, plus flucloxacillin, 250 mg 6-hourly iv • If penicillin-allergic, give clindamycin, 600 mg 8-hourly iv • The leg should be supported on a footstool or on pillows • It is useful to draw around the area of erythema with an indelible marker so that the progress of the cellulitis can be assessed.

▶ **Arterial embolism** • This constitutes a surgical emergency: either you or your SHO/registrar should contact the on-call vascular surgical team immediately. The patient may well need to go to theatre, so check that he/she has had a recent FBC, U&E and ECG and take blood for 'group and save' • Begin anticoagulation with iv heparin, 5000 u as a bolus injection, followed by 1400 u per hour.

▶ **Ruptured knee joint** • Initially (before the diagnosis is proven) give analgesics, which may be continued as needed after the arthrogram • If you think that someone may have had either a DVT or a ruptured knee joint, remember that heparin is contraindicated in cases of ruptured joint • The treatment is analgesics and rest initially, followed by mobilization with a supportive elastic stocking.

EXCESSIVE BRUISING OR BLEEDING

Causes • (→ Table 16.20)

History The most important questions relating to the haemorrhagic disorder are: • Have you ever had a problem with excessive bleeding before, eg after dental extraction? • Have you lost weight? • Have you been feverish or otherwise generally unwell? • What drugs or medicines have you had recently? (a full, detailed drug history, including over-the-counter medications, is essential (Table 16.21) • How much alcohol do you drink? • Is there a family history of any similar problem?

Examination Look especially for: • Evidence of anaemia • Bruising or bleeding inside the mouth • The pattern of bruising in the skin • Lymph-node enlargement • Signs of chronic liver disease (spider naevi, palmar erythema, Dupuytren's contracture, oedema, ascites, splenomegaly, testicular atrophy) • Enlargement of the liver or spleen • It is also wise to examine the eyes for signs of fundal haemorrhage as this has important implications for the management of the patient.

Clinical patterns • Purpura and bleeding from mucous membranes are common in platelet and blood vessel disorders

Table 16.20
Causes of excessive bruising or bleeding (in order of frequency)

Diagnosis	Causes
Connective-tissue atrophy	Old age
	Steroid therapy
	Wasting
Thrombocytopenia	Viral infections
	Drug-induced (inc. alcohol)
	B_{12} or folate deficiency
	Bone-marrow dyscrasias
	Increased consumption (idiopathic thrombocytopenic purpura (ITP), DIC, hypersplenism)
	Systemic lupus erythematosus (SLE)
Clotting-factor deficiency	Liver disease
	Drug-induced (heparin, warfarin)
	Excess consumption (DIC)
	Dilution (large blood transfusion)
	Congenital (haemophilia, etc.)
	Vitamin K deficiency (eg malabsorption)
Vessel-wall disorders	Aspirin
	Osler-Weber-Rendu disease
	Angiodysplasia

Table 16.21
Drugs causing thrombocytopenia

Cytotoxic therapy
Diuretics (thiazides, furosemide (frusemide))
NSAIDs (including aspirin)
Sulphonamides
Rifampicin
Quinidine
Methyldopa
Penicillins

Table 16.22
Causes of DIC

Septicaemia, especially Gram-negative or meningococcal
Obstetric causes
   intrauterine death
   abruption placentae
   amniotic fluid embolism
Incompatible blood transfusion
Pancreatitis
Anaphylaxis
Malignancy, especially promyelocytic leukaemia
Major surgery, especially with extra-corporeal shunts
Severe trauma or burns

but rare in diseases affecting clotting factors • In platelet disorders bruising is usually multiple and superficial, while in coagulopathies it is deeper and often single • Vascular and platelet disorders (Table 16.20) lead to prolonged bleeding from superficial cuts, whereas clotting factor abnormalities produce delayed bleeding from deeper structures such as muscles, joints, gastrointestinal tract (GIT) • Bleeding from needle puncture sites should make you think of DIC.

Investigations • FBC, platelet count and blood film • PT and KCCT (APTT) • If DIC is suspected (→ Table 16.22), ask for a fibrinogen titre and/or a measure of fibrin degradation products such as D-dimer; your local haematology laboratory will advise you if you are unsure • Remember to take blood for group and cross-match • Laboratory features of DIC include the following: reduced platelet count, prolonged PT, KCCT and thrombin time, reduced fibrinogen titre, increased fibrin degradation products (or D-dimer), fragmented red cells on blood film.

Management box

You will almost certainly want to involve your SHO/registrar in the patient's management. However, a few basic principles can be stated.

▶ im injections are absolutely contraindicated in someone with a clotting disorder: it is best to write, in red, on the drug prescription sheet: 'No im injections'. By the same token, invasive vascular procedures such as CVP line insertion should be undertaken with great caution, if at all, in patients with clotting defects.

→

▶ Transfused platelets are rapidly consumed and repeated transfusion can give rise to platelet antibodies which would make subsequent transfusion of platelets impossible. Platelet transfusion should not, therefore, be undertaken on the basis of the count alone unless this is very low (less than 25×10^9/l). The indications for platelet transfusion are related to active bleeding, as judged by:
  – externally visible bleeding (GIT, etc)
  – new bleeding into the skin (petechiae or purpura)
  – CNS bleeding (including fundal haemorrhage)
  – cover for intercurrent surgery.

It is vital, therefore, to examine the skin and the optic fundi daily in any patient with moderate or severe thrombocytopenia.

▶ If the patient has a deficiency of clotting factors (liver disease, overtreatment with warfarin, DIC, etc) and is actively bleeding, FFP should be given in order to replace them. A cross-match will need to be performed before FFP is given. It is usually administered in a dose of 2 or 4 units at a time (run in fairly quickly). If the patient is volume-depleted or is actively bleeding, fresh blood should be given. The coagulation defect may be corrected by giving the patient vitamin K as phytomenadione, 5 mg iv, given slowly.

▶ Patients with haemophilia who present with an acute bleed will require factor VIII concentrate or cryoprecipitate. Consult your local haematologist.

HEADACHE

Causes → Table 16.23

History • Prodrome preceding the headache: migraine attacks often begin with changes in mood (euphoria or depression), arousal (feeling full of energy or lethargic) or appetite (food preferences) • The onset of the headache (those marked A in Table 16.23 come on relatively acutely, whereas the other disorders cause chronic headache) • Tension headaches can be acute or chronic • Is the headache continuous or episodic? • Severity of the headache and impact on daily activities • Site, migraine headache is usually unilateral at its onset, though it may become bilateral later • Occipital headache coming on suddenly must raise the suspicion of subarachnoid haemorrhage or meningitis, *even if there is no definite meningism on examination* • Previous history of headaches or migraine; migraine rarely begins after the age of 35 • Associated symptoms, eg nausea, photophobia, disorientation.

Table 16.23
Causes of headache

Common
　Tension headache – A
　Cervical spine disease
　Trauma
　Migraine – A
　Subarachnoid haemorrhage – A
　Intracerebral haemorrhage – A
　Intracranial tumour
　Raised ICP
　Meningitis – A
　Encephalitis – A
　Temporal arteritis – A
　Post-ictal
Uncommon
　Hypercapnia
　Stroke – A
　Subdural haematoma
　Cerebral artery aneurysm
　Carbon monoxide poisoning
　Hypertensive encephalopathy – A
　Acute glaucoma – A
　Sinusitis
　Trigeminal neuralgia – A

Examination • Assess the patient's level of consciousness and orientation (GCS, → p 417). If there is depression of consciousness or disorientation, you are obviously dealing with a serious cause of headache such as meningitis, encephalitis, subarachnoid haemorrhage, poisoning, trauma or raised ICP • Check the patient's temperature, pulse and BP • Look for evidence of trauma to the head • Examine the eyes for signs of glaucoma (red eye, oval pupil) • Check for a rash (meningitis) • Temporal arteritis is a disease of the over-60s: in this age group, check to see whether the temporal arteries are palpable and tender • Perform a quick neurological examination, checking especially for signs of meningism, that the pupils are equal and reactive, that there is no papilloedema and that there is no obvious hemiparesis. Note that hypercapnia may cause papilloedema • It is useful to look for papilloedema, but its absence does not mean that raised ICP can be excluded • In subarachnoid haemorrhage, you may see subhyaloid haemorrhages • In malignant hypertension there may be exudates or haemorrhages in the fundi.

Investigations and management

▶ If you suspect **temporal arteritis**, ask for a blood count and ESR – this need not be obtained as an emergency. Temporal artery biopsy, which can be performed after treatment has started, may be needed later. Treat suspected temporal arteritis with prednisolone, beginning with a dose of 60 mg/day. If the diagnosis of temporal arteritis is correct, the response to steroids is usually dramatic within 24–48 hours.

▶ If **meningitis or subarachnoid haemorrhage** is suspected, a decision needs to be made as to whether lumbar puncture (LP) or urgent CT scanning is indicated: blind LP is not acceptable nowadays, so consult your SHO or registrar. If subarachnoid haemorrhage is a serious possibility, give nimodipine orally or (if the patient cannot swallow) iv via a central vein. Give analgesia in the form of dihydrocodeine or pethidine and anti-emetics (metoclopramide or prochlorperazine). If a CT scan is thought unnecessary or has been done and is negative, LP should be performed to look for evidence of meningitis or encephalitis and also to exclude SAH if the clinical index of suspicion is high (→ p 497). Send cerebrospinal fluid (CSF) samples for microscopy and culture, protein and glucose and remember to send a blood sample for glucose at the same time (Table 16.24).

▶ If **meningitis** is suspected clinically, antibiotics must be started immediately. Do not wait for the CSF results. In adults, give iv benzylpenicillin, 2.4 g every 4 hours; if the patient is allergic to penicillin, give chloramphenicol, 12.5 mg/kg every 6 hours. If **TB meningitis** is suspected, consult a senior colleague or your local microbiologist.

▶ If a patient has meningitis due to either *Haemophilus influenzae or meningococcus*, family and close friends should be offered prophylaxis, usually with rifampicin; if in doubt consult your local microbiologist. Remember also that meningitis is a notifiable disease.

▶ **Migraine** should in the first instance be treated with simple analgesics (aspirin or paracetamol) and anti-emetics; ergotamine derivatives are not usually necessary. In severe cases, consider sumatriptan (oral or sc) or a similar drug.

▶ Investigate and treat other types of headache according to their cause.

▶ Except in cases of trauma, a skull X-ray is usually unhelpful in making a diagnosis of the cause of headache.

Table 16.24
CSF values in meningitis

	Normal	Bacterial	Viral	TB
Appearance	Clear	Turbid	Clear or turbid	Turbid (may be fibrinous)
Polymorphs (per mm³)	0	> 200	< 100	< 100
Mononuclear cells (per mm³)	0	< 100	10–1000	100–300
Protein (g/l)	< 0.5 g/l	> 1 g/l	0.5–1 g/l	1–5 g/l
Glucose	2/3 of blood glucose	< 50% of blood glucose	2/3 of blood glucose	< 1/3 of blood glucose

HYPERTENSION

Hypertension may be defined as a blood pressure consistently above 160/100 mmHg (lower pressures may define hypertension in many cases). It may present a problem to the junior physician in one of three ways:

- a patient is admitted electively for investigation and treatment of known hypertension
- a patient is admitted as an emergency for treatment of severe hypertension or its complications (left ventricular failure, visual disturbance, renal failure, hypertensive encephalopathy, aortic dissection)
- hypertension discovered in the course of managing a patient with a related condition (stroke, MI) or an unrelated one.

If hypertension has not been diagnosed before, it is important to measure the BP yourself and to see several readings over 2 or 3 days before coming to a decision. The only exception to this is if the BP is very high (over 200 systolic or 120 diastolic) *and* is definitely causing acute complications such as papilloedema, fits, left ventricular failure (LVF), renal failure or aortic dissection.

Usually there are no underlying causes, but it is obviously worth looking for one.

History • Ask about personal or family history of renal disease
• Previous history of hypertension, eg during pregnancy
• Symptoms which might suggest a phaeochromocytoma, eg palpitations, headache, attacks of pallor.

Examination • In patients under 50, check the femoral pulses for radiofemoral delay • Examine the heart for cardiomegaly and for 3rd or 4th heart sounds • Examine the chest for evidence of left ventricular failure • Examine the abdomen for renal masses and bruits • Examine the optic fundi for arteriovenous nipping (significant only in patients under 65), exudates, haemorrhages and papilloedema. If you find retinopathy this indicates that the hypertension has been present for months or years rather than coming on acutely • Finally, be on the lookout for signs of Cushing's syndrome, eg central obesity, livid striae in the skin, thinning of skin over the hands, moon face, proximal myopathy.

Grading of hypertensive retinopathy • Stage I = arteriolar narrowing • Stage II = arteriolar irregularity, arterio-venous nipping • Stage III = 'blot' and 'flame' haemorrhages and 'cotton wool' exudates • Stage IV = papilloedema, associated with malignant hypertension.

Investigations • Every patient with hypertension should have the urine examined for casts, protein and blood • Take blood for U&E and have it performed quickly; if there is proteinuria or oedema, ask for a serum albumin • A low serum potassium in someone who has not been taking diuretics, particularly if accompanied by a raised bicarbonate, should make you think of Conn's syndrome • Ask for an ECG and chest X-ray to look for evidence of left ventricular hypertrophy and strain and of left ventricular failure • In patients under 60 you should consider the possibility of a phaeochromocytoma, so send off two 24-hour urine samples for catecholamines (metanephrines, VMA, etc). Putting the patient on a vanilla-free diet is not necessary • Resist the temptation to treat hypertension in the context of an acute stroke • A high proportion of patients with phaeochromocytoma have sustained hypertension, not intermittent as is often suggested in textbooks • In younger patients or where there is a suggestive history, renal function should be investigated by means of an isotope renogram, intravenous urogram (IVU) or renal angiogram (renal ultrasound is not sufficient as you need to know about function and not just structure).

Management box
▶ **Non-urgent treatment** Your chief may have a particular favourite drug or drugs for treating hypertension. If not, consider using the following:
– **Thiazide diuretics** These are effective both at reducing BP and at lessening the risks of hypertension-associated diseases. They do not reduce BP very much so are suitable only for patients with mild to moderate hypertension (180/110 or less). Supplementary potassium may need to be given. →

- **β-blockers** They reduce BP and are particularly suitable for patients who also have angina; they may be combined with diuretics. They should be used with great caution, if at all, in patients with peripheral vascular disease and are contraindicated in patients with a history of airways obstruction or heart block. Some authorities now regard β-blockers as a poor choice for the treatment of hypertension because of their tendency to cause side-effects. β-blockers must not be used alone in patients suspected of having a phaeochromocytoma, who require combined alpha- and beta-blockade.

- **Angiotensin converting enzyme (ACE) inhibitors** These have a good side-effect profile and often need to be taken only once daily. They are particularly useful in patients with associated heart failure. ACE inhibitors can cause worsening of renal function in the presence of renal artery stenosis and renal function should be carefully monitored (at least every 48 hours) after an ACE inhibitor has been introduced. This is especially true of patients who have widespread atherosclerotic vascular disease, in whom clinically silent renal artery stenosis is common. ACE inhibitors may cause first-dose hypotension, especially in patients who have been taking diuretics, so the first dose should be given with the patient lying in bed and BP should be measured every 10-15 min for the first 2 hours. Many so-called 'once daily' ACE inhibitors do not actually control blood pressure for 24 hours and should therefore be given in divided doses.

- **Calcium-channel blockers** These also have a good side-effect profile and are useful in people with angina. Verapamil and diltiazem should not be used in people who have, or who are at risk of, heart failure and should only be combined with a β-blocker with great caution. Combinations of CCBs and diuretics are not as effective as other anti-hypertensive combinations.

- **Non-drug methods of controlling BP** These should not be forgotten, especially weight reduction and reducing alcohol consumption.

▶ **Emergency and urgent treatment** → Chapter 17 p 432.

LYMPH-NODE ENLARGEMENT

Minor lymph-node enlargement is common in certain circumstances, for example in children with upper respiratory infections and in the inguinal nodes of many adults.

You should check specifically for lymph-node enlargement in the following circumstances:

- unexplained fever or weight-loss
- persistent cough or shortness of breath
- unexplained anaemia or bruising
- patients who are jaundiced
- patients with an abdominal mass
- patients with finger clubbing
- suspected breast cancer
- increased risk of TB, eg immigrants, socially deprived, homeless, alcoholics, those who are HIV-positive.

History Review the history, asking specifically about: • Weight-loss • Respiratory symptoms • Abnormal bleeding and bruising • Infections in the relevant area • Contact with unusual infections, eg farm animals (brucellosis), domestic animals (toxoplasmosis) • Risk factors for HIV infection.

Examination • If the enlarged nodes are in the neck, check the head and neck carefully, including the mouth and throat • Check for finger clubbing • In women, be sure to check for breast lumps • Examine the chest for signs of reduced movement, consolidation, pleural effusions or a fixed rhonchus (a sign of bronchial obstruction) • Examine for abdominal masses, especially the liver and spleen.

Investigations • Virtually every patient with lymphadenopathy should have a blood count and erythrocyte sedimentation rate (ESR) or plasma viscosity (PV), LFTs and a CXR • If an infectious cause is suspected (Table 16.25), ask for a glandular fever screening test and appropriate serology, eg brucella, toxoplasma • If TB is suspected, obtain sputum for smear and culture and early morning urines (the *whole* of the specimen passed first thing in the morning) for culture • Tuberculin test (Mantoux or Heaf test) may be useful, especially by excluding TB if the test is negative • If there is a pleural effusion a diagnostic aspiration should be performed: withdraw 20 ml of fluid using a standard venepuncture needle and syringe and send the sample to the laboratory for cytology, protein concentration, culture and sensitivity • Fluid specimens for cytology must be sent to the laboratory fresh: the cells will be unrecognizable if the sample is stored in the refrigerator overnight • A pleural biopsy may be needed – consult your SHO or registrar • Aspiration cytology or biopsy of an enlarged lymph node may be required – consult your SHO or registrar.

LIVER ENLARGEMENT

A liver edge that is palpable is not always enlarged and may be due to displacement in patients with pulmonary

Table 16.25
Differential diagnosis of lymphadenopathy

Neoplastic	Haematological
	    Acute leukaemias, lymphomas, CLL,
	    histiocytosis
	Non-haematological
	    Carcinoma: lung, breast, kidneys

Infection	Viral
	    EBV, CMV, HIV, hepatitis A, rubella
	Bacterial
	    TB, syphilis
	Fungal
	    Histoplasmosis
	Protozoal
	    Malaria, toxoplasmosis

Immune conditions	SLE, RA
Metabolic	Lipid storage disorders
Others	Sarcoidosis, drugs (eg phenytoin), histiocytosis X

hyperinflation. It is therefore essential to identify the upper border of the liver by percussion, which is usually at the 5th rib or 5th intercostal space in the mid-clavicular line. Hepatomegaly can be defined as a liver with a span of more than 12 cm in the mid-clavicular line. Enlargement of the liver might be found in the course of examining a patient where you are already expecting such a finding (for example a patient with alcoholic liver disease or advanced malignancy) or it may be a chance observation.

Causes → Table 16.26 • A patient with cirrhosis may have an enlarged liver. It is only in advanced cirrhosis that the liver becomes small and shrunken.

History Review the history, asking about: • Alcohol intake • Previous history of liver disease • Previous history of heart disease • Weight-loss • Contact with infectious disease.

Examination • General examination: look for evidence of chronic liver disease (jaundice, palmar erythema, spider naevi, Dupuytren's contracture) • Check for enlarged lymph nodes • Examine the heart and chest, looking for evidence of heart

Table 16.26
Causes of liver enlargement

Process	Disease
Congestion	CCF*
	Budd–Chiari syndrome
Infective	Viral hepatitis
	Bacterial (Weil's disease)
	Parasites (Hydatid disease)
Malignancy	Hepatoma
	Metastatic*
Myeloproliferative	Myelofibrosis
	Leukaemia
Infiltrative	Fatty liver (NASH), alcohol*
	Amyloidosis
Anatomical	Reidel's lobe
Displacement	COPD*
Fibrosis	Cirrhosis
Biliary obstruction	Choledocholithiasis
	Pancreatic carcinoma

*Common causes

failure, hyper-inflation of the lungs, abnormal or asymmetrical chest movement • Re-check the abdomen and try to answer the following questions:

Is the liver: smooth or nodular? tender or non-tender? pulsatile? Is the spleen enlarged? Is there ascites? Are there any other abdominal masses?

Investigations • Basic blood tests: blood count, LFTs, clotting screen, hepatitis, A, B and C • Further blood tests: anti-nuclear factor, auto-antibodies, glandular fever screening test (Paul-Bunnell, Monospot), alpha-fetoprotein (if hepatoma is suspected) • CXR, liver ultrasound • Where indicated, abdominal CT scan, liver biopsy.

SPLENOMEGALY

An enlarged spleen may be found in the context of other clinical signs (for example chronic liver disease or subacute bacterial endocarditis), or may be an isolated finding (for example infectious mononucleosis).

Causes → Table 16.27

Table 16.27
Causes of splenomegaly

Myeloproliferative disorders:
   myelofibrosis*, chronic myeloid leukaemia*, essential
   thrombocythaemia, primary polycythaemia
Portal hypertension
Lymphoma
Leukaemias
Haemolytic anaemias
Haemoglobinopathies
Bacterial infections:
   subacute bacterial endocarditis, septicaemia, tuberculosis,
   brucellosis, salmonellosis
Viral infections:
   infectious mononucleosis, acute viral hepatitis
Protozoal infections:
   chronic malaria*, Kala-azar*
Inflammatory disorders:
   Felty's syndrome, SLE, sarcoidosis
Storage disorders:
   Gaucher's disease
Amyloid

*massive enlargement

History • Easy bruising • Foreign travel • Previous history of liver disease • Previous history of connective tissue disease • Previous history of heart disease • Contact with infectious disease • Weight-loss.

Examination • Stigmata of chronic liver disease • Stigmata of subacute bacterial endocarditis • Enlarged lymph nodes • Bruises • Pallor • Examine heart for new murmurs • Examine abdomen for hepatomegaly and ascites.

Investigations • Full blood count and blood film (thick film required if recent foreign travel and malaria suspected) • LFTs and clotting screen • Anti-nuclear factor; rheumatoid factor; haemolysis screen if indicated • Consider CXR, abdominal US or CT scan, echocardiogram, bone marrow aspirate and trephine.

ASCITES

Causes • → Table 16.28 • You should ask yourself: • Is it ascites? Be sure to differentiate the swelling from other causes of

Table 16.28
Causes of ascites

Common	Less common	Rare
Cirrhosis	Nephrotic syndrome	TB
CCF	Hypoproteinaemia	Constrictive pericarditis
Malignancy	Abdominal trauma	Budd–Chiari syndrome

abdominal distension such as fat, faeces or a mass • *Careful percussion is needed* • Are there any abdominal masses (including the liver and spleen)? Paracentesis may be performed either for diagnostic purposes or to relieve symptoms (pain from severe distension, or breathlessness) ($\rightarrow$ p 148).

Equipment • Minor dressing pack • Antiseptic • Lignocaine • For a diagnostic tap, 20 ml syringe and 21-gauge needle (green) • For a therapeutic tap, 60 ml Luer-lock syringe, 3-way tap, 18-gauge cannula (Venflon, etc) • Drainage tube and a 2 l measuring jug to act as receiver (or one-piece drain and collecting bag if the ascites is to be drained slowly) • Specimen bottles for biochemistry (protein content), microbiology and cytology.

Procedure • Ask the patient to lie supine, as flat as is comfortably possible • Percuss carefully and locate the site of maximum dullness • Clean the skin over this area with antiseptic • Infiltrate the skin and subcutaneous tissues with lignocaine • For a diagnostic tap, pass the needle through the abdominal wall, aspirating gently as you do so. Withdraw about 20 ml of fluid and note the colour. Remove the needle and put a dressing over the wound. Put the specimens into the respective bottles • Diagnostic aspirations should be done reasonably early in the day: fluid for cytology must be processed within a short time as the cells will degenerate if the specimen is kept in the fridge overnight • If the fluid is cloudy and there are more than 250 polymorphs/mm^3, infection is likely to be present even if subsequent culture is negative. Start antibiotics (eg a cephalosporin and metronidazole) while waiting for the laboratory results.

Management box
$\rightarrow$ Chapter 6 p 148.

FOCAL NEUROLOGICAL DEFICIT (INCLUDING STROKE)

Causes → Table 16.29.

History • The speed of onset of the deficit is important: disorders which come on instantaneously or over a few minutes are likely to be vascular in origin • Talk to relatives about the patient's intellectual abilities and any history of even a minor

Table 16.29
Causes of focal neurological deficit

Brain disorders
  Stroke/TIA
  Epilepsy
  Subarachnoid haemorrhage
  Head injury
  Tumour or abscess
  Hypoglycaemia
  Encephalitis
  Subdural haematoma
  Migraine
Spinal cord disorders
  Embolism to spinal artery (more common after surgery for aortic aneurysm)
  Cervical spondylosis
  Rheumatoid arthritis of the cervical spine (atlanto-axial subluxation)
  Paraspinal abscess or tumour
  Vertebral collapse secondary to tumour or osteomyelitis
  Epidural or intramedullary haemorrhage (esp. with platelet or clotting disorders)
  Paget's disease of vertebrae
Combined disorders
  Demyelination
Peripheral nerve disorders
  Carpal tunnel syndrome
  Diabetes (cranial mononeuropathy)
  Guillain-Barré syndrome
  B_{12} or folate deficiency
  Alcoholism
  Drugs: cisplatin, vincristine, isoniazid, nitrofurantoin, etc
  Uraemia
  Trauma
  (Rarely) vasculitis, lead poisoning, prophyria, amyloidosis, etc

head injury or fall – these may give clues to the presence of a subdural haematoma • Distribution of the weakness or sensory disturbance: the deficit in Guillain-Barré syndrome begins in the feet and/or hands and progresses proximally. In the case of stroke, involvement of the face, arm and leg on one side suggest a lesion in the internal capsule, whereas if the face alone is involved (or the face and arm), the lesion is more likely to be cortical • Bilateral weakness, such as a paraparesis, is unlikely to be the result of a stroke • Ask about a past history of stroke, heart disease, hypertension, diabetes or hyperlipidaemia • Look for associated symptoms such as headache, mental clouding, nausea or vomiting, speech disturbance • A history of sudden-onset of occipital or retro-orbital headache, particularly if preceded by episodes of headache over the previous few days or weeks, is suspicious of subarachnoid haemorrhage *even if there is no neck stiffness.*

Examination • If consciousness is impaired, assess conscious level formally using the GCS (p 417) • If the patient appears to have intracranial disease (such as stroke), assess orientation (day, month, year, place) and check for the presence of dysphasia, both receptive (obeying simple commands) and expressive (naming objects) • When testing for receptive dysphasia, do not demonstrate by gesture what you want the patient to do – the whole point is to assess his/her language abilities! • Examine the nervous system carefully, including sensory testing and the level of any boundary between normal and abnormal sensation • In the case of patients with *stroke*, check BP and examine for the presence of carotid bruits and cardiac murmurs • *Make sure you have checked for the presence of a gag reflex*; if at all possible the adequacy of the patient's swallowing should be assessed by a speech therapist • If the patient appears to have spinal cord disease, check perianal sensation and do a rectal examination to check sphincter tone.

Investigations and management

Stroke patients: • check blood count, ESR, U&E and glucose, ECG • ask for a sickle test in black subjects • if the patient is anything other than mildly ill, these tests will need to be done urgently • CXR can be ordered routinely • syphilis serology is ordered by some teams: check with your consultant • skull X-ray should be requested if there is a history of trauma • further investigations should include CT scan (within 24 hours of onset of symptoms), ECG, carotid artery Doppler scans, serum lipids, tests for an abnormal clotting tendency such as lupus anticoagulant or factor V Leiden, ANA and other tests for vasculitis • cerebellar haemorrhage can be a cause of brain-stem compression and raised ICP requiring urgent surgery - if a stroke patient with cerebellar signs starts to deteriorate, he/she will require an urgent

CT scan and/or neurosurgical opinion • fluid should be replaced orally if possible but only if the patient has a gag reflex and can be seen to swallow water without problems • feeding does not need to be instituted immediately but can wait until the patient can swallow or until it is clear that nasogastric feeding will be necessary. If in doubt, consult the speech therapist • good nursing care and physiotherapy are important to prevent pressure sores and contractures and to encourage mobilization. It is unwise, therefore, to lodge disabled patients with stroke on non-medical wards • patients who are incontinent of urine may need to be catheterized in order to prevent damage to the skin • patients with stroke may benefit from aspirin or anti-coagulation but these should be started only after a CT scan has been done to exclude a haemorrhage as the cause of the stroke: for this reason it is routine practice in most hospitals for all stroke patients (except those who are likely to die quickly) to have a CT scan • if haemorrhage has been excluded and the patient is in sinus rhythm, give aspirin 75–150 mg daily plus dipyridamole as Persantin Retard, 200 mg bd • for patients in atrial fibrillation there is now good evidence that warfarin reduces future stroke risk substantially, so such patients should be treated with warfarin; this is usually started about 1–2 weeks after the stroke, as early anticoagulation carries the risk of bleeding into the infarct. If warfarin is contra-indicated consider aspirin, 300 mg daily, plus dipyridamole. While waiting for a decision about aspirin and/or warfarin, put the patient on sc heparin or LMW heparin • hypertension should be treated if it is persistent, but BP should not be lowered rapidly unless it is causing a major problem such as papilloedema or cardiac failure. If you are tempted to lower BP rapidly, *consult a more senior colleague first*.

Encephalitis: • as well as routine blood tests, blood cultures, etc, you should ask for a CT scan and an EEG • lumbar puncture should be performed: the typical findings are a raised cell count (mononuclear cells), normal CSF glucose (ie more than 50% of the blood glucose) and raised protein of 0.4–0.8 g/l. Detection of *Herpes simplex* viral antigen in the CSF is available in some hospitals • treatment: aciclovir 10 mg/kg iv every 8 hours for 10 days.

Demyelination: • the most helpful investigation is an MRI scan to look for plaques • visual evoked responses may also be helpful and a lumbar puncture is usually performed to look for oligoclonal immunoglobulin bands in the CSF • treatment should be decided by a neurologist but may include steroids or ACTH • patients with disability will require full supportive care including physiotherapy and occupational therapy, bladder catheterization where appropriate, etc.

Spinal cord disorders: • X-rays of the cervical, dorsal or lumbar spine should be ordered as required • for more detailed imaging, MRI scanning is the investigation of choice • management will depend on the cause; remember, however, that *acute-onset* paraparesis is a *neurosurgical emergency*: improvement will occur only if the spinal cord is decompressed within a few hours of the onset • therefore in such a case, contact your SHO or registrar with a view to urgent neurosurgical referral.

Peripheral neuropathy: • check serum B_{12} and folate and consider tests for rare disorders such as blood lead level, porphyrin screen, etc (Table 16.29) • lumbar puncture should be performed in suspected Guillain-Barré syndrome: the CSF may be normal initially; later on the typical findings are of a raised CSF protein (> 1 gm/l) but with a normal cell count • if Guillain-Barré syndrome is suspected the greatest risk to the patient is from respiratory failure • therefore, although treatment is largely supportive with physiotherapy and nursing care, these patients must be monitored regularly by means of vital capacity measurements or blood gases; mechanical ventilation is occasionally needed • as in any case of immobilization, these patients should receive sc heparin or LMW equivalent.

Diabetic mononeuritis: this requires no specific treatment other than strict control of blood glucose, which may require starting the patient on insulin • if the patient has an oculomotor weakness with diplopia, refer to an orthoptist • if a foot drop is present, refer for physiotherapy and consider the provision of a splint • the patient should be warned that it may take up to 3 months for the weakness to resolve.

ANAEMIA

Although anaemia has many causes, the most common in the UK in adults are:

- iron deficiency due to menstrual losses with inadequate replacement
- anaemia of chronic disease (eg rheumatoid arthritis, cancer, chronic inflammation)
- iron deficiency due to a colonic carcinoma
- oesophagitis secondary to a hiatus hernia.

Peptic ulcer is an uncommon cause of anaemia as such, though it is of course a common cause of haematemesis. Other important but less common causes of anaemia include pernicious anaemia, bone marrow dyscrasias (aplastic anaemia, leukaemia, etc), haemoglobinopathies (thalassaemia in Asian and Mediterranean people and sickle-cell disease in black people), blood-loss due to inflammatory bowel disease, malabsorption (especially coeliac disease), gastric carcinoma and chronic renal failure. Dietary deficiency is a rare cause of anaemia in the UK, except perhaps in the elderly (combined iron and folate deficiency). Haemolytic diseases are also rare as causes of anaemia.

History • Take a detailed menstrual history in any woman of reproductive years or who is within 2 years of the menopause • Ask about appetite, abdominal pain, nausea and vomiting • Ask about bowel habit and changes in habit, also about the character of the stool • Ask about weight-loss.

Examination • Look especially for evidence of weight-loss or abnormal bruising • Check for lymphadenopathy • In the abdomen, check for enlargement of liver or spleen and for any masses • Make sure to perform a rectal examination: it is *negligent* not to do this.

Investigations

Full blood count and ESR: • a low mean corpuscular volume (MCV) and mean corpuscular haemoglobin concentration (MCHC) usually indicate iron deficiency, though the anaemia of chronic disease may also sometimes be hypochromic • conversely, anaemia resulting from blood loss may be normochromic in the early stages and people with combined iron and folate deficiency (eg the elderly) may have normal red cell indices; the anaemia of chronic disease is usually normochromic • macrocytosis (high MCV) is often a sign of B_{12} or folate deficiency but can also occur with liver disease, alcohol abuse, hypothyroidism and occasionally in other circumstances such as haemolytic states • the blood count and film may give a clue to other diagnoses such as haemolysis or leukaemia • the ESR will show a progressive rise with greater degrees of anaemia but very high values (over 100) suggest a collagen-vascular disease (think of temporal arteritis/polymyalgia rheumatica in older patients) or malignancy.

Haematinics: • send samples for: • serum ferritin or iron and total iron-binding capacity (TIBC) • serum B_{12} and folate • red cell folate • if haemolysis is suspected, send blood for LFTs, reticulocyte count, haptoglobins and Coombs' test • if a haemoglobinopathy is suspected, ask for HbA_2 and F, sickle test and Hb electrophoresis • it is also wise to discuss the case with your local haematologist.

Radiology/lower GI endoscopy: • colonoscopy or a barium enema is essential in any patient who might have a colonic carcinoma • if a barium enema is to be done then, prior to the X-ray, a sigmoidoscopy should be performed to check the lowest 10 cm of the rectum to ensure that there is not a stenosing lesion which would render a barium enema dangerous • if malabsorption or Crohn's disease is suspected, a small bowel meal or small bowel enema might be appropriate • discuss the exact requirement with the X-ray department or a more senior colleague • all men over 50 and all post-menopausal women, if presenting with unexplained anaemia, have a carcinoma of the colon until proved otherwise • oral iron should be withheld for a week before barium enema or colonoscopy as it makes the stool sticky and it is then very hard to achieve good bowel preparation.

Upper GI endoscopy: • this is the preferred method for investigating the upper gastrointestinal (GI) tract. It is at least as accurate as radiology and allows lesions to be biopsied • in older patients, beware of attributing the anaemia to peptic ulceration or oesophagitis. These may well co-exist with a more sinister lesion in the colon.

Biopsy: • request an endoscopic small bowel (usually duodenal) biopsy if coeliac disease is suspected • aspiration and/or biopsy of bone marrow is indicated in suspected pernicious anaemia or bone marrow dyscrasias • if you are unsure whether there is an indication for bone marrow examination in a particular case, ask your local haematologist.

Other tests • in suspected pernicious anaemia or in a patient with B_{12} deficiency of unknown cause, a test of B_{12} absorption, such as a Schilling test, is required • you should also ask for an auto-antibody screen with particular reference to gastric parietal cells, intrinsic factor and thyroid antigens.

Management box

This will depend on the underlying cause: it is rarely possible to justify blood transfusion without a diagnosis of the cause of the anaemia.

▶ **Iron** This should almost always be given orally and usually as ferrous sulphate tablets. Side-effects, such as abdominal discomfort and constipation, are dose-related so that the precise formulation is unimportant; however, a once-daily preparation may be useful in the elderly to aid compliance, while in those who have trouble swallowing tablets, a syrup may be prescribed. Treatment should continue until the haemoglobin level is normal and for about 3 months thereafter to replenish body iron stores. Where a patient is severely intolerant of oral iron or compliance is a major problem, a total-dose intravenous infusion may be given. This must be undertaken with care, beginning with a test dose, and under medical supervision with facilities to hand to treat anaphylaxis (→ p 455).

→

- Oral iron should be withheld for a week before barium enema or colonoscopy as it makes the stool sticky and it is then very hard to achieve good bowel preparation.
- The Hb does not rise any more quickly after intramuscular or intravenous iron than with oral iron therapy.
- **Vitamin B$_{12}$** This is given intramuscularly in a dose of 0.25–1 mg of hydroxocobalamin every other day for 1–2 weeks, then 250g weekly until the blood count is normal, followed by 1 mg every 2–3 months. In a patient with severe B$_{12}$-deficiency anaemia the myocardium is abnormal due to a sort of 'B$_{12}$-deficient cardiomyopathy'; when treatment with B$_{12}$ is started the serum potassium will fall rapidly, so regular measurements of serum potassium, and supplements of potassium, are essential.
- **Folic acid** This is given orally, usually in a dose of 5 mg daily. If a patient has, or might have, B$_{12}$ deficiency as well as folate deficiency, he/she must be given a dose of vitamin B$_{12}$ before starting folic acid, to avoid possible neurological complications of B$_{12}$ deficiency.
- **Blood transfusion** ($\rightarrow$ also p 519) In the treatment of anaemia, as distinct from acute blood loss, transfusion is indicated if the patient has symptoms from his/her anaemia or the Hb is less than 8 g/dl. You should take all necessary blood samples for investigations before transfusing the patient. Replacement of blood should normally be with packed red cells, aiming to bring the Hb level up to around 10–11 g/dl. Each unit of blood will raise the Hb level by about 1 g/dl. In the elderly or in someone with heart failure, give 20 mg of furosemide (frusemide) with each alternate unit of packed cells in order to avoid fluid overload. Patients with pernicious anaemia should **not** be transfused as they are very sensitive to fluid overloading and because transfusion may cause the bone marrow to 'shut down'. In chronic renal failure, transfusion is not usually necessary unless the Hb is less than 7 g/dl and also carries a high risk of fluid overload. Consult a more senior colleague.

RENAL IMPAIRMENT OR POOR URINE OUTPUT

A poor urine output and/or renal function is particularly likely in association with:

- pre-existing renal disease
- widespread atherosclerosis
- diabetes
- recent surgery
- dehydration

- hypotension or a poor cardiac output
- nephrotoxic drugs such as gentamicin, gold, penicillamine, cytotoxic drugs, paracetamol, tetracyclines
- septicaemia and DIC
- bladder or pelvic tumours (including prostate).

The problem will usually declare itself in the form of a rising urea or creatinine or an evident fall-off in urine output: a healthy person should pass more than 30 ml urine/hour. Sometimes it may be noticed because of progressive symptoms (drowsiness, apathy, anorexia, nausea, oedema). When faced with a patient whose urine output/renal function are deteriorating, the normal diagnostic process is reversed, as the priorities are:

- to assess the causes and treatment of the *immediate* deterioration
- to consider underlying causes of renal impairment.

Management box

▶ Immediate management → Table 16.30.
▶ Management of acute renal failure → Chapter 17, p 473.

Table 16.30
Management of renal impairment or poor urine output

Question	Action
Is the patient dehydrated?	• Assess skin turgor, venous pressure and BP, lying and standing or lying and sitting: if the systolic pressure falls by more than 20 mmHg (more than 10 mm going from lying to sitting) or falls below 100 mmHg when the patient stands up, this is good evidence of volume depletion
	• If the patient appears to be dehydrated and the risk of provoking pulmonary oedema is low, it is reasonable to give a fluid challenge in the form of 250 ml normal saline over a few minutes, under constant supervision; if there is no clinical deterioration the process may be repeated

Table 16.30
Management of renal impairment or poor urine output
(Cont'd)

Question	Action
	• If there is postural hypotension, give a unit of plasma expander (Haemaccel, Gelofusin)
	• Look for other treatable causes of hypotension ($\rightarrow$ pp 470–471)
	• If blood loss has occurred (remember to check drains if the patient has had a recent operation) replace with whole blood (not packed cells)
Is there outflow obstruction?	• Examine the abdomen to see if the bladder is distended
	• Perform a rectal examination
	• Catheterize the patient (pp 495–497) so that urine flow can be measured; if the patient is already catheterized ask nursing staff to wash the catheter out to check that it is not blocked
	• Ask for a plain KUB X-ray to look for stones
	• Consider an ultrasound scan to look for evidence of obstruction
Is the patient receiving any nephrotoxic drugs?	• Review admission drug history and the current prescription sheet
Is the patient septicaemic?	• Review history and examination
	• Take blood for culture if pyrexial
	• Check coagulation screen, platelet count and fibrinogen titre (or D-dimer)
Is the patient hyperkalaemic?	• If serum potassium is > 5.5 mmol, give calcium resonium by mouth or by enema and do an ECG
	• If > 6.5 mmol, see pp 409 and 475 and *inform your SHO or registrar*

Table 16.30
Management of renal impairment or poor urine output (Cont'd)

Question	Action
Is there any evidence of underlying renal disease or nephropathic illness?	• Ask about previous kidney diseases, haematuria, hypertension • Consider myeloma in the elderly • Consider hypercalcaemia, especially in patients with malignancy

ELECTROLYTE IMBALANCE

ACIDOSIS

Acidosis, the presence of excessive hydrogen ions in body fluids, can be divided into two varieties: respiratory and metabolic (Fig. 16.2).

Respiratory acidosis
This occurs due to accumulation of CO_2 secondary to reduced respiratory clearance. Causes include COPD, sedatives, CVA, chronic lung disease, airway obstruction, severe acute asthma and neuromuscular disease.

Clinical features Include confusion, vasodilatation with warm peripheries, papilloedema and asterixis.

> *Management box*
> ▶ Improve ventilation by treatment of bronchospasm or airways obstruction, reversal of sedation or neuromuscular relaxants. Intubation and artificial ventilation may be required in severe cases.

Metabolic acidosis
This is due to reduction in bicarbonate ions in body fluids usually due to neutralization of bicarbonate by acids such as lactic acid or ketones or exogenous substances such as salicylates, ethylene glycol or ethanol. In such circumstances an increased anion gap $(Na-(Cl+HCO_3))$ <12 mmol/l exists. In certain

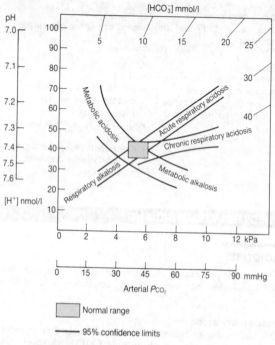

Fig. 16.2 Acid-base diagram.

circumstances metabolic acidosis exists with a normal anion gap and is due to loss of HCO_3 from the renal or GI tract.

Clinical features Hyperventilation, shock, nausea, vomiting, anorexia and coma.

Management box

▶ Correct the underlying abnormality such as diarrhoea, ketoacidosis, or renal failure by treating dehydration with iv fluids and instituting dialysis or insulin therapy whichever is appropriate.

▶ In only a minority of situations where acidosis is severe (pH < 7.1) should bicarbonate treatment (1.26%) be considered and only the minimum administered to correct the acidosis (ie raise pH to > 7.2).

→

▶ During the administration of HCO_3 the serum K falls and should be closely monitored.
▶ Administration of 8.4% HCO_3 is indicated only during cardiac arrest.

ALKALOSIS

Respiratory alkalosis

Respiratory ventilation over and above that required to remove CO_2 will result in respiratory alkalosis by reducing $PaCO_2$. The causes are listed in Table 16.31. A mixed picture of metabolic acidosis and respiratory alkalosis is common in sepsis, salicylate poisoning and hepatic failure.

Clinical features • Rapid deep respiration, tetany, paraesthesia particularly perioral and peripheral, light-headedness and collapse.

Metabolic alkalosis

An increase in serum HCO_3 usually occurs due to loss of acid from the stomach or renal tract. Volume contraction due to excessive diuretic administration results in alkalosis as does hypokalaemia by increasing HCO_3 reabsorption. Excessive

Management box
▶ This should be directed towards the cause.
▶ Sedation or rebreathing into a paper bag should be considered in those with psychogenic hyperventilation.

Table 16.31
Causes of respiratory alkalosis

Acute	• hyperventilation
	• CNS disorders: trauma, infection, CNS tumours, CVA
	• salicylates
	• heat stroke
	• fever, sepsis
Chronic	• all of the above
	• pregnancy
	• hepatic encephalopathy
	• severe anaemia
	• long-term residence at high altitudes

mineralocorticoids, either endogenous or exogenous results in metabolic alkalosis.

Clinical features • Usually non-specific • Tetany, neuromuscular excitability, lethargy and delirium occur in acute, severe cases.

Management box
▸ Again treat the underlying cause, eg pyloric obstruction, potassium supplementation or stop overzealous diuretic administration.
▸ Occasionally administration of acidic fluids containing ammonium chloride 70 mmol/l may be indicated.

HYPERCALCAEMIA

The physiologically important calcium in blood is the ionized form but this is rarely assayed. The total calcium when associated with hypoalbuminaemia should be corrected by adding 0.1 mmol/l to the calcium for every 5 g/l the albumin is below 40 g/l.

Aetiology • Over 90% of cases are due to primary hyperparathyroidism or malignancy, eg squamous cell bronchial carcinoma • Most tumour-related hypercalcaemia is caused by a peptide with PTH-like activity, although bone metastases and rarely ectopic PTH may be responsible • Other causes of hypercalcaemia include sarcoidosis, thyrotoxicosis, Addison's disease, milk-alkali syndrome, Paget's disease (if immobilized) and iatrogenic (vitamin D therapy and drugs, eg thiazides).

Clinical features • Often asymptomatic, discovered on biochemical screening • Weakness, constipation, confusion, anorexia, renal colic, polyuria, nocturia, polydipsia and proximal myopathy.

Investigations • Ionized calcium if available • Serum calcium and albumin • Skeletal survey • Isotopic bone scan • 24-hour urinary calcium • PTH assay • Parathyroid US or selective cervical vein canalization with PTH assay • Screen for malignancy.

Management box
▸ Mild hypercalcaemia responds well to oral phosphate 1–2 g/day but may cause diarrhoea.
▸ Moderate or severe hypercalcaemia should be treated with iv fluids (6–8 l/day); potassium supplements are usually required.
▸ Intravenous diphosphonates (ie pamidronate 30–90 mg) is effective for hypercalcaemia of malignancy.

→

▶ Hypercalcaemia due to myeloma, sarcoidosis or vitamin D excess is responsive to prednisolone 20–40 mg/day.
▶ Additional therapy with iv furosemide (frusemide), and phosphates may be needed.
▶ Treatment of the underlying disease may reverse the hypercalcaemia.

HYPERKALAEMIA

A serum potassium above 5.5 mmol/l represents a medical emergency and may be due to impaired potassium excretion, eg acute renal failure, potassium-sparing diuretics in those with renal impairment, ACE inhibitors, hypoaldosteronism, adrenal insufficiency, excessive potassium intake in those with renal impairment or imbalance in internal potassium balance, eg diabetic keto-acidosis, haemolysis and rhabdomyolysis.

Clinical features • Often asymptomatic • Muscle weakness may be present but the most important features are cardiac with arrhythmias and conduction defects leading to asystole.

Investigations • Serum potassium • ABG analysis • ECG • Creatinine clearance • Urinary potassium excretion • Low urinary excretion in those with hyperkalaemia suggests renal failure, normal excretion hypoaldosteronism and high excretion tissue potassium leakage.

Management box
▶ Attach a cardiac monitor.
▶ If there are ECG changes (bradycardia; tall, peaked T-waves, widened QRS complexes), give 10 ml of 10% calcium gluconate iv immediately, followed by iv glucose and insulin (see below).
▶ For all patients with serum K > 6.5 mmol/l, whether ECG is abnormal or not, give iv injection of 50 g of glucose plus 15 units of soluble insulin, continue with iv infusion of 10% or 20% glucose (if you have good venous access), plus iv insulin, adjusted according to hourly measurements of blood sugar.
▶ Then *inform your SHO or registrar.*
▶ Identification and treatment of the cause, such as removal of spironolactone in those with moderate renal impairment, is essential.

HYPOKALAEMIA

A serum potassium (< 3.5 mmol/l) may result from excessive renal loss, eg diuretic therapy or magnesium deficiency, GI loss, eg diarrhoea, vomiting, metabolic imbalance such as occurs in alkalosis, insulin therapy or in periodic paralysis, and endocrine causes such as hyperaldosteronism, Bartter's syndrome or Cushing's syndrome (severe hypokalaemia with ectopic ACTH).

Clinical features • Muscular weakness • Polyuria • ECG changes with U-waves and flattened T-waves • Ileus.

Investigations • Serum potassium • 24-hour urinary potassium (if low suggests low intake or GI losses cf a high output which indicates a renal cause or hyperaldosteronism) • ECG.

> *Management box*
> ▶ Treat the underlying cause such as vomiting.
> ▶ Discontinue diuretic therapy or supplement with KCl or a potassium-sparing diuretic.
> ▶ If hypokalaemia is severe, or if vomiting precludes oral potassium supplements, iv KCl should be administered but at a rate not to exceed 20 mmol/hour.

HYPONATRAEMIA

Clinically significant hyponatraemia usually means a serum sodium concentration of less than 130 mmol/l. Problems become more severe when the serum sodium is less than 125, potentially critical when it is less than 120 and life-threatening below 115.

Causes Hyponatraemia may be spurious, eg blood taken downstream from a glucose drip! Causes of true hyponatraemia can be grouped according to whether there is overall hyper-volaemia, normovolaemia or hypovolaemia, as follows:

Hypervolaemic • cirrhosis of the liver • congestive cardiac failure • nephrotic syndrome • psychogenic polydipsia (uncommon) • in these conditions urinary sodium concentration is low (< 10 mmol/l).

Hypovolaemic • diuretics, especially thiazides, amiloride or spironolactone • excessive salt-loss, eg renal disease (especially after relief of lower urinary tract obstruction) • diarrhoea • loss from gastrointestinal stomas or fistulae • adrenal insufficiency (primary or secondary) – the hyponatraemia is not usually severe, ie serum sodium is usually >120 mmol/l • blood loss with inappropriate crystalloid replacement • with diarrhoea, fistula loss or blood loss urinary sodium will be low • with adrenal insufficiency, diuretic therapy or after relief of urinary tract obstruction urinary sodium will be high (> 20 mmol/l).

Normovolaemic • inappropriate ADH secretion, often referred to as SIADH (Table 16.32) • drugs, especially antidepressants, also chlorpropamide, carbamazepine, phenothiazines, ACE inhibitors (some of these cause SIADH) • some cases of adrenal insufficiency • pseudohyponatraemia secondary to hyper-lipidaemia (rare) • with these causes urinary sodium is usually high.

History • Ask especially: • How long has the patient been unwell? • Any history of previous renal disease/urinary tract obstruction? • What drugs has he/she been taking?

Physical examination Check for: • Level of consciousness/alertness (→ Glasgow Coma Scale, p 417) • Whether the patient is over- or under-hydrated • Blood pressure, including change

Table 16.32
Causes of SIADH

Carcinoma of lung
Numerous other malignancies, eg lymphoma, Ca prostate or
   pancreas
Cerebral causes
  cerebral abscess
  meningitis/encephalitis
  subarachnoid haemorrhage
  subdural haematoma
  cerebral tumour
  post-operative
Pulmonary causes
  pneumonia
  lung abscess
  tuberculosis
Drugs
  tricyclic antidepressants
  SSRIs
  carbamazepine
  chlorpropamide
  phenothiazines
  cytotoxic drugs: cyclophosphamide, vincristine
Others
  hypothyroidism

from lying to sitting: a drop in systolic pressure of more than 10 mmHg or to a pressure less than 100 mm is significant (Table 16.29) • Focal signs in the chest • Focal neurological signs.

Investigations • CXR • If the patient is fluid overloaded, check LFTs and serum magnesium • If the patient is not fluid overloaded, take blood for random serum cortisol (can be stored and analysed later if the patient is admitted out of hours), blood for magnesium estimation (potassium and magnesium depletion enhance ADH release), plasma and urine osmolality and urine for sodium concentration (these last two will be high if the patient has recently been on diuretics) • In SIADH the plasma osmolality will be reduced (<280 mOsm/kg), urine osmolality will be >200 and the urinary Na concentration will be >20 mmol/l • These measurements are only reliable if the patient is not dehydrated, not hypoadrenal and has not recently received diuretics • As soon as is convenient (ie not in the middle of the night), and provided the patient is not on treatment with hydrocortisone, do a short tetracosactrin (Synacthen) test (→ p 487) • A peak cortisol level of more than 600 nmol/l, with a rise from 0–30 mins of >330 nmol/l, excludes primary and secondary adrenal insufficiency.

Management box

▶ If there is a possibility of adrenal insufficiency, give iv hydrocortisone, 100 mg 6-hourly, together with iv normal saline, 1 l 8-hourly, with supplementary potassium. You can always stop the hydrocortisone later if the diagnosis of adrenal insufficiency is discarded.

▶ Withdraw any potentially responsible drugs.

▶ If the patient is dehydrated and/or hypotensive, give iv normal saline, with supplementary potassium.

▶ If the patient is not dehydrated and has mild to moderate hyponatraemia without serious neurological impairment (serum sodium usually > 120) the treatment of choice is fluid restriction to a total of 750–1000 ml per 24 hours. If this is ineffective or the patient finds it very uncomfortable, selective water diuresis can be encouraged by giving demeclocycline, 300 mg tid • If the hyponatraemia is more severe (serum sodium < 120) OR the patient is more severely ill, ie there is marked depression of consciousness or fits, consider iv hypertonic (1.8%) saline. This treatment must be given carefully, as there is said to be a risk of damage to myelin sheaths in the brain stem (central pontine myelinolysis) from the resultant osmotic changes, so *consult your SHO or registrar* • There is little point in giving furosemide (frusemide) in order to remove water as this usually results in at least as much sodium loss as water excretion. Give furosemide (frusemide) only if there is generalized fluid overload.

HIRSUTISM

Hirsutism means excessive growth of body hair in a woman, in a pattern which is more typical of a man (face, thighs, abdomen, between the breasts). There is often a fear that removal of the hair, especially by shaving, will accelerate hair growth or make the hair coarser. The normal spectrum of hair growth in women is quite wide and body hair is obviously more noticeable if it is dark. There is a greater natural tendency to body-hair growth in women from certain ethnic groups, ie those of Mediterranean or Indo-Asian origin (→ also Ch. 13, p 312).

Causes (→ Table 16.33) At one end of the spectrum are women with excessive body consciousness, whose degree and extent of body hair growth is normal but who are unhappy with their lot; these women usually have no other clinical features of endocrine disorder. Women with idiopathic hirsutism have abnormal hair growth but fairly regular periods while those with polycystic ovary syndrome (PCOS) have oligo- or amenorrhoea. At the other end of the spectrum are women who have severe endocrine disturbance with features of *virilization*: male-pattern baldness, clitoral enlargement, masculine pattern of muscle development, deepening of the voice.

Table 16.33
Causes of hirsutism

Common	Idiopathic hirsutism, polycystic ovary syndrome, drugs (cyclosporin, danazol, phenytoin, minoxidil, progestagens), excessive body consciousness
Less common	Cushing's syndrome, late-onset congenital adrenal hyperplasia
Rare	Ovarian hyperthecosis, tumours of ovary, adrenal carcinoma, disorders of sexual differentiation
Adrenal	Cushing's syndrome, virilizing tumours, congenital adrenal hyperplasia
Pituitary	Acromegaly
Ovarian	Polycystic disease, virilizing tumours, gonadal dysgenesis
Turner's syndrome	
Iatrogenic	Due to androgenic drugs
Idiopathic	Target organ hypersensitivity

History • Duration of the problem • Menstrual history (amenorrhoea or severe oligomenorrhoea suggests PCOS or a more severe endocrine abnormality) • Weight gain (a feature of PCOS and Cushing's syndrome) • Drug history • Are there any features of virilization?

Examination   • Extent of body-hair growth • Is the hair fine or coarse? • Are there any clinical features to suggest Cushing's syndrome? • External genitalia – is there clitoral enlargement?

Investigations • Almost all patients should have a measurement of serum testosterone, SHBG (sex-hormone-binding globulin), FSH and LH • In idiopathic hirsutism and PCOS the serum testosterone is high-normal or slightly raised and SHBG is low • In PCOS the FSH is usually normal but LH is often high, with a LH:FSH ratio of 2:1 or greater • Patients with PCOS are often obese and usually insulin-resistant so the urine should be checked for glucose or a random blood glucose should be estimated • Ovarian ultrasound may support the diagnosis of PCOS, however, many teenage girls and young women have multi-cystic ovaries on scan without having PCOS • If Cushing's syndrome is suspected, ask for 24-hour urine cortisol and arrange an overnight dexamethasone suppression test (p 189) • If the patient is under 25, especially if there are any features of virilization, consider late-onset congenital adrenal hyperplasia or a disorder of sexual differentiation – such patients should have blood taken for karyotyping and for a 9 am measurement of 17-hydroxyprogesterone and should be referred to an endocrinologist • If there is virilization in an older subject, consider adrenal or ovarian tumours – ask for ovarian ultrasound/pelvic CT/CT of adrenals.

Management box

▶ Treat specific cause if found, eg withdrawal of any offending drugs.

▶ For idiopathic hirsutism cosmetic measures and reassurance may be enough, otherwise use Dianette (a combination of oestrogen with cyproterone, an anti-androgen) or spironolactone (caution: an unlicensed indication; metabolic products of the drug cause tumours in rodents).

▶ For PCOS, Dianette or spironolactone can again be used.

▶ There is increasing interest in the possibility that insulin-sensitizing drugs may help in the treatment of idiopathic hirsutism and PCOS.

▶ In difficult cases or if infertility is an issue, refer to an endo-crinologist or infertility clinic.

17

Medical emergencies

416

CONFUSION AND COMA

Science basics Confusion is an impairment in the thought processes, while coma and stupor are abnormalities in the level of consciousness. The two patterns of abnormality not infrequently exist in the same patient. Many patients with severe illnesses become confused, which commonly makes their assessment and management more difficult. In the elderly relatively minor illnesses may make the patient confused and care must be taken to look for a cause and not label the individual 'demented'. The history from relatives or neighbours is invaluable in the assessment of confused or comatose patients. Treatment of such patients should be made with a clear understanding of the likely underlying disorder and blanket sedation should be avoided.

Confusion

Aetiology • Infection (may be occult especially in the elderly) • Alcohol abuse – delirium tremens is the most severe form and is relatively unusual • Metabolic – hypo- and hyperglycaemia, uraemia, hypo- and hyperthroidism, hypercalcaemia • Drugs, especially sedatives • Hypoxaemia • Hypotension • Subdural haematoma • Night-time disorientation • Deafness • Dementia.

Coma

Aetiology • Hypoglycaemia – sweaty, tachycardia, fits • Hyperglycaemia – less often comatose, dehydrated, air-hunger • Head injury • Post-ictal • CVA especially cerebral haemorrhage • Drugs • Hepatic failure • Hysteria.

A formal assessment of the level of consciousness should be performed to allow changes to be identified. The Glasgow coma scale is the best known and has prognostic significance (Table 17.1).

Table 17.1
Glasgow coma scale

Score	Motor response	Verbal response	Eye opening
6	Obeys simple commands	–	–
5	Attempts to remove source of painful stimuli to head or trunk	Orientated	–

Table 17.1
Glasgow coma scale (*Cont'd*)

Score	Motor response	Verbal response	Eye opening
4	Attempts to withdraw from source of pain	Disorientated	Eyes open
3	Flexes arm at elbow and wrist in response to nail bed pressure	Random speech	Open to speech
2	Extends arms at elbow and wrist in response to nail bed pressure	Mumbling	Open to pain
1	No motor response to painful stimuli	No speech	No opening

Add the individual scores: best = 15, worst = 3.

The investigation and treatment of certain of these causes of coma is described under the appropriate section. Irrespective of the cause the adequacy of ventilation should be ensured by ABG and assisted ventilation introduced when necessary.

CARDIORESPIRATORY ARREST

Science basics This should be recognized in a patient who has collapsed without respiratory effort and in whom the carotid or femoral pulses are absent. The brain suffers irreversible damage within minutes of circulatory failure and throughout resuscitation an adequate cardiac output should be maintained.

Management box
- After diagnosing a cardiac arrest, call for assistance.
- If a monitor and defibrillator are not immediately available, commence basic life-support.
- Clear airway of vomit, foreign objects, etc.
- Open airway by the dual manoeuvres of head tilt and chin lift.
- *Breathing* Commence mouth-to-mouth or mask-to-mouth ventilation ensuring the chest rises with each breath. Use of a →

self-inflating bag and valve to ventilate allows the delivery of high-flow oxygen, especially with a reservoir bag attached. Laryngoscopy should only be attempted by the experienced and should take no longer than 30 seconds. With two resuscitators present one ventilation should be given to five chest compressions.

▶ *Circulation* A precordial thump should be given to witnessed or monitored cardiac arrests. Chest compressions (two finger breadths above xiphisternum) should be given at a rate of 80/min.

▶ *Advanced life-support* This assumes the underlying rhythm disturbance can be determined and that intravenous access, drugs, and a defibrillator will be available ($\rightarrow$ Fig. 17.1 p 420).

▶ New Guidelines in Fig. 17.2.

UNSTABLE ANGINA

Science basics This is defined as angina ● of recent onset which is severe ● present with minimal exertion or at rest ● with recent rapid increase in severity and duration or rapid decrease in exercise tolerance. Aggressive management is indicated to reduce the otherwise high risk of infarction.

Management box
▶ Bed-rest.
▶ Aspirin 75–300 mg daily.
▶ Removal of exacerbating factors such as cardiac failure, infection, hypertension, arrhythmias and anaemia.
▶ Maximal therapy with β-blockers, calcium antagonists and nitrates (often intravenous).
▶ Intravenous heparin anticoagulation (APTT-2 × normal), or subcutaneous low molecular weight heparin (ie enoxaparin 1 mg/kg bd).
▶ Anti-platelet drugs such as glycoprotein IIb/IIIa inhibitors may be used in specialized units.
▶ Angiography in those whose pain does not settle, with subsequent options of angioplasty or CABG.

MYOCARDIAL INFARCTION

Science basics Myocardial infarction, death of part of the cardiac muscle, is the commonest cause of death in the UK and affects 1 in 200 people per year.

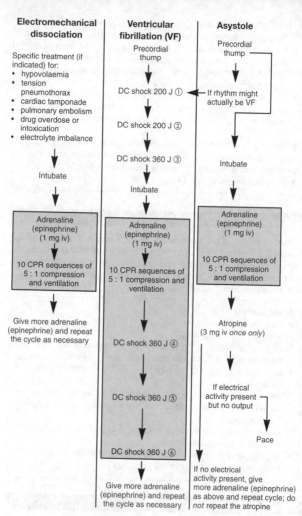

Fig. 17.1 Emergency resuscitation procedure.

Adult Advanced Life Support
1998 guidelines

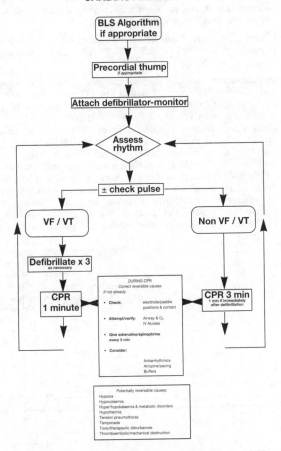

In accordance with the 1998 ERC and Resuscitation Council (UK)
Guidelines for Resuscitation

Fig. 17.2 Adult Advanced Life Support:1998 ERC and
Resuscitation Council (UK) Guidelines.

Clinical features

Symptoms: severe, crushing, central chest pain, often radiating into the neck and down the arms, which is prolonged and not relieved by nitrates. Commonly associated with sweating, nausea, vomiting and dyspnoea. Many infarcts are associated with lesser or no chest pain, the so-called silent infarct.

Signs: pallor, peripheral shut-down, tachycardia, change in BP, cyanosis, gallop rhythm and if LVF exists basal crepitations, raised JVP and S_3.

Investigations   • ECG: classical changes are early ST elevation and T-wave inversion followed by Q-wave development. However ECG may be normal in the early stages • In sub-endocardial (non Q-wave) infarcts ST depression and T-wave changes only occur • Cardiac enzymes – these develop serially: first increases in creatine kinase MB (peaks 18–24 hours), then aspartate transaminase (peaks 24 hours) and lastly lactate dehydrogenase (peaks day 3). None of the enzymes are specific for MI but the pattern of change is highly suggestive. The peak of the creatine kinase rise correlates approximately with the size of the infarct • An elevated troponin level is consistent with myocardial damage and gives useful prognostic information • Thrombolysis therapy may modify the pattern of enzyme

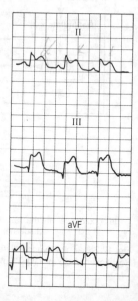

Fig. 17.3   Acute inferior myocardial infarction.

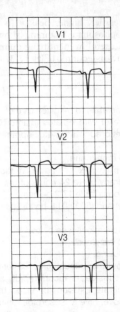

Fig. 17.4 Established anteroseptal myocardial infarction.

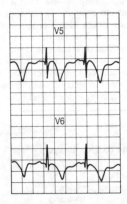

Fig. 17.5 Subendocardial lateral myocardial infarction.

release causing an earlier, higher peak • In cases where doubt exists 99m Tc-pyrophosphate scanning shows the infarct as a 'hot spot' • CXR is useful in identifying pulmonary oedema and a proportion of aortic dissections. (Figs 17.3, 17.4 and 17.5)

Management box

▶ Obtain iv access.
▶ Aspirin (300 mg soluble) to be given as early as possible.
▶ Adequate pain relief with opiates (diamorphine 2.5–5 mg iv, with an anti-emetic such as metoclopramide 10 mg iv) and transfer to CCU.
▶ Continuous ECG monitoring.
▶ Bed-rest and high-flow oxygen administration.
▶ Thrombolytic therapy up to 24 hours of the onset of pain and no contraindications (Table 17.2 below).
▶ Subcutaneous heparin (5000 IU 8-hourly) if iv heparin not given after alteplase.
▶ Look out for complications (see below).
▶ Blood for cardiac enzymes.
▶ Prohibition of smoking.
▶ If pain subsides but then recurs, give further diamorphine.
▶ If pain does not subside, or recurs rapidly after diamorphine, consider an iv nitrate infusion, provided the systolic BP is 100 mmHg or above, give iv isosorbide dinitrate, beginning at 2 mg/hour and increasing until pain is controlled. Do not continue increasing if systolic BP falls below 100 mm.
▶ If initial serum potassium is less than 4.0 mmol/l give an infusion of potassium chloride, 40 mmol diluted in 500 ml of 5% glucose over 4 hours. Use a programmable controller to ensure that the infusion does not run in too quickly.
▶ If the patient develops ventricular ectopics these are likely to cause considerable anxiety to the nursing staff. Do not allow yourself to be persuaded to treat ectopics just because they are frequent or R-on-T in nature. The prognostic value of these features has been grossly exaggerated.

Table 17.2
Contra-indications to thrombolysis

Known bleeding diathesis
Treatment with oral anticoagulants
Recent significant or severe bleeding
CNS disease with risk of bleeding (stroke within last 6 months, intracranial aneurysm, recent spinal surgery)
Unconsciousness without known cause

Table 17.2
Contra-indications to thrombolysis (Cont'd)

Possible aortic dissection
Recent prolonged or traumatic external cardiac massage
Pregnancy or recent delivery
Recent arterial or large vein puncture
Severe uncontrolled arterial hypertension (systolic pressure > 200 mmHg)
Bacterial endocarditis
Pericarditis
Acute pancreatitis
Documented upper GI ulceration during the last three months
Severe liver disease with increased bleeding risk
Major surgery or trauma in last 3 months

Complications

Tachyarrhythmias: sinus tachycardia is common and may be a sign of incipient cardiac failure. AF is not uncommon and is usually adequately treated with digoxin. If cardiovascular collapse develops DC cardioversion is indicated. Ventricular tachycardia requires treatment with iv lignocaine 100 mg over 2 minutes followed by 4 mg/minute initially then reducing slowly over 36 hours. Second-line agents include mexiletine, disopyramide and amiodarone. Cardioversion is indicated for VT if hypotension or heart failure develops and is always immediately indicated for VF.

Bradyarrhythmias: sinus bradycardia and AV block is common following infarction, especially an inferior MI. If it is symptomatic, treatment with atropine is usually sufficient, although insertion of a pacemaker is required for resistant and haemodynamically significant bradycardia. Bradyarrhythmias associated with anterior MI signify major myocardial damage and pacing is indicated for any bradycardia associated with hypotension, and prophylactically for 2nd-degree heart block (Mobitz type II), complete heart block and bifascicular block.

Cardiogenic shock: hypotension with peripheral and renal shut-down is a serious prognostic event following MI. A Swan-Ganz catheter should be inserted and the pulmonary wedge pressure maintained at 15–20 mmHg by vasodilator and inotrope therapy. A right ventricular infarct may cause hypotension with a low LA filling pressure and appropriate fluid replacement may reverse the shock. Inotropic agents are important in increasing cardiac output and tissue perfusion. Any arrhythmia which may make the hypotension worse should be treated, avoiding negatively inotropic agents if possible.

NARROW COMPLEX TACHYARRHYTHMIA

If not already done, give oxygen and establish iv access
Doses based on adult of average body weight

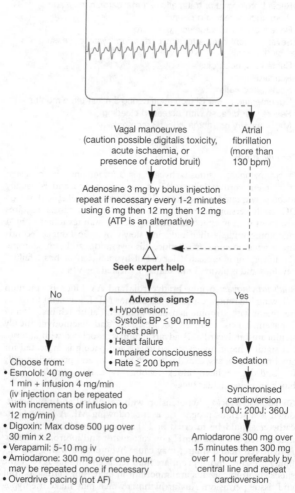

Vagal manoeuvres
(caution possible digitalis toxicity,
acute ischaemia, or
presence of carotid bruit)

Atrial
fibrillation
(more than
130 bpm)

Adenosine 3 mg by bolus injection
repeat if necessary every 1-2 minutes
using 6 mg then 12 mg then 12 mg
(ATP is an alternative)

Seek expert help

No

Adverse signs?
- Hypotension:
  Systolic BP ≤ 90 mmHg
- Chest pain
- Heart failure
- Impaired consciousness
- Rate ≥ 200 bpm

Yes

Choose from:
- Esmolol: 40 mg over
  1 min + infusion 4 mg/min
  (iv injection can be repeated
  with increments of infusion to
  12 mg/min)
- Digoxin: Max dose 500 µg over
  30 min x 2
- Verapamil: 5-10 mg iv
- Amiodarone: 300 mg over one hour,
  may be repeated once if necessary
- Overdrive pacing (not AF)

Sedation

Synchronised
cardioversion
100J: 200J: 360J

Amiodarone 300 mg over
15 minutes then 300 mg
over 1 hour preferably by
central line and repeat
cardioversion

In accordance with the 1998 ERC and Resuscitation Council (UK)
Guidelines for Resuscitation

Fig. 17.6   Narrow complex tachyarrhythmia.

BROAD COMPLEX TACHYARRHYTHMIA

If not already done, give oxygen and establish iv access
Doses based on adult of average body weight

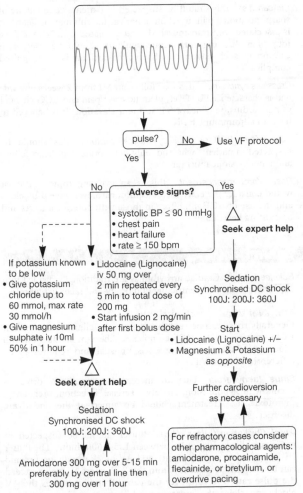

pulse? — No → Use VF protocol

Yes

Adverse signs?

No ← → Yes

Seek expert help

- systolic BP ≤ 90 mmHg
- chest pain
- heart failure
- rate ≥ 150 bpm

If potassium known to be low
- Give potassium chloride up to 60 mmol, max rate 30 mmol/h
- Give magnesium sulphate iv 10ml 50% in 1 hour

- Lidocaine (Lignocaine) iv 50 mg over 2 min repeated every 5 min to total dose of 200 mg
- Start infusion 2 mg/min after first bolus dose

Sedation
Synchronised DC shock
100J: 200J: 360J

Start
- Lidocaine (Lignocaine) +/–
- Magnesium & Potassium
  as opposite

Seek expert help

Further cardioversion as necessary

Sedation
Synchronised DC shock
100J: 200J: 360J

For refractory cases consider other pharmacological agents: amiodarone, procainamide, flecainide, or bretylium, or overdrive pacing

Amiodarone 300 mg over 5-15 min preferably by central line then 300 mg over 1 hour

In accordance with the 1998 ERC and Resuscitation Council (UK)
Guidelines for Resuscitation

Fig. 17.7 Broad complex tachyarrhythmia.

Pulmonary oedema: this is common and is usually responsive to diuretic therapy. If resistant, vasodilators such as iv nitrates should be added and the pulmonary capillary wedge pressure monitored. Occasionally positive pressure ventilation is required.

Pericarditis: this should be suspected in patients complaining of sharp, positional pain in whom a pericardial rub may be heard. It is associated with transmural MI and is treated with NSAIDs (eg ibuprofen 400 mg tid). Anticoagulants should be used with caution in such patients as haemopericardium is a recognized complication.

Dressler's syndrome: this may follow an MI from 2 weeks onwards and is characterized by fever, pleuritic chest pain and ECG changes of pericarditis, ie concave ST segment elevation. It is believed to have an autoimmune basis.

Post infarct VSD or papillary muscle rupture: this should be suspected in patients who suddenly deteriorate with heart failure and a new systolic murmur.

Post infarct management: this is an evolving topic but most would consider the early use of aspirin, cardioselective β-blockers and the use of ACE inhibitors in those with anterior infarcts and co-existing heart failure.

ARRHYTHMIAS

Science basics Cardiac arrhythmias are traditionally divided into supraventricular and ventricular and brady-and tachyarrhythmias.

Supraventricular tachyarrhythmias
Generally these can be recognized from the clinical signs and an ECG showing narrow QRS complexes. Aberrant conduction with widening of the QRS complex is unusual and requires to be differentiated from VT.

Sinus tachycardia Due to increased sympathetic drive as occurs with hypotension, anxiety, exercise, infection, pregnancy, thyrotoxicosis. Treatment should be aimed at the underlying disorder.

Atrial fibrillation/flutter Atrial flutter should be suspected in patients with a regular pulse between 125–160/minute. The flutter (F) waves occur at 300/minute and AV block usually occurs and can be recognized clinically from the JVP where 'a' waves exceed the pulse rate. Pressure over the carotid sinus increases the AV block and slows the pulse rate while pressure is maintained. Atrial fibrillation should be suspected in an individual with an irregular pulse (Fig. 17.8). Carotid sinus compression does not

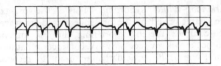

Fig. 17.8 Atrial fibrillation.

influence the heart rate and the 'a' waves are absent from the JVP.

Treatment of acute atrial fibrillation/flutter (<48 hours) aims to achieve sinus rhythm. This may be achieved 'chemically' with intravenous amiodarone (5 mg/kg over 20–120 minutes up to 15 mg/kg for 24 hours) or flecanide (2 mg/kg up to a total dose of 150 mg iv over 10–30 minutes) if there is no evidence of cardiac failure or structural heart disease, or by electrical cardioversion.

Atrial fibrillation/flutter of greater than 48 hours duration (persistent) can be treated with digoxin (see Chapter 19) or β-blockade (atenolol 50–100 mg/day) to slow the ventricular rate. Patients with persistent (>48 hours) atrial fibrillation/flutter should be considered for electrical cardioversion only after 4 weeks of anticoagulation and the anticoagulation continued for 4 weeks thereafter. Digoxin should be withheld before electrical cardioversion.

Permanent atrial fibrillation/flutter should be rate controlled with digoxin.

Paroxysmal atrial fibrillation/flutter may be treated with β-blockade (atenolol 50–100 mg/day), sotalol, or propafenone.

Anti-coagulation should be considered in all patients presenting with acute or chronic atrial fibrillation/flutter. It is particularly indicated if there is evidence of valvular heart disease, an enlarged left atrium, left ventricular dysfunction, or a history of thromboembolic cerebrovascular disease.

Paroxysmal supraventricular tachycardia This disorder is characterized by episodes of atrial or nodal tachycardia, with a heart rate of 140–220/minute, which may be self-limiting or require treatment. There is often a past history of arrhythmias or palpitations. In a minority, pre-excitation syndromes such as Wolff-Parkinson-White or Lown-Ganong-Levine (short PR interval without the delta wave) syndrome can be identified. The patient can often be taught to treat their own attacks by the Valsalva manoeuvre. Carotid sinus pressure frequently terminates an attack. In others treatment with intravenous adenosine, verapamil or β-blocker may be required or, more rarely, cardioversion. Prophylaxis against further attacks may be obtained with verapamil, β-blockers, disopyramide or digoxin.

Wolff-Parkinson-White syndrome This is a pre-excitation syndrome characterized by the presence of a delta wave before the QRS complex thereby shortening the PR interval. Pre-excitation occurs via an accessory AV conduction pathway – the bundle of Kent. It is particularly important to recognize this disorder because the supraventricular arrhythmias which occur (including SVT and AF) should not be treated with digoxin which may worsen the problem. Treatment is by cardioversion if shocked or disopyramide or amiodarone.

Ventricular tachyarrhythmias

Generally these are more sinister arrhythmias recognized by an ECG with wide QRS complexes.

Ventricular tachycardia This is a serious arrhythmia usually signifying serious underlying cardiac disease (Fig. 17.9). The heart rate is from 140–220 and carotid sinus pressure has no influence on the rate. The commonest causes include acute MI, cardiomyopathies and ventricular aneurysm. With the exception of an idioventricular rhythm, which arises from an ectopic focus high within the ventricular conducting system and which is common following acute MI, all ventricular tachycardias require urgent treatment. The treatment of recurrent arrhythmias in those with an adequate BP is intravenous lidocaine (lignocaine) (100 mg over 2 min followed by 4 mg/min initially then reducing slowly over 36 h) or amiodarone (5 mg/kg via a slow central infusion up to a maximum dose of 1.2 g in 24 hours) or mexiletine (100–250 mg over 10 min followed by 250 mg infusion over 60 min) may sometimes be required. In hypotensive patients DC cardioversion followed by iv lidocaine (lignocaine) should be carried out urgently.

Ventricular fibrillation This is the commonest cause of death following acute MI (Fig. 17.10). It is generally a reversible condition with adequate treatment and its recognition is the basis for cardiac monitoring in CCU. Risk factors include hypokalaemia, acid-base imbalance and catecholamines such as iv adrenaline (epinephrine). It should be recognized by cardiovascular collapse and an ECG showing chaotic QRS complexes. Treatment is by

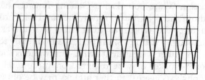

Fig. 17.9   Ventricular tachycardia.

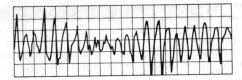

Fig. 17.10   Ventricular fibrillation.

immediate DC cardioversion (see Fig. 17.1). Oral therapy to reduce the risk of recurrence is the same as for VT.

Bradycardias

Sinus bradycardia   A heart rate below 60/min is usually due to increased vagal tone. It occurs in athletes, post inferior MI, hypothyroidism and with β-blocker treatment. It is rarely symptomatic but if it does require treatment atropine 0.6 mg iv is usually effective.

Sinoatrial block   When this occurs a complete cardiac cycle is missing on the ECG and is a common feature of the sick sinus syndrome. Treatment, when symptomatic, is by pacemaker insertion.

First-degree heart block   Manifested by a prolongation of the PR interval (>0.2 seconds), does not produce bradycardia and is an electrocardiographic phenomenon.

Second-degree heart block   Is divided into two types: Mobitz type I (Wenkebach), where the PR interval progressively lengthens until a beat is omitted and the cycle repeated and Mobitz type II, a more serious disorder, where QRS complexes are dropped every 2, 3 or 4 beats but where the PR interval is constant.

Third-degree or complete heart block   Exists where there is no association between the p wave and the QRS complexes and the ventricular rate is maintained by an escape rhythm originating in the ventricular conducting system or ventricles (Fig. 17.11). Treatment of second- and third-degree heart block is with iv atropine followed by insertion of a temporary or permanent pacemaker.

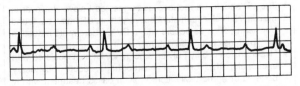

Fig. 17.11   Complete heart block.

PULMONARY OEDEMA

Management box

▶ Establish an iv line and give furosemide (frusemide), 50 mg as a bolus; enormous doses are not necessary. Consider giving regular iv diuretics.

▶ Give oxygen by face mask. If a venturi-type mask is to be used, give 10 l/min. If there is a previous history of chest disease, give 4 l/min. If the patient has definite pulmonary oedema, give high-flow oxygen (10 l/min) regardless of previous chest history.

▶ Give diamorphine, 5 mg iv.

▶ If the condition is severe, give isosorbide dinitrate or glyceryl trinitrate by intravenous infusion, 5 mg/hour (increased to 10 mg/hour if needed).

▶ If the patient is in fast atrial fibrillation, check serum potassium; once you know that the serum potassium is above 4.0 mmol/l, give digoxin, 0.5–0.75 mg by iv infusion in 100 ml of 5% glucose (*not* saline) over 20 min. If the patient has some other form of tachyarrhythmia this may need urgent treatment: consult your SHO or registrar.

▶ If the patient is hypotensive (systolic BP less than 100 mmHg), consider iv dobutamine infusion.

▶ Consider (CVP) monitoring and urinary catheterization.

MALIGNANT HYPERTENSION

Science basics In malignant hypertension there is diastolic BP >120 mmHg with symptoms such as encephalopathy, cardiac failure and/or deteriorating renal function. • Treatment of malignant hypertension is essential as the 12–month survival untreated is only 10%. It is nearly always more dangerous to reduce BP rapidly than to leave it untreated or to reduce it slowly.

Signs: progressive hypertensive retinopathy: flame-shaped haemorrhages, 'cotton-wool' exudates, papilloedema.

Management box

▶ The BP should be reduced as suggested below. However in certain clinical circumstances very high BP may be found transiently, such as occurs with a CVA, where rapid reduction of hypertension may be detrimental.

▶ Hypertension is only truly an emergency if it is associated with encephalopathy, cerebral haemorrhage, acute pulmonary oedema or aortic dissection. In such cases treatment with iv labetalol or sodium nitroprusside may be required – consult →

your SHO or registrar. If the BP is > 220/140 or there is renal failure, grade III or IV retinopathy or myocardial ischaemia associated with the hypertension, the situation is urgent but not an emergency – these patients can nearly always be managed with oral rather than parenteral therapy. The treatment of hypertensive urgencies is with bed-rest together with drugs such as:

- nifedipine, 10 mg sublingually (by biting a capsule) followed by a long-acting calcium channel blocker such as amlodipine or nifedipine MR. Such treatment is often combined with furosemide (frusemide)
- labetalol, 100–300 mg stat, then 200 mg bd. Caution required if patient is at risk of LVF
- an ACE inhibitor – watch carefully for evidence of renal failure.

▶ In urgent cases the aim of treatment is to reduce blood pressure to 100–110 mmHg over 24–48 hours; do not allow yourself to be persuaded by the nursing staff to reduce the BP any more rapidly.

RESPIRATORY FAILURE

Science basics This is defined as a respiratory disorder of such extent that respiratory function is inadequate for the individual's metabolic requirements. It is divided into two types (Table 17.3):

Table 17.3
Types and causes of respiratory failure

Type I		Type II	
Acute	*Chronic*	*Acute*	*Chronic*
$PaO_2\downarrow\downarrow$	$PaO_2\downarrow$	$PaO_2\downarrow$	$PaO_2\downarrow$
$PaCO_2\leftrightarrow$	$PaCO_2\leftrightarrow$	$PaCO_2\leftrightarrow$	$PaCO_2\uparrow$
$pH\leftrightarrow$	$pH\leftrightarrow$	$pH\downarrow$	$pH\downarrow$ or $\leftrightarrow$
$HCO_3\leftrightarrow$	$HCO_3\leftrightarrow$	$HCO_3\leftrightarrow$	$HCO_3\uparrow$
Asthma	Emphysema 'pink puffer'	Acute epiglottitis	Chronic bronchitis 'blue bloater'
Pul oedema	Thrombo-embolic pul HT	Severe acute asthma	Primary alveolar hypoventilation
Pul embolus	Lymphatic carcinomatosis	Respiratory muscle paralysis	
ARDS			
Pul fibrosis			

Type I: hypoxaemia (PaO_2 <8.0 kPa) without CO_2 retention due to ventilation/perfusion mismatch.

Type II: hypoxaemia and hypercapnia ($PaCO_2$ >6.0 kPa) due to hypoventilation.

Clinical features   Look for signs of the underlying disease. In both types of respiratory failure hypoxia may be accompanied by central cyanosis, breathlessness and confusion, while hypercapnia may be associated with a coarse flapping tremor (asterixis), warm peripheries, a bounding pulse, peripheral oedema and papilloedema. Ultimately coma and death may ensue.

Investigations   • Clinical examination • ABG • CXR • PEFR • Spirometry • FBC and biochemical profile • Sputum culture may help establish the cause.

Management box

▶ Type I failure – treat hypoxia with unrestricted oxygen therapy (35% +) and repeat gases after 20 min to ensure correction of PaO_2 and absence of a significant rise in $PaCO_2$.

▶ Type II failure – 24% or at the most 28% oxygen should be administered and close monitoring of the $PaCO_2$ maintained.

▶ Since many patients with COPD maintain adequate ventilation by stimulation from hypoxia rather than the $PaCO_2$ level, correction of hypoxia with high-flow oxygen may depress respiration resulting in CO_2 narcosis and death.

▶ If adequate correction of hypoxia cannot be achieved without worsening hypercapnia, mechanical ventilation may be indicated if the underlying pathology is reversible. In those patients where this is not considered appropriate respiratory stimulants such as iv doxapram 1–4 mg/min may have some value.

▶ Other treatment depends upon the cause.

▶ Nasal intermittent positive pressure (NIPPV) ventilation has a useful role if tolerated.

▶ Physiotherapy is important in the management of exacerbations of COPD as is appropriate antibiotic therapy.

▶ Bronchodilators and steroids are indicated if airways obstruction exists.

ACUTE ASTHMA

Science basics   This requires urgent assessment and aggressive management as it is life-threatening. Figure 17.12 outlines the management procedure. Indications for mechanical ventilation are summarized in Table 17.4.

Table 17.4
Indications for mechanical ventilation in asthma

Do not delay until the patient is moribund
- $PaO_2 < 6.5$ kPa and falling
- $PaCO_2 > 6.5$ kPa and rising
- pH < 7.3 and falling ($H^+ > 50$ nmol/l and rising)
- Increasing exhaustion and respiratory distress
- Cardiorespiratory arrest

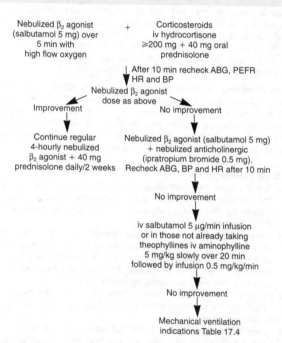

Fig. 17.12 The management of severe acute asthma.

PNEUMOTHORAX

Science basics Pneumothorax, the presence of air within the pleural cavity, may be due either to a penetrating injury letting air in from the outside or be spontaneous with air leaking from the lung. The primary causes of spontaneous pneumothorax in the UK are rupture of a subpleural bulla or due to a pleural adhesion.

Three types of pneumothorax are recognized: *closed* where the leak spontaneously closes off; *open* where the communication between the lung and pleural space remains open; and *tension* where a small communication remains open but only during inspiration so that the volume of air in the pleural space slowly or rapidly increases compressing the adjacent lung.

Clinical features

Symptoms: rapid onset of sharp chest pain and breathlessness which is seldom severe.

Signs: may be few but include cyanosis, tachypnoea, hyper-resonance, reduced expansion and reduced air-entry on the affected side. In tension pneumothorax breathlessness may rapidly increase with evidence of mediastinal shift (deviated trachea and apex beat towards the opposite side) causing severe respiratory and CVS embarrassment and death if left untreated.

Investigations • Inspiratory and expiratory CXR, small leaks may only be identified on the expiratory film • CXRs may need to be repeated within a short period to assess change in size, especially where a tension pneumothorax is considered • ABG analysis is essential if pre-existing lung disease exists since respiratory failure may be precipitated by even a small pneumothorax.

Management box

▶ Small closed pneumothoraces (< 20%) should be left unless the patient has compromised respiratory function from underlying lung disease although a repeat CXR is essential if the patient deteriorates.

▶ Larger ones require drainage either by aspiration or by insertion of a large-bore catheter through either the 2nd intercostal space anteriorly or laterally in the 4th or 5th intercostal space, which is connected to an underwater drainage system which acts as a one-way valve allowing air out but not in.

▶ Open pneumothoraces usually indicate a broncho-pleural fistula and are susceptible to infection. Surgical intervention is usually indicated.

▶ A tension pneumothorax is a medical emergency and requires rapid treatment ideally with the insertion of an intercostal drain but where not available a large 'intravenous' cannula should be inserted to relieve intrapleural pressure.

▶ In patients who suffer repeated spontaneous pneumothoraces pleurodesis is indicated. This can be achieved by inserting irritant substances such as kaolin which provokes an inflammatory reaction resulting in adhesions between the two pleural surfaces. Alternatively a surgical procedure involving the stripping of one layer of pleura thus obliterating the pleural space can be performed (pleurectomy).

PULMONARY EMBOLISM

Science basics This is due to the passage of a venous thrombosis usually from the deep veins in the leg or pelvis to the pulmonary artery. In many situations obvious DVT is absent. The diagnosis often relies on a high degree of clinical suspicion ($\rightarrow$ p 93). See also Chapter 4, p 93 and Chapter 16, p 355.

Clinical features Collapse, hypotension, sweating and tachycardia. Haemoptysis if present is suggestive.

Investigations • ABG analysis usually demonstrates hypoxia and hypocapnia • CXR is often normal although classically reveals wedge-shaped collapse, bilateral abnormalities or a pleural effusion • A ventilation/perfusion scan usually reveals numerous mismatched ventilation perfusion abnormalities • ECG may show sinus tachycardia, R heart strain, RBBB or a S_1, Q_3, T_3 pattern • Pulmonary angiography is occasionally required and is the 'gold standard' investigation.

Management box

▶ Give oxygen, 35% (8 l/min) if there is a previous history of chronic obstructive pulmonary disease, otherwise 60–100% (35 l/min). Aim to keep the patient's oxygen saturation (by pulse oximeter) above 90% and the arterial pO_2 above 8 kPa, preferably above 10 kPa.

▶ Make sure the patient is receiving plenty of iv fluid so as to increase right ventricular filling (and hopefully, therefore, right ventricular output) and commence treatment with a low molecular weight heparin (LMWH), eg tinzaparin, 175 u/kg by once-daily sc injection ($\rightarrow$ Table 19.7). Monitoring of dose by blood testing is not required. If, for some reason, your chief does not like LMWH in this situation, check APTT then give unfractionated heparin, 5000 u bolus injection followed by 17 500 u per 12 hours. Re-check KCCT (APTT) after 10 hours' treatment and adjust heparin dose accordingly ($\rightarrow$ p 572).

▶ Give pain relief as needed. Do not be afraid to give diamorphine if the pain is severe.

▶ If the lung scan confirms the diagnosis, start warfarin: check prothrombin time (PT), then give a dose of 10 mg warfarin and repeat the PT 18 hours later. Give subsequent doses of warfarin according to Table 19.5.

▶ If the lung scan is equivocal but the clinical suspicion of PE is strong, consider spiral CT scan, MRI scan or bilateral venography.

▶ If the patient is shocked, give plasma expander and consider thrombolysis. Ask for help from a more senior person.

▶ Have the patient fitted with anti-embolism stockings.

$\rightarrow$

▶ Consider investigating the patient for a thrombotic tendency, especially if the thromboembolism is recurrent or if the pulmonary embolism is large (these investigations can only be done when the patient is not on anticoagulants).

▶ If a patient presents with a PE without any apparent cause, an underlying malignancy should be considered. Likely primary tumours include carcinomas of the pancreas and liver and brain tumours. There is also an association with cancers of the prostate, ovary and uterus, also non-Hodgkin's lymphoma and leukaemia.

UPPER GASTROINTESTINAL HAEMORRHAGE

Science basics   Presentation is with haematemesis, melaena (with bleeding in GI tract down to ascending colon), iron-deficiency anaemia.

Aetiology   (Table 17.5) Other causes include: swallowed blood from epistaxis, blood dyscrasia, haemorrhagic telangiectasia, pseudoxanthoma elasticum, Ehlers-Danlos' syndrome, Ménétrier's disease, AV malformations and haemobilia.

Clinical features

Symptoms: ask about dyspepsia, alcohol abuse, analgesic ingestion, family history, syncope, dizziness and antecedent retching.

Signs: blood pressure (systolic BP <100 = >30% blood-volume reduction), heart rate, pallor, sweating and stigmata of liver disease.

Table 17.5
Causes of gastrointestinal bleeding

Cause	%
Duodenal ulcer	40
Gastric ulcer	15
Erosions	10
Varices	10
Oesophagitis	5
Mallory-Weiss	5
Carcinoma	5
Other	10

Investigations

Haematology: haemoglobin and haematocrit (may be normal until haemodilution occurs), leukocytosis and thrombocythaemia common.

Biochemistry: raised urea (protein load), abnormal LFTs in liver disease, serum iron, transferrin.

Nasogastric aspirate: if history of bleeding unclear (some false-negatives).

Endoscopy: allows identification of cause in >90% and means of treatment of varices by sclerotherapy. Sclerotherapy with 1:100 000 adrenaline (epinephrine) may also be useful in stopping bleeding from some peptic ulcers. Risk of rebleeding higher if a 'visible vessel' is seen in ulcer crater.

Barium radiology: identifies bleeding site in 80%. Useful in convalescent phase or with chronic blood loss.

Angiography: useful if bleeding still active but site unknown.

Radiolabelled RBCs: useful in determining low-grade bleeding from GI tract, especially if the pathology is out of reach of the endoscope.

Management box

▸ An iv line should be established in all patients and blood transfusion given to those with a systolic BP <100 or HR >100.

▸ The majority of patients stop bleeding spontaneously. Those who continue to bleed, identified by persistent hypotension or continuous transfusion requirement, should be referred for surgery or early endoscopy with sclerotherapy of the ulcer with adrenaline (epinephrine) following resuscitation.

▸ Where variceal bleeding is considered urgent endoscopy and sclerotherapy or band ligation is indicated. Those in whom bleeding has stopped should undergo endoscopy on the next available list. Ulcers with adherent clot or a visible vessel at the base are at increased risk of rebleeding and should be treated by sclerotherapy where available. Those who rebleed should be referred for surgery.

▸ Ulcers without stigmata associated with a high risk of rebleeding or where sources such as erosions are found should receive H_2-antagonists, eg ranitidine 300 mg bd orally and remain in hospital for 3–5 days.

▸ Evidence of *H. pylori* infection should be sought, and eradication therapy given. Confirmation of success of eradication therapy should be obtained by urea breath test or repeat upper GI endoscopy after 6–8 weeks.

▸ Those with Mallory-Weiss tears require no specific therapy and can be discharged early.

OESOPHAGEAL VARICES

Science basics Portal hypertension develops as a consequence of increased splanchnic bloodflow and increased hepatic vascular resistance in patients with liver disease. This leads to the opening up and dilatation of portosystemic anastomoses, the most important of which are at the lower end of the oesophagus. Only 30% of patients with varices ever bleed and this is commonest in those with the largest varices. Other risk factors are poorly understood.

Clinical features Brisk haematemesis is the commonest presentation although occasionally varices may bleed slowly with melaena or anaemia. In many stigmata of chronic liver disease are present.

Investigations The diagnosis should be made at endoscopy which should be undertaken urgently in patients with known or presumed liver disease. Endoscopy allows identification of the bleeding site as well as a means of treatment.

Management box

▸ Acute bleeding: resuscitation followed by injection sclerotherapy by a skilled operator. Where unavailable or unsuccessful iv octreotide (50 µg bolus, 50 µg/hour infusion) or the vasopressin analogue glypressin (2 mg 6-hourly) should be introduced. This latter drug is less toxic than vasopressin and has improved efficacy. If bleeding continues balloon tamponade with a Sengstaken tube is usually successful. Transjugular intrahepatic portosystemic stent shunt (TIPSS) or oesophageal transection should be considered in those who do not respond to such measures.

▸ Rebleeding: this is common after all the above medical procedures and can be reduced by injection sclerotherapy or band ligation to obliterate varices. Propranolol 160 mg LA/day also reduces the risk of rebleeding. A TIPSS should be considered in those who continue to rebleed.

▸ Prophylactic: many patients with varices never bleed and sclerotherapy for all patients with varices is not appropriate. Propranolol 160 mg LA/day reduces the risk of bleeding and should be used in those with large varices without contraindications to β-blockade.

Prognosis The overall mortality from acute upper GI haemorrhage remains unchanged over the last 40 years at around 10%. Adverse prognostic factors include old age, shock at presentation, rebleeding and varices. Early and aggressive resuscitation and treatment, particularly of the at-risk group, is essential.

ACUTE PANCREATITIS

Aetiology → Table 17.6

Clinical features

Symptoms: pain, usually severe, is almost always present and maximal in the epigastrium and radiating to the back. The pain may be relieved by sitting forward. Nausea and vomiting are also common.

Signs: include epigastric tenderness and guarding, abdominal distension, pyrexia, jaundice, peri-umbilical or flank bruising (Cullen's and Grey-Turner's signs respectively), shock and coma.

Investigations • Serum amylase levels are high in the vast majority. Normal levels occasionally occur because the patient presents late. In these cases high urinary amylase levels may be detected. Other disorders may give rise to hyperamylasaemia (Table 17.7). Although amylase may be raised in a variety of other disorders such as perforated peptic ulcer or cholecystitis, a value more than 4 times the upper limit of the reference range (ie above 400 iu/l) is virtually diagnostic of acute pancreatitis. Peritoneal lavage reveals fluid with high amylase and transaminase levels in severe pancreatitis • Pancreatic calcification on the abdominal X-ray is characteristic of alcoholic pancreatitis; a sentinel duodenal loop due to regional ileus may be present • CXR may show elevation of the L hemidiaphragm with atelectasis and pleural effusion • FBC, U&E, glucose, serum calcium, LFT, clotting screen and 'group and save' • FBC often shows a leukocytosis and

Table 17.6
Aetiology of pancreatitis

Acute	Chronic
Alcohol	Alcohol
Gallstones	Obstruction of pancreatic duct
Drugs eg thiazides, azathioprine, oestrogen, furosemide (frusemide)	Hyperparathyroidism
Trauma	Haemochromatosis
Post-operative, post ERCP	Idiopathic
Pancreatic carcinoma	Hereditary
Hyperparathyroidism	Tropical calcific pancreatitis
Viral infection eg mumps, coxsackie, E-B virus	

Table 17.7
Causes of hyperamylasaemia

Acute pancreatitis
Intestinal perforation or obstruction
Laparotomy
Morphine
Posterior penetrating DU
Renal failure
Mumps
Mesenteric ischaemia
Hepatitis
Pancreatic cancer
Burns
Congenital hyperamylasaemia

rise in Hb due to haemoconcentration • Hyperglycaemia, hypo-calcaemia, hypoxaemia and methaemalbuminaemia indicate severe pancreatitis • AXR may be needed to exclude other causes of the patient's symptoms • US scanning may detect swelling of the inflamed gland and may also identify gallstones in the gallbladder or dilatation of the CBD; US is particularly useful in identifying pancreatic pseudocysts, a common complication of acute pancreatitis (CT or MRI scanning may also be used).

Complications These are common and include shock, pancreatic pseudocysts and abscesses, ARDS, diabetes mellitus, renal and hepatic failure and DIC.

Management box

▸ No definitive treatment is available and supportive measures such as correcting electrolyte disturbances, fluid replacement and adequate pain relief are important. Recognition and early treatment of renal and respiratory failure, and infection including abscesses is essential.

▸ The patient should be nil by mouth and should receive iv fluids, usually saline and a plasma expander such as Haemaccel. Nasogastric suction may be needed. Adequate analgesia (using pethidine or buprenorphine, not morphine) should be given. Peritoneal lavage and protease inhibitors are, in general, **not** necessary. In all but the mildest cases, be sure to inform your SHO or registrar.

▸ Other treatment such as reducing pancreatic secretion by nasogastric aspiration or glucagon, early surgery for severe necrotic pancreatitis and early ERCP with sphincterotomy to allow passage of bile duct stones have all been shown in some studies to be beneficial.

Table 17.8
Features predicting the severity of an attack of acute pancreatitis

Age >55 yrs
WCC >15 × 10^9/l
Glucose >10 mmol/l
LDH >600 iu/l
AST >200 iu/l
Blood urea >16 mmol/l
Serum Ca$^+$ <2.0 mmol/l
Serum albumin <32 g/l
Arterial pO$_2$ <8kPa

Prognosis The mortality from acute pancreatitis is approximately 15% and acute haemorrhagic pancreatitis has a mortality of over 50%. Predictive factors of a poor prognosis include fever, hypotension, tachycardia and respiratory problems on admission. The later development of hypocalcaemia, hypoxaemia and hyperglycaemia are all poor prognostic indices (Table 17.8).

ACUTE OR FULMINANT HEPATIC FAILURE

Science basics This is defined as the development of encephalopathy within 8 weeks of the onset of symptoms in patients without prior liver disease. The commonest causes in the UK are paracetamol poisoning, viral hepatitis due to hepatitis A, B and non-A, non-B viruses and drug toxicity including halothane hepatitis.

Clinical features The most obvious clinical abnormality in fulminant hepatic failure is encephalopathy which can be divided into four stages: grade I – confusion; grade II – drowsiness; grade III – severe confusion and drowsiness; and grade IV – coma. Other features include bruising, GI bleeding, jaundice and oliguria.

Investigations and complications

Cerebral oedema: this may develop in patients with grade IV encephalopathy and is characterized by systemic hypertension, bradycardia, pupillary dilatation and opisthotonus.

Renal failure: this is common and can be divided into acute tubular necrosis with a high urinary sodium with low osmolality, and functional renal failure with low urinary sodium and high osmolality.

Sepsis: this is also common and due to either bacteria or fungi and may develop without obvious signs other than deterioration in clinical condition.

Bleeding: due to coagulopathy secondary to impaired hepatic synthetic function and DIC. Bleeding may be subcutaneous, gastrointestinal, renal or intracerebral.

Cardiopulmonary disturbance: characterized by shock and ARDS.

Metabolic: derangement in metabolism is usual with hypoglycaemia, hyponatraemia, hyperkalaemia, metabolic alkalosis and hypoxia being common. Metabolic acidosis in patients with paracetamol poisoning indicates a poor progress.

Management box

▶ Prophylactic measures which are appropriate in all patients include: skilled nursing with patients semirecumbant and head-up position, dextrose infusion, H_2-antagonist therapy and broad-spectrum antibiotics. Where appropriate the following should be instituted: mechanical ventilation to correct hypoxia and treat cerebral oedema, haemodialysis and/or ultrafiltration to treat renal failure and volume overload, Swan-Ganz pressure monitoring to ensure adequate cardiac filling volumes to cardiac output, 10% mannitol administration 100 ml over 20 min to treat intracranial hypertension and the administration of FFP and platelets to correct coagulopathy associated with haemorrhage. Liver transplantation should be considered in patients who are deteriorating and in whom recovery is predicted as being unlikely.

Prognosis This is poor but is greatly influenced by skilled intensive-care management. Overall the mortality for patients who develop grade IV encephalopathy is around 70%. However, the cause is important with the mortality in such patients with paracetamol poisoning and hepatitis A and B being approximately 50% compared with a mortality of 90% in those due to non-A, non-B hepatitis or halothane hepatitis with grade IV encephalopathy. However it should be remembered that those patients who survive usually make a full and complete recovery.

MENINGITIS

Science basics Inflammation of the meninges may be due to bacterial, viral, spirochaetal, protozoal or fungal infection. Viral infection is the commonest while syphilis and tuberculous infection are rare though increasing with AIDS.

Clinical features These may develop rapidly or, in tuberculous and fungal infection, over weeks and consist of features due to infection, meningism and raised intracranial pressure.

History of travel is important to differential diagnosis.

Symptoms: include lethargy, headache, neck pain, photophobia, fever and vomiting.

Signs: meningeal irritation, neck stiffness (inability to bend the patient's head so that the chin touches the chest), Kernig's sign (inability to straighten the leg below the knee once the hip is flexed to 90°) (NB may be absent in elderly), drowsiness and rarely papilloedema. A rash may accompany meningitis from a variety of organisms but a purpuric rash is characteristic of meningococcal meningitis (occurs in about 50%).

Investigations • Lumbar puncture with examination of the CSF preceded by CT if indicated • Blood cultures • Pneumococcal antigen • Consider borrelia, syphilis and rickettsial serology, CSF cryptococcal antigen, tuberculin test and PCR for tuberculin, thick and thin blood smears (malaria). (Table 17.9)

Management box

▶ Specific antibiotic treatment for bacterial meningitis depends upon identification of the organism and local strain. Meningococcus and pneumococcus, iv benzylpenicillin 1.2–2.4 g 4-hourly. *H. influenzae*, 3rd generation cephalosporin (cefotaxime or ceftriaxone). TB, rifampicin, isoniazid, streptomycin and pyrazinamide. Cryptococcus, iv amphotericin and oral flucytosine. Treatment of presumed bacterial meningitis before microbiological confirmation is usually with a 3rd generation cephalosporin for young adults, plus ampicillin in those over 50 years old. Treatment of viral meningitis is generally symptomatic except for herpes simplex treated with aciclovir and CMV treated with ganciclovir.

Table 17.9
Causes of CNS infections and CSF abnormalities

Cause	Microscopy	Biochemistry
Bacteria	Polymorphs > 100's per mm^3 and organisms e.g. Gram-negative diplococci	Low glucose (< a third of plasma) High protein
Viral	Lymphocytes 500–1000 mm^3 no organisms	Normal glucose Mild protein ↑

Table 17.9
Causes of CNS infections and CSF abnormalities (*Cont'd*)

Cause	Microscopy	Biochemistry
TB	Lymphocytes 100's per mm^3 (can be polymorphs initially) and TB bacilli on Z-N or auramine stain	Low glucose normal in 20% of cases High protein

Prognosis This depends upon the cause, with worse survival in pneumococcal than *H. influenzae* or meningococcal, and in bacterial meningitis the delay before diagnosis and treatment is crucial to survival.

SUBARACHNOID HAEMORRHAGE

Science basics: Spontaneous bleeding into the subarachnoid space: 70% due to intracranial aneurysms, 10% arteriovenous malformation (AVM).

Clinical features Sudden severe headache associated with vomiting. Often followed by loss of consciousness. Neck stiffness and Kernig's sign present indicating meningeal irritation. Papilloedema and retinal and subhyaloid haemorrhages may be present on fundoscopy.

Investigations • CT scanning 95% sensitive • LP if diagnosis still in doubt (shows blood-stained CSF and xanthochromia) • Cerebral angiography to localize vascular lesion.

> *Management box*
> ▶ Nimodipine (60 mg 4-hourly) reduced to cerebral ischaemia. Surgery to clip aneurysm or excise AVM.

ENCEPHALITIS

Science basics The majority of viruses which cause meningitis can cause encephalitis (infection of the brain tissue). The commonest cause in the UK is herpes simplex. HIV infection is increasing and other types include measles, mumps, varicella, poliomyelitis, rarely EBV, CMV, arboviruses, rabies and malaria.

Clinical features

Symptoms: these often include a prodromal illness followed by headache, drowsiness and fits.

Signs: focal neurological deficit, eg marked deterioration in conscious level, aphasia, hemiplegia, cranial nerve lesions and pyrexia.

Investigations • Differentiation from encephalopathy, cerebral abscess and CNS tumours • Lumbar puncture after CT scanning, CSF pressure is usually increased with raised protein and lymphocytic pleocytosis (10–1000s) • EEG shows non-specific diffuse slowing with epileptiform discharges in herpetic encephalitis • Virological and immunological studies of the CSF and serum may be useful in confirming the diagnosis but the results are not available in the acute phase, though early PCR detection of viral antigen is becoming available • Blood film for malaria.

Management box
▶ With the exception of herpes simplex encephalitis treatment is symptomatic. Aciclovir iv 5–10 mg/kg infusion tid for 10 days with dexamethasone 4 mg tid is indicated if herpetic encephalitis is suspected. Vaccination against poliomyelitis has virtually eliminated polio encephalo-myelitis.

Prognosis This is good in most patients although neurological deficit may remain (the poorest outlook of the more common causes occurs in herpes simplex with a mortality rate of 15–20%).

STATUS EPILEPTICUS

Science basics This is defined as repeated episodes of epilepsy without the patient having recovered consciousness from the previous attack. Repeated generalized seizures are readily apparent but non-convulsive status may require EEG monitoring to diagnose. In pseudostatus there may be a psychiatric background, movements tend to be random rather than rhythmic, often writhing, with alternating side-to-side head movements and pelvic thrusting. Cyanosis is unusual, eye opening resisted and corneal and pupillary reflexes are retained with flexor plantars; incontinence is rare.

Management box
▶ The first priority here is to make sure that the patient is 'safe' when you arrive, ie that the fit has stopped, the patient has a clear airway and a normal pulse rate and BP.
  – **If the patient is not 'safe' when you arrive, you should bleep your SHO or registrar urgently.**
  – If you arrive during the fit, do not restrain the patient at all; simply wait for the fit to end and protect the patient from injury. If possible remove false teeth, put on a face mask and give 100% oxygen. Ask for suction and suck out saliva, etc. →

from the mouth. If the fit is continuing (more than 3 minutes), give Diazemuls, 10–20 mg intravenously *slowly* (5 mg/min) or diazepam 10–20 mg rectally. An alternative is a slow iv injection of clonazepam, 1 mg.

▶ Try to establish from witnesses the exact nature of the attack:
 – Did the patient actually convulse?
 – Did the attack begin focally or with generalized rigidity?
 – Did the patient appear to lose consciousness?
 – Was the patient aware of any aura or did he/she behave oddly or cry out just before the attack?
 – Is the patient pregnant (eclampsia)?

▶ **A typical *grand mal*** or generalized fit begins with a tonic phase, with rigidity of the whole body, followed by convulsive jerking of the limbs and trunk. During the attack the patient may become pale or cyanosed. Afterwards the patient will often be drowsy and disoriented for several minutes and there may be a short-lived focal weakness (Todd's paresis).

▶ Find out if there is a past history of epilepsy.

▶ Once the fit has stopped, check the patient's state of consciousness (GCS, Table 17.1) and carry out a quick neurological review: check especially for meningism, that the pupils are equal and reactive, that there is no papilloedema and that there is no obvious hemiparesis. If the patient is not fully conscious, nurse in the recovery position

▶ Consider secondary causes of fitting (Table 17.10).

Investigations In someone who has an unexpected fit with no definite cause it is wise to check the blood glucose at the bedside using a finger-prick blood sample and also to send blood to the laboratory for urgent U&E, serum calcium, glucose and blood count. If there is any suggestion of hypoxia or if the patient is having fits in quick succession, check blood gases and give 100% oxygen by face mask.

Table 17.10
Secondary causes of fitting

Metabolic
 Hypoglycaemia*
 Hypocalcaemia
 Hypoxia*
 Water intoxication
 Hypo- or hypernatraemia
 Liver failure*

Table 17.10
Secondary causes of fitting (*Cont'd*)

Structural
    Head injury*
    Stroke*
    Intracranial tumour*
    A-V malformations
Infective
    Encephalitis*
    Meningitis
    Cerebral abscess
    Cerebral toxoplasmosis (in AIDS patients)
Toxic
    Phenothiazines
    Tricyclic antidepressants
    Amphetamines (ecstasy)
    Alcohol or benzodiazepine withdrawal*
Degenerative
    Alzheimer's disease

*The most common causes

Management box

▶ **To terminate a seizure** It is often best to wait for a few moments and simply allow the fit to subside (see above). If, however, the fit is continuing remove false teeth, put on a face mask and give 100% oxygen. Ask for suction and suck out saliva, etc, from the mouth. Give Diazemuls, 10–20 mg intravenously *slowly* (5 mg/min) or diazepam, 10–20 mg rectally. An alternative is a slow iv injection of clonazepam, 1 mg.

▶ **Hypoglycaemia** If the bedside glucose test suggests hypoglycaemia, give 25–50 ml of 50% glucose into a large vein, followed by a saline flush; if venous access is difficult, give 1 mg glucagon intramuscularly. You may need to follow this up with a glucose infusion. Consult your SHO or registrar.

▶ **Alcohol withdrawal and liver disease** Give intravenous thiamine (as Pabrinex – note *risk of anaphylaxis*), followed by an infusion of 10% glucose, 50 ml/hour. Regular blood glucose monitoring (2–4 hourly by a bedside method) is advisable.

▶ **Seizures without known cause** Nurse the patient in the recovery position and ensure that oxygenation and BP are adequate. Ask the nursing staff to do regular observations ('neuro. obs.') every half hour or every hour.

→

▶ **Recurrent fits** You should not give more than two bolus doses of Diazemuls. If fitting recurs after two doses connect the patient to an ECG monitor and prepare a phenytoin infusion by diluting 250 mg of phenytoin solution in 100 ml of normal saline; give a loading dose of 15 mg/kg at a rate of not more than 50 mg/min (20 ml/min) (Table 17.11). This may be followed by doses of 100 mg (40 ml), given by infusion over 30 mins every 6–8 hours as maintenance therapy. When phenytoin is diluted for iv infusion the solution should be used within an hour of being made up and should not be refrigerated. The iv line should be flushed with normal saline before and after the infusion.

Table 17.11
Phenytoin dosage

Body weight (kg)	Volume of phenytoin solution needed to give 15 mg/kg (ml)
40	240
45	270
50	300
55	330
60	360
65	390
70	420
75	450
80	480
85	510
90	540
95	570
100	600

SEPTICAEMIA

Science basics Bacteraemia is the spread of infection into the bloodstream and if organisms multiply there it is known as septicaemia. The primary site of infection is often unknown but is commonly the gall bladder, bowel, lungs, meninges or urinary tract. Dissemination may result in the formation of abscesses in multiple organs. A number of predisposing factors often exist including multiple trauma, surgery, diabetes, alcoholism, immunosuppression or malignancy. Any infective organism can produce septicaemia but the commonest cause is the Gram-negative group of bacteria.

Clinical features The classical features of septic shock are fever, hypotension, vasodilatation, tachycardia and tachypnoea. Multiple organ failure may result, eg kidneys, heart, lungs (ARDS), DIC, pancreas, bowel, liver and brain.

Investigations FBC • Clotting screen, fibrinogen level, fibrin degradation products • Urea and electrolytes, creatinine • LFTs • Urinary electrolytes • Creatinine clearance • Glucose • ABG • ECG • CXR • Multiple blood cultures (aerobic and anaerobic culture) • MSU • CSF • Drain fluid • Sputum Gram stain and culture.

Management box

▶ Reverse hypotension, hypoxaemia, treat infection and improve tissue perfusion. Ensure adequate oxygenation (supplemental oxygen by face-mask or nasal cannulae or endotracheal intubation and artificial ventilation if necessary). Pending the results of blood gas estimation, give 60–100% oxygen (35% if the patient has a history of COPD).

▶ Establish iv access. Monitor pulse, BP, temperature and urine output hourly. Neurological observations may be needed. Central venous or pulmonary artery wedge pressure measurements are helpful.

▶ Septicaemic patients are severely ill, so fluid balance and throughput should be monitored by inserting a central venous pressure line and a urinary catheter. In patients with evidence of DIC fresh frozen plasma (to replace clotting factors) or platelets may be needed.

▶ Blood pressure should be maintained with crystalloids, colloids or a combination of both. Dopamine, dobutamine or noradrenaline (norepinephrine) may be needed to maintain adequate cardiac and urinary outputs. Surgical drainage of any suspected areas of sepsis should be undertaken.

▶ Antimicrobial therapy should be commenced immediately (after blood cultures have been taken), and should be effective against a wide variety of organisms. The combination of a broad-spectrum penicillin/ cephalosporin, an aminoglycoside and an anti-anaerobic agent is often used, eg azlocillin/cefotaxime and gentamicin/tobramycin and metronidazole. This regimen can be altered once culture results become available. Individual types of organ failure are treated conventionally.

▶ Sepsis may result in myocardial depression so if the patient remains hypotensive despite having a normal central venous pressure, consider using an inotropic agent (dobutamine, adrenaline (epinephrine)). If urine output is poor despite a normal CVP, consider low-dose dopamine infusion; this drug **must not** be given into a peripheral vein.

▶ Corticosteroids, often in high doses, have been extensively used in the treatment of septicaemic shock but research has shown that they are of no value.

Prognosis   Approximately 50% survival.

HYPOGLYCAEMIA

Science basics   The biochemical definition of hypoglycaemia is a blood glucose < 2.2 mmol/l although symptoms may begin at higher blood-sugar levels. Causes include diabetes treated with excessive insulin or sulphonylureas, liver failure, hepatoma, Addison's disease, and hypopituitarism.

Clinical features   Hunger, sweating, tremor, confusion, tachycardia, and, if prolonged, coma, focal CNS signs including hemiparesis or, most serious, cerebral cortical infarction.

Investigations   Immediate diagnosis and treatment is important. A blood glucose on finger-prick testing should be obtained whenever possible and a sample taken for laboratory confirmation.

Management box

▶ Should not be delayed waiting for the blood glucose result. If the patient is conscious 20–30 g of readily absorbable carbohydrate (Lucozade, milk) should be given orally. If the patient is unable to take oral fluid iv glucose in the form of 50% dextrose (50 ml) or 10% glucose (250 ml) should be administered through a large venflon. Glucagon 0.5–1 mg im raises the blood sugar more slowly than iv glucose and should only be used in those where iv access is difficult or by relatives while awaiting medical attention. In unusual situations where iv access cannot be obtained and glucagon is unavailable or contraindicated (eg sulphonylurea-induced hypoglycaemia) glucose should be administered via nasogastric tube.

▶ Recurrent hypoglycaemia is common in diabetics taking long-acting insulin preparations or sulphonylureas and hospital admission is required for monitoring in such cases.

KETOACIDOSIS

Science basics   This is a true medical emergency with a mortality of 10–20% and may present in a known diabetic or those not previously known to be diabetic.

Clinical features   These are dominated by: • dehydration characterized by tachycardia, hypotension and dry, slack skin • acidosis with deep rapid respiration (air hunger) • ketosis with vomiting, fetor and abdominal pain. Drowsiness is common but, unlike hypoglycaemia, coma is uncommon. Precipitating features such as infection, eg pneumonia, MI or surgery may be obvious. Consider also missed insulin or a faulty insulin injection pen.

Investigations • Blood glucose • U&E and osmolality • Arterial blood gases • Urinalysis • CXR • Blood and urine cultures.

Management box

▶ Establish iv line.

▶ Administer 2 l normal saline over 4 hours, then 2 l over the next 8 hours, then 1 l every 8 hours. The CVP should be monitored in elderly patients and those with IHD.

▶ Start iv insulin infusion: initially 6 units/hour, 2–4 units/hour thereafter. Aim to gently lower blood glucose to 12–15 mmol/l.

▶ Monitor urine output.

▶ Administer iv potassium unless plasma potassium >5 mmol/l. Even when the initial blood potassium is high, 20 mmol K/l of fluid replaced will be required to maintain normokalaemia. Continuous ECG monitoring is useful.

▶ Bicarbonate replacement to correct the acidosis is rarely required. If the arterial pH is < 6.9 a slow infusion of 100 mmol $NaHCO$, (1.26%) with 20 mmol K may be given over 30 min. Blood gases and serum K should be repeated 30 min later. Bicarbonate therapy has been associated with cerebral oedema and many authorities discourage its use.

▶ In comatose patients, where vomiting is prominent or a succussion splash is present, a nasogastric tube should be passed to empty the stomach since gastroparesis and ileus are common.

▶ Once the blood glucose is below 15 mmol/l, 10% glucose should be substituted for iv saline to avoid hypernatraemia. Reduce insulin infusion rate to around 2–3 units per hour (higher rates if serum bicarbonate still <10).

▶ Regular reanalysis of U&E, glucose, and arterial blood gases. Manual blood-glucose strip testing may be inaccurate in the presence of hyperglycaemia and ketonaemia.

▶ The precipitating cause of ketoacidosis should be sought. This may be obvious from the history, eg omission of insulin, but is commonly due to infection. Routine administration of broad-spectrum antibiotics, eg cefuroxime, 750 mg iv every 6–8 hours recommended by some authorities.

Complications Avoid cerebral oedema (due to too-rapid lowering of blood glucose, injudicious use of bicarbonate or excess hypotonic fluids), hypoglycaemia and hypokalaemia. Cerebral oedema is a significant cause of mortality, particularly in children, as is aspiration pneumonia if a nasogastric tube is not inserted. Return to subcutaneous insulin should be delayed until the bowel sounds have reappeared, the serum bicarbonate ≥ 20 and the patient has been able to tolerate light solid food without vomiting.

HYPEROSMOLAR NON-KETOTIC COMA

Science basics Severe hyperglycaemia without ketosis is a medical emergency of non-insulin dependent diabetes. It may be precipitated by an intercurrent illness, drugs (thiazide diuretics, steroids), or high glucose intake.

Clinical features Dehydration, confusion or coma. The hyperosmolar state predisposes to thrombotic episodes (myocardial infarction, CVA, peripheral vascular insufficiency).

Management box

▶ Investigations are the same as for diabetic ketoacidosis (DKA).
▶ Initial fluid replacement is with 0.9% saline, although 0.45% saline may be used in severe cases and if blood sodium is greater than 150 mmol/l. Close monitoring of fluid balance is required as patients are often elderly.
▶ Less insulin may be required than for DKA, and after the acute episode there is no absolute need for insulin therapy.
▶ Give iv heparin, 5000 u stat, then 1400 u/hour.
▶ Precipitating causes should be sought and treated.

ACUTE ADRENAL CRISIS

This condition is characterised by profound hypotension, abdominal pain and hyperkalaemia. A blood sample should be taken for later analysis (cortisol measurement), then iv normal saline should be given, as well as iv hydrocortisone (100–200 mg 6-hourly). Clinical improvement is usually dramatic and steroid therapy should never be withheld in those in whom the diagnosis has been considered whilst the results of tests are awaited. An urgent tetracosactrin (Synacthen) test is **not** required – this can be done later.

HYPOTHERMIA

Science basics This is particularly likely to occur in the elderly, alcoholics and in those unexpectedly exposed to low temperature, eg immersion in cold water. The diagnosis may be missed unless low-reading thermometers are used in those at risk who have a low reading on an ordinary mercury thermometer. Risk factors include hypothyroidism, pituitary and adrenal insufficiency, CVA and drug/alcohol abuse.

Clinical features Cold peripheries, hypotension, pallor, confusion, cyanosis, coma, respiratory depression and bradycardia.

Investigations • Rectal temperature using a low-reading thermometer • U&E, FBC, TFTs • ABG (metabolic acidosis) • CXR and ECG (J waves may be present) • Overdosage with drugs, eg antidepressants, benzodiazepines, should be considered.

Management box

▶ Rewarm by 1°C per hour
▶ Maintain an adequate airway, administer oxygen, iv fluids, monitor blood potassium and cardiac rhythm. If the arterial pH < 7.2 consider $NaHCO_3$ 1.26% administration.
▶ Rewarming can usually be achieved by passive means by wrapping the patient in a space blanket in a warm room. Failure to rewarm passively should suggest hypothyroidism.
▶ Consider active rewarming, eg pleural/peritoneal lavage, cardiopulmonary bypass.
▶ Persistent hypotension on rewarming may result in renal failure requiring peritoneal or haemodialysis.
▶ Pneumonia is a common complication and many would advocate prophylactic antibiotics, eg iv cefuroxime 750 mg tid and metronidazole 500 mg tid.
▶ Resuscitation of patients with hypothermia complicated by asystole should be continued until the patient has been rewarmed to normal temperatures. Rapid rewarming of patients by warm water baths is appropriate when they have been exposed to profound low temperatures, eg immersion in cold water.

ANAPHYLAXIS

Science basics This occurs in the clinical setting of the introduction, usually in the form of an injection, of antigen in patients already hypersensitive to the allergen, eg penicillin, antisera or insect sting.

Clinical features Rapid onset (within minutes) of laryngeal spasm, pruritus, nausea and vomiting, hypotension, urticaria, cyanosis and dyspnoea.

Management box

▶ Adrenaline (epinephrine) 500–1000 µg im and an antihistamine such as chlorphenamine (chlorpheniramine) 10 mg slow iv infusion. In those with severe reactions systemic steroids, eg

→

hydrocortisone 200 mg iv, followed by further steroids is indicated. In hereditary angioneurotic oedema due to C1 esterase inhibitor deficiency (an autosomal dominant trait) FFP followed by danazol 200–800 mg/day prophylaxis is effective.

▸ This condition is characterized by profound hypotension, abdominal pain and hyperkalaemia.

▸ A blood sample should be taken for later analysis (cortisol measurement), then iv normal saline should be given, as well as iv hydrocortisone (100 mg 6-hourly).

▸ Clinical improvement is usually dramatic and steroid therapy should never be withheld in those in whom the diagnosis has been considered while the results of tests are awaited.

▸ An urgent tetracosactrin (Synacthen) test is **not** required – this can be done later.

▸ Consider provision of an adrenaline pen (Epipen) for early treatment of future attacks.

OVERDOSE

Deliberate self-poisoning is a very common medical emergency. A few basic observations ● Most people who take an overdose are not psychiatrically ill. Many ODs are impulsive, precipitated by alcohol excess, or related to social problems ● Patients who attempt suicide, often repeatedly, have a high rate of successful suicide whether they are psychiatrically ill or not. Repeated overdosage is, therefore, a bad prognostic sign and must be taken seriously.

In summary, therefore, you have a responsibility to assess the self-poisoned patient in two ways: in terms of drug toxicity, and in psychiatric terms.

Basic approach

If the patient is semi-conscious, unconscious or incoherent, before doing anything else you should ● Make sure that you are not dealing with a cardiac arrest, i.e. check that the patient has a palpable carotid or femoral pulse ● Note whether the patient is cyanosed or appears to have an abnormal breathing pattern (eg Cheyne-Stokes breathing). Check that the airway is clear ● Check the BP ● If the patient's immediate survival seems in danger, call for help from someone more senior ● If the patient's immediate survival is not threatened, try to obtain the answers to the following questions from a relative, friend or other witness.

If the patient is conscious and coherent ask: ● What has been taken? ● When was it taken? ● Was anything else taken apart

Table 17.12
Psychological and personal backgrounds

1. Why did they do it?
2. Was the act premeditated or impulsive?
3. Did the patient intend to die?
4. Did the patient intend to be discovered?
5. Is there continuing suicidal intent?
6. Has the precipitating crisis resolved?
7. What are the patient's social circumstances and potential supports?
8. Are there any young children at home who might be at risk?
9. Can they identify anything which makes life worth living?
10. Have they harmed themselves before?
11. Is there a family history of suicide?
12. What are the main psychiatric symptoms (if any)?
13. Do they currently have a problem with alcohol or drug abuse?
14. Does the patient have a history of psychiatric disorder?
15. Are they expressing hopelessness?

from the main poison? • What is the psychological and personal background? (Table 17.12) • All patients should have some form of assessment by psychiatrist or psychiatric nurse liaison.

Risk factors for serious suicide attempts • Clinical depression present • Psychosis (delusions/ hallucinations/bizarre behaviour, etc) • Evidence of clear premeditation or continuing suicidal intent (the more detailed the plans the more serious the risk) • Violent method chosen • Alcoholics and drug addicts • Older (over 45) and younger (under 16) age • Serious or chronic physical illness present • Those in a major life crisis which has not yet resolved • Deliberate self-harm (DSH) recidivists and those who have harmed themselves recently, often recurrent offenders with personality disorder.

Examination • Look for needle-marks, skin-blistering, dilated pupils, eg amfetamines/MDMA/anticholinergics/TCAs etc • Assess the patient's level of consciousness in terms of the GCS (Table 17.1, pp 417–418) • Examine each system in turn, looking especially for: Tachycardia, eg anticholinergics, amfetamines, ecstasy, β-agonists, MAOIs phenothiazines, theophylline, tricyclics, sympathomimetics; Bradycardia, eg β-blockers/cyanide/digoxin/ organophosphates; Hypertension, eg amfetamines/ ecstasy/ cocaine/MAOIs; Hypotension (common in severe poisoning from any cause); Hypertonia/ hyperflexia, eg amfetamines/ecstasy/ anticholinergics/ cabamazepine/MAOIs/theophylline/TCAs/

carbon monoxide; Hypotonia, eg alcohol/barbiturates/ benzo-diazepines/haloperidol/opiates/organophosphates/phenothiazines; Tachypnoea, eg amfetamines/ecstasy/ethyleneglycol/methanol/salicylates/theophylline/cyanide.

Investigations • Take blood for salicylate and paracetamol levels in all patients (the history may be unreliable) • If you know that the patient has taken paracetamol or a paracetamol-containing compound preparation (eg co-proxamol, co-dydramol), do not take blood until after 4 hours from the time of ingestion • Take blood for U&E and blood glucose in paracetamol, salicylates, TCAS/ecstasy, etc • Check CK in SSRI/phenothiazines • In cases of paracetamol poisoning take blood for INR and LFTs • In appropriate cases, take blood for levels of specific poisons, eg lithium, digoxin, theophylline, paraquat, phenytoin, carbamazepine • LFTs not usually done at baseline unless late presentation • Check LFTs and INR in all patients at end of Rx with NAC • If possible obtain a urine sample for toxicology screening, particularly for drugs of abuse and for measurement of paraquat levels • ECG in *all* tricyclics/phenothiazines/carbamazepine/phenytoin/antihistamines • If the patient is un-conscious ask for a CXR (together with X-rays of any injured parts) • Monitor pulse, BP, oxygen saturation, urine output.

Management

General measures If you are not familiar with the poison, consult the *Toxbase*, available to most hospitals, or National Poisons Information Service – New number 0870 600 6266 will direct you to the centre responsible for your area.

Gastric lavage: this is rarely performed nowadays and is only of value if a potentially life-threatening amount of drug was ingested and if undertaken within 1 hour of ingestion. Consider if the patient has taken salicylates, iron salts or theophyllines. It must *not* be undertaken in those who have swallowed a corrosive or a petroleum product or organic solvent. If the patient is semi-conscious or unconscious the airway must be protected by means of an endotracheal tube (passed by an *experienced* person) before lavage is attempted. For the technique of gastric lavage, see Table 17.13.

Activated charcoal: this is of value for the elimination of several drugs but is not of value for others. This is preferred for the majority of poisons since many poisons are adsorbed by activated charcoal and it compares favourably with gastric emptying techniques. Patient with depressed conscious level should only be given charcoal once the airway has been adequately protected because of risk of aspiration pneumonitis • Substances for which charcoal is not of value: ethanol, methanol, ethylene glycol

Table 17.13
Technique of gastric lavage

- Have a suction apparatus ready to hand (check that it is working)
- Lay the patient in the left lateral position
- Raise the foot of the bed
- Pass the lavage tube, asking the patient to swallow (get someone to show you how to do this before you make your first solo attempt)
- Check that the tube is in place by blowing air down it and listening over the stomach
- Wash out the gastric contents using 300 ml volumes of tepid water
- Repeat until no more tablets are retrieved and the fluid is clear
- When pulling out the tube, pinch the top end to prevent aspiration of fluid from the tube.

(antifreeze), cyanide, iron salts, lithium, petroleum distillates, mercury, lead or strong acids or alkalis.

Charcoal should, if possible, be given within an hour of ingestion: its effect becomes less after that. The recommended dose of charcoal for an adult is 50 g or 1 g/kg body weight for children. For salicylate poisoning a single dose of 50 g, given within 1 hour of ingestion, is appropriate. For certain other poisons repeated dosing is recommended, ie 50 g stat, then 50 g every 4 hours. Drugs for which multiple doses of charcoal are recommended include: carbamazepine, dapsone, phenobarb, quinine and theophylline.

Whole bowel irrigation   This technique, in which the bowel is washed out with polyethylene glycol, is sometimes used in serious poisoning with sustained-release or enteric-coated preparations. It may also be of value in poisoning with lithium, iron, or cocaine body-packers.

ANTIDOTES FOR SPECIFIC DRUGS

Paracetamol

This drug is freely available over the counter and is also present in many compound analgesics (co-proxamol, co-dydramol, etc). It is highly toxic in overdosage. Risk of severe liver damage is based on dose ingested: < 150 mg/kg unlikely, > 250 mg/kg likely, > 12 g potentially fatal.

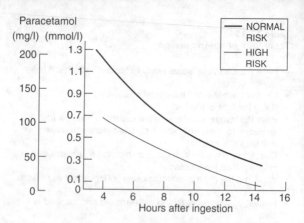

Fig. 17.13   Paracetamol venous blood levels following overdose.

Initial measures • Take blood for U&E, glucose, clotting screen, paracetamol level and LFTs (note that the paracetamol level is only interpretable if it is measured 4 hours or more after ingestion) • Check the patient's paracetamol level against the 'treatment lines' on Fig 17.13. People with alcoholic liver disease, malnutrition, on enzyme-inducing drugs or who are HIV positive, are at increased risk of toxicity. If the level is *well below* the relevant line, no specific antidote is required; if, however, the level is close to or above the line, give acetylcysteine (Parvolex) by iv infusion • If the paracetamol level is doubtful, ie near the treatment line, it is safer to give acetylcysteine than not to give it • Make up the acetylcysteine in 5% glucose (see the package insert in the box) and give 150 mg/kg in 200 ml over 15 min, followed by 50 mg/kg in 500 ml over 4 hours, then 100 mg/kg in 1000 ml over 16 hours. Treatment should be started within 8 hours to give maximum protection • Methionine may be a suitable alternative in remote areas where there may be considerable delay in transfer to hospital.

Further measures • After completion of NAC check U&E, LFT, INR – if normal no further Rx required and patient can be discharged • If bloods abnormal or late presentation check INR daily (more frequently in severe poisoning). The INR is the best overall guide to the extent of liver damage. If the INR exceeds 4.0 within the first 48 hours or exceeds 6.0 within the first 72 hours, ask for help from someone more senior. If the INR remains above 2.0, continue with acetylcysteine infusion at the maintenance rate • Review the patient carefully each day for signs of liver failure and check LFT, U&E, INR daily

• Monitor glucose regularly • Monitor urine output (catheterize if necessary).

Poor prognostic features • Prolonged prothrombin time, ↑ plasma creatinine, metabolic acidosis, hypoglycaemia, encephalopathy. Peak liver and renal necrosis will be reached 72–96 hours post-ingestion. Some patients with severe liver damage may be candidates for liver transplantation.

Aspirin

This drug is freely available over the counter and is found in many compound analgesics. Symptoms of aspirin poisoning include tinnitus, hyperventilation, deafness, vasodilatation and sweating. Aspirin poisoning does not cause coma until a very late stage. Therefore severe poisoning can be present in a patient who is fully conscious.

Initial measures • Measure salicylate concentration at least 2 hours after ingestion, may need to repeat levels 2 hourly until no longer rising • Take blood for U&E, acid/base state, clotting screen and salicylate level and blood glucose • If the patient presents within an hour of ingestion, give activated charcoal, 50 g by mouth if > 250 mg/kg ingested.

Further measures • Check ABGs in significant poisoning • If the plasma salicylate level is greater than 500 mg/l (3.6 mmol/l), elimination can be enhanced by iv fluid: deficits or losses should be replaced and alkalinization of the urine may then be promoted by the giving of iv 1.26% sodium bicarbonate at approximately 100 ml/hour • Monitor urinary pH every 4 hours (try to keep it in the range 7.5–8.5) and plasma U&E every 4 hours. • Haemodialysis may be necessary in severe poisoning (level > 700 mg/l) or in patients with renal failure, cardiac failure; convulsions or severe acidosis • Give vitamin K, 10 mg iv, if the PT is prolonged.

Non-steroidal anti-inflammatory drugs

Ibuprofen may cause nausea, vomiting and tinnitus but serious poisoning is uncommon. Mefenamic acid is quite often taken in overdosage; the main hazard is convulsions which should be treated with diazepam.

Tricyclic antidepressants

The main dangers from these drugs when taken in overdosage are cardiac arrhythmias and conduction defects; there may also be metabolic acidosis in cases of severe poisoning. Other effects include dry mouth, urinary retention, coma, hypotension, hypothermia, convulsions and respiratory failure.

Initial measures • Take blood for U&E, blood gases and acid/base state • Arrange a cardiac monitor • If the patient presents within 1 hour of ingestion, give 50 g activated charcoal by mouth or nasogastric tube if the patient is conscious: A second dose of 50 g should be considered after 2 hours in patients with central features of toxicity.

Further treatment • Correct hypoxia – apart from any other benefits, this will lessen the tendency to fits or cardiac arrhythmias • Correct acidosis (pH <7.2) with iv 1.26% sodium bicarbonate, 500 ml initially (or 50 ml 8.4%) also used to correct ECG abnormalities if evidence of broad QRS complexes or arrhythmias • If the patient convulses, give iv diazemuls, 10–20 mg • Correct hypotension by raising foot of bed and expanding intravascular volume. If this is not successful, inotropes such as dobutamine, may be needed • Do not use anti-arrhythmic drugs, ask for help.

Benzodiazepines

This group includes diazepam (Valium), lorazepam (Ativan), nitrazepam (Mogadon), etc. They do not, as a rule, cause life-threatening effects unless the patient has chest disease or is in some other way at special risk from respiratory depression.

Management   Treatment is essentially supportive; however, if you are concerned about respiratory depression check arterial blood gases. Flumazenil, a benzo antagonist, is rarely required and should *not* be used as a 'diagnostic test' or in mixed over-doses. It may precipitate convulsions in epileptics or in patients who have taken tricyclic antidepressants and arrhythmias in patients who have taken cardiotoxic drugs.

Iron

Poisoning is commonest in children and is usually accidental. Symptoms include: nausea, vomiting, diarrhoea, haematemesis, rectal bleeding. Hypotension, coma and hepatic necrosis may occur later. Features likely if >20 mg/kg body weight ingested, severe toxicity with 150–300 mg/kg body weight.

Initial management   • Consider gastric lavage if ingestion >60 mg/kg has occurred within 1 hour of presentation (<55 μmol/l = mild poisoning, >55 μmol/l = moderate poisoning, >90 μmol/l = severe poisoning) • Take blood for urgent serum iron measurement 4 hours after ingestion.

Further measures   Give desferrioxamine by iv infusion at a rate of 15 mg/kg/hour (maximum 80 mg/kg in 24 hours). If severe iron poisoning is suspected, start the desferrioxamine infusion as soon as you have taken blood for serum iron – do not wait for the result • If the patient is shocked or unconscious, check ABG and correct acidosis • Monitor renal and liver function • Observe for evidence of gut perforation/infarction.

Opiates

These drugs cause coma and respiratory depression. Overdosage can be recognized by the presence of pinpoint pupils.

Management • Carefully assess pulse, BP and rate and depth of respiration • Give naloxone, 0.8–2 mg iv as a bolus. The plasma half-life of naloxone is shorter than that of most opioid analgesics, therefore repeat dose may be necessary • If ventilation appears inadequate, check ABG • Make sure that the patient is going to be closely supervised by a nurse or doctor • Repeat naloxone every 2–3 min until breathing is adequate (up to a maximum dose of 10 mg). Alternatively, naloxone can be given by continuous iv infusion: dilute 2 mg in 500 ml of 5% glucose and give at a rate of 25 ml/min, adjusted according to response • Naloxone may precipitate symptoms of opiate withdrawal in addicts, eg tremor, sweating, abdominal pain, hallucinations: sedation with diazepam or droperidol may be required.

Overdosage of co-proxamol (distalgesic): this drug contains an opiate (dextropropoxyphene) combined with paracetamol. It is very dangerous if taken in overdose. The initial features are those of opiate toxicity with coma, respiratory depression and pinpoint pupils. In severe cases cardiovascular collapse may occur. Naloxone may be required. Paracetamol toxicity may occur later and acetylcysteine should be used when appropriate (see above).

Phenothiazines

These drugs cause less depression of consciousness than other sedative drugs. Hypotension, hypothermia, sinus tachycardia and arrhythmias may occur. Dystonic reactions (rigidity, oculogyric crises, etc.) may occur even with quite small doses. In severe poisoning convulsions may occur, as phenothiazines lower the fit threshold.

Management This is largely supportive, paying special attention to respiration, airway and BP. Patients should be connected to a cardiac monitor if they are: • over 40 or tachycardic • have taken a large overdose • have any history of heart disease. Severe dystonic reactions can be treated with procyclidine, 5–10 mg im, repeated if necessary after 20 min, or 5 mg iv; it is usually effective within 5 min. Alternatively, give benzatropine, 1–2 mg im or iv, repeated if symptoms reappear.

Adverse reaction Neuroleptic malignant syndrome is not a consequence of overdosage of phenothiazines as such but is a rare, very serious, idiosyncratic reaction to neuroleptic drugs, including haloperidol, chlorpromazine and flupentixol (Depixol). It consists of hyperthermia, fluctuating consciousness, muscular rigidity and altered autonomic function with pallor, tachycardia, labile BP, sweating and urinary incontinence. It is potentially fatal so if you think that a patient has the syndrome consult your SHO or registrar immediately.

Paraquat

Concentrated liquid paraquat (Gramoxone) is used by farmers and commercial gardeners. It is extremely toxic. The granular form (Weedol), used by amateur gardeners, contains only 2.5% paraquat and is less dangerous. Ingestion of liquid paraquat is followed by nausea, vomiting and diarrhoea, then by painful ulceration of the tongue, lips and throat. Renal failure may ensue at this stage. Dyspnoea due to proliferative pneumonitis occurs after several days. If you need to confirm the absorption of paraquat this can be done by means of a simple urine test. If urine test is positive, measure plasma paraquat concentration.

Management   Treatment should be begun immediately, with administration of 100 g of activated charcoal which should be given with a laxative such as magnesium sulphate. Follow this up with charcoal, 50 g every 4 hours (or more frequently if tolerated) until the charcoal is seen in the stool. Vomiting may be a problem and an antiemetic may be needed. Oxygen should be avoided in the early stages as it can exacerbate the damage to the lungs.

Amphetamines

These cause wakefulness, excessive activity, paranoia, hallucinations and hypertension, followed by exhaustion, hyperthermia, convulsions and coma. Diazepam recommended for agitation rather than chlorpromazine. Risk of hyperpyrexia with amphetamines/MDMA; fans, tepid sponging, cooled iv fluids and ice baths to correct hyperthermia; dantrolene occasionally required.

Ecstasy (a mixture of amphetamine derivatives, chiefly MDMA) can cause delirium, coma, convulsions, ventricular arrhythmias, hyperpyrexia, rhabdomyolysis, acute renal failure, hyponatraemia and liver failure. Treatment is essentially supportive; close monitoring (including the ECG) is required. Diazepam should be given to control severe agitation or convulsions.

Carbon monoxide

CO poisoning usually results from inhalation of vehicle exhaust or fumes from a gas heater which is inadequately ventilated or where a flue is blocked. The person affected should be removed into fresh air and 100% oxygen given as soon as possible. Note that, although severely poisoned, the person *will not be cyanosed* because carboxyhaemoglobin is bright red. Admission to hospital is almost always necessary because of the risk of delayed complications such as cerebral oedema.

Management   • Carefully assess pulse, BP and rate and depth of respiration • Take blood for FBC, U&E and carboxyhaemoglobin level • Check ABG • Make sure that the patient is going to be closely supervised by a nurse or doctor • Cerebral oedema should be anticipated in the severely poisoned person and treated with mannitol – if you are unsure about this, consult a more senior person • Hyperbaric oxygen treatment should be considered (no definite evidence of benefit) if: he/she is or has been unconscious; the patient is a pregnant woman; the carboxyhaemoglobin level is greater than 40%; there are neurological or psychiatric features.

Digoxin

Digoxin overdosage is usually accidental but can nevertheless be serious. Minor degrees of toxicity produce anorexia, nausea, diarrhoea, abdominal pain, headache, fatigue and confusion. More severe toxicity may produce atrioventricular block, ventricular ectopics or ventricular tachycardia, QRS prolongation or atrial tachycardia with block.

Management If you suspect digoxin toxicity, obtain an urgent ECG with rhythm strip and ask for a U&E and digoxin level. If the patient presents less than an hour after ingestion, give activated charcoal, 50 g stat, than 50 g every 4 hours. If the degree of toxicity is minor, simply withdrawing digoxin, ensuring adequate hydration and correcting hypokalaemia may be enough (use iv potassium if the serum potassium is less than 3.0 mmol/l). If there is more severe poisoning as judged by the severity of the dysrhythmia, the treatment of choice is with digoxin-specific monoclonal antibodies ('Digibind'). *You should consult an experienced person before using this treatment.*

Other measures include hydration to maintain a good urine output (as digoxin is mainly excreted by the renal route) and prophylactic pacing in cases of heart block/bradycardia.

Lithium

Most cases of lithium toxicity occur as the result of long-term treatment associated with accumulation of the drug due to reduced renal excretion. The early features of overdosage include apathy and restlessness; later the patient may develop vomiting, diarrhoea, weakness, ataxia, dysarthria, muscle twitching or tremor. In severe poisoning there may be convulsions, coma, renal failure, dehydration or hypotension. The ECG may show non-specific ST-segment depression, T wave inversion, AV block or prolongation of the QRS or QT intervals.

Therapeutic concentrations of lithium are between 0.4 and 1.0 mmol/l; concentrations above 2.0 mmol/l are usually associated with severe toxicity.

Management This is largely supportive: iv fluid may be needed so as to maintain a good urine output. Diuretics should be avoided. In severe cases haemodialysis may be needed.

Theophyllines

These drugs can cause vomiting, agitation, restlessness, dilated pupils, sinus tachycardia and hyperglycaemia. Severe hypokalaemia can develop rapidly. More serious effects include haematemesis, convulsions and arrhythmias.

Initial measures • Take blood for U&E and theophylline level • Give activated charcoal, 50 g by mouth (then 25 g every 2 hours) or 50 g every 4 hours.

Further measures • Attach an ECG monitor if the patient is over 50, has a history of heart disease or has a serum potassium less than 4.0 mmol/l • Correct hypokalaemia by giving iv potassium; up to 60 mmol/hour may be needed in severe cases • Treat convulsions with iv diazemuls. Diazepam can also be used to treat agitation • Provided the patient does not suffer from asthma or airways obstruction, extreme tachycardia, hypokalaemia and hyperglycaemia may be treated with a short-acting β-blocker given iv; if propranolol is contraindicated verapamil may be used to treat arrhythmias • In severe poisoning consider haemo-perfusion or repeated administration of charcoal.

Antimalarials

Poisoning with chloroquine and hydroxychloroquine is extremely dangerous and is difficult to treat. **Contact the Poisons Information Centre immediately**.

Organophosphorus insecticides

These compounds may be absorbed either though the skin or via the gut or bronchi. Common symptoms of poisoning include anxiety, restlessness, dizziness, headache, pupillary constriction, nausea, hypersalivation, vomiting, abdominal colic, diarrhoea, bradycardia and sweating. Muscle weakness and fasciculation may develop and progress to generalized flaccid paralysis, which may affect the ocular and respiratory muscles. Hyperglycaemia and glycosuria may also be seen.

Management • Consider gastric lavage if substantial amount ingested within 1 hour • Remove the patient to fresh air • Remove contaminated clothing and wash contaminated skin • In severe poisoning make sure that the airway is clear and that the patient is adequately oxygenated. Have a sucker handy to remove bronchial secretions • Specific antagonism of the poisons can be achieved using atropine, 2 mg im or iv, repeated every 20–30 mins until the skin becomes flushed and dry, the pupils dilate and the patient develops a tachycardia. Another drug which is sometimes used is pralidoxime mesilate: consult a more senior person or the Poisons Information Centre before you give this compound.

ACUTE DISTURBANCE OF HAEMODYNAMIC FUNCTION (SHOCK)

Science basics This term describes acute circulatory failure producing cellular hypoxia due to inadequate or disturbed tissue perfusion. ($\rightarrow$ Table 17.14).

Pathophysiology Shock produces hypotension which leads to stimulation of baroreceptors and chemoreceptors raising sympathetic nervous tone and stimulating release of catecholamines from the adrenal medulla. This produces a rise in heart rate, myocardial contractility and systemic resistance and a decrease in venous capacitance in an attempt to maintain venous return and cardiac output and thus the maintenance of BP. Various hormones are also released in response to shock including ACTH, GH, ADH, endorphins, cortisol, aldosterone and glucagon, as well as a variety of prostacyclin and liposomal enzymes. These mediators are beneficial only when targeted locally against infection or tissue damage, but when their release is uncontrolled and disseminated widespread tissue damage can occur leading to multiple organ failure (lungs, ARDS, heart, kidneys, GI tract and brain).

Clinical features The features depend upon the underlying cause of the shock, but usually include poor skin perfusion (cold, pale, clammy, cyanosis). Confusion, restlessness, oliguria, tachycardia, hypotension, sweating, pyrexia, and rigors may be present. Increasing acidosis occurs as the shock progresses with accelerating multi-organ failure. BP may be maintained initially, especially in young people, but hypotension occurs as shock progresses.

Table 17.14
Causes of shock

Cardiogenic	Usually secondary to IHD Failure of peripheral circulation
Hypovolaemic	Haemorrhage, burns, sepsis, anaphylaxis
Normovolaemic	Arteriovenous shunts, diffuse venous dilatation
Mechanical	Massive pulmonary embolism, cardiac tamponade

Investigations • Invasive monitoring is often required • Arterial cannulation • Central venous access • Urinary catheterization • Measurement of cardiac output, oxygen delivery and uptake • Mixed venous oxygenation • Baseline haematological clotting studies • U&E and creatinine • Liver function • Glucose, lactate • Blood cultures • CXR, ECG.

Management box

▶ Early and aggressive resuscitation is necessary. A patent airway must be maintained and supplemental oxygen provided to ensure adequate tissue oxygenation and ventilation. The underlying cause of the shock should be corrected, eg haemorrhage stemmed or infection treated. Broad-spectrum antibiotics are often necessary, but should be tailored once culture results and sensitivities are available. Volume fluid replacement is necessary via wide-bore cannulae, and their effect is monitored. Thus cardiac output and BP are restored. The choice of fluid for volume replacement is usually via colloids or blood if necessary. Crystalloid solutions are rapidly lost from the circulation.

▶ Inotropic agents, eg adrenaline (epinephrine), noradrenaline (norepinephrine) or dobutamine, are used to maintain cardiac contractility. Dopamine or dopexamine are used to improve renal blood flow.

▶ Vasodilator therapy, eg sodium nitroprusside, nitroglycerine, hydrallazine or isosorbide dinitrate, may be used in cardiogenic shock to increase stroke volume and improve coronary flow but their use requires careful monitoring.

▶ The critically ill patient usually requires artificial ventilation and haemodialysis. TPN may be necessary. Estimation of trans-mucosal pH allows the adequacy of tissue oxygenation to be assessed. DVT prophylaxis and lowering of the gastric pH (eg H_2-blocking agents) are commonly employed. Close nursing supervision is vital.

ADULT RESPIRATORY DISTRESS SYNDROME

Science basics ARDS is a common and serious disorder characterized by acute respiratory failure due to pulmonary injury and accompanied by hypoxia and respiratory distress. The precise pathogenesis is unclear but a leaky alveolar epithelial/endothelial membrane develops and is followed by fibrous tissue deposition. Precipitating factors are shown in Table 4.11, p 90.

Clinical features The usual presentation is a few days after the recognition of a serious underlying disease and not uncommonly during convalescence.

Symptoms: include breathlessness and deterioration in clinical condition.

Signs: tachypnoea, cyanosis, intercostal indrawing and hypotension.

Investigations • CXR shows a 'white-out' with sparing of the costophrenic angles in the early stages. This helps in the differentiation from LVF in which a more central infiltration occurs associated with cardiomegaly • ABG: hypoxia with hypocapnia and respiratory alkalosis; the hypoxia is relatively resistant to oxygen administration and progressive • Swan-Ganz catheterization shows a PCWP <18 mm/kg (with normal plasma oncotic pressure).

Management box

▶ This can be divided into two parts; treatment of the underlying disorder and treatment of the lung problem.

▶ The underlying disease may not be obvious. Shock, if present, should be corrected aggressively but once an adequate circulation has been restored fluid administration, particularly crystalloids, must be administered with care as pulmonary oedema develops readily. Inotropic support (eg dobutamine) is commonly required. The use of high-dose steroid therapy is controversial particularly in septic shock, but is recommended in fat embolism and following aspiration. Sepsis when present should be treated aggressively with intravenous antibiotics and surgical drainage or resection of septic foci. Where large volumes of blood are required, filters to remove particulate material reduce the risk of ARDS.

▶ The pulmonary problem requires mechanical ventilation with sufficient oxygen to maintain an adequate but not increased PaO_2. High concentrations of oxygen may lead to further lung damage. Control of respiration with increased tidal and minute volumes and PEEP are usually required with careful monitoring of the cardiac output and blood pressure. Prevention of pulmonary oedema by careful fluid balance, loop diuretics and salt-poor colloid administration is important. Early recognition and adequate treatment of ARDS greatly improves survival. The mortality remains around 70% due most often to multi-organ failure and many patients are left with permanent restrictive lung damage.

LOW BLOOD PRESSURE

Science basics As with most measurements in medicine, it is a change in BP which is more significant than the absolute value: an elderly man whose BP is usually 170/100 but who suddenly drops down to 110/70 is likely to need further investigation. Remember also that, at least in advanced societies, average BP rises progressively with age, so a reading of 95/50 might be quite normal in a 17-year-old girl but would not be at all normal in a middle-aged subject.

Hypotension impairs vital organ function by:

- reducing coronary perfusion
- reducing renal bloodflow and therefore urine output
- reducing cerebral perfusion and thereby impairing consciousness.

Causes The three principal causes of hypotension are summarized in Table 17.15. Uncommon but important causes include adrenal insufficiency, self-poisoning with drugs, eg phenothiazines or antidepressants, tension pneumothorax, aortic

Table 17.15
Causes of hypotension

Diagnosis	Cause
Volume depletion	Blood loss (gastrointestinal, trauma, into a fracture, leaking aortic aneurysm)
	Loss of crystalloid or colloid (diarrhoea, vomiting, drains, diabetic ketoacidosis, burns, polyuric renal failure, adrenal insufficiency, over-vigorous use of diuretics)
Pump failure	MI
	Major arrhythmias (fast atrial fibrillation, supra-ventricular tachycardia (SVT), ventricular tachycardia, complete heart block)
	Pulmonary embolism (large)
	Myocardial depression due to septicaemia or acidosis
	Myocardial depressant drugs, eg β-blockers, antiarrhythmics
	Over-vigorous treatment of hypertension
Fall in peripheral vascular resistance	Septicaemia
	Peritonitis
	Pancreatitis
	Over-vigorous use of vasodilators to treat angina or heart failure

dissection, pericardial effusion (tamponade), anaphylaxis. Gynaecological causes such as rupture of an ectopic pregnancy should be considered in appropriate patients.

Diagnosis

History • Ask about: • pain (chest, abdominal or back) • breathlessness • any indications of blood-loss, especially melaena. In young women, ask about the date of the last period • Review the drug history. Could there be a pharmacological cause?

Examination Remember to check the following: • Does the patient look dehydrated? • Is the patient cold, clammy and peripherally shut-down? • Does the patient look as though he is suffering? • Is the patient fully conscious? • Is the patient pyrexial? • Is the JVP visibly distended or collapsed? • Is the patient sweating? • Check the patient's pulse and BP yourself. Measure the BP with the patient supine and also sitting upright: a fall in systolic pressure of more than 10 mmHg (or a fall to less than 100 mm) makes it likely that the patient is volume-depleted • Examine the heart, looking for a gallop rhythm, pericardial friction rub, new murmurs. If the patient has interscapular pain (which is suggestive of an aortic dissection) check both carotid and both brachial pulses to look for inequality of pulse volume and measure the BP in both arms • Examine the respiratory system, looking for reduced chest movement on one side, tracheal deviation (both of these would occur with a tension pneumothorax), markedly reduced breath sounds or a pleural rub (which would suggest pulmonary embolism) • Examine the abdomen, looking for evidence of peritonitis or ileus and for an aortic aneurysm; if you suspect leakage from an aneurysm make sure you check the femoral pulses • Check any drains for evidence of bleeding and be sure to perform a rectal examination if gastrointestinal bleeding is suspected.

Investigations and management

Volume depletion

Suspected bleeding Take blood for full blood count, U&E and blood grouping. Insert one or, in severe cases, two large-bore iv cannulae and give plasma expander (eg Haemaccel) until blood is available. Losses should be replaced as whole blood; concentrated red cells should only be used in frail or elderly patients where there is a major risk of overload from over-transfusion. Grouped, uncrossmatched blood can be obtained quickly and should be given in patients who are peripherally shut-down, oliguric or semi-conscious. If whole blood is not available to you, give concentrated red cells together with saline. You may need to squeeze the bag or compress it with an inflatable cuff in order to increase the rate of fluid flow. Insert a urinary catheter to monitor urine output.

Other causes of fluid loss   Take blood for FBC and U&E, then give intravenous fluids such as plasma expanders (Gelofusin, Haemaccel, etc) or saline. If the loss seems to be of water more than solutes, ie if the patient is dry as the result of poor drinking or perspiration, the iv fluid of choice is 5% glucose. Remember, however, that water depletion rarely results in hypotension of more than mild degree. (For a fuller discussion of intravenous fluid therapy → p 510) Insert a urinary catheter to monitor urine output.

When treating hypovolaemia remember the possible risk of overloading the patient with fluid; if you are at all concerned about this a central venous line should be put in to monitor central venous pressure (CVP).

Pump failure   Arrange an *ECG* and look for: • tachycardia • rhythm disorder or heart block • pathological Q waves, ST segment elevation and other evidence of MI • signs of PE, namely, right axis deviation and deep, slurred S waves in lead I, QRS widening in VI, V2, ST segment depression and T wave inversion in V1 and V2 • If you are not sure how to interpret the ECG ask the duty medical SHO or registrar • Arrange a CXR to look for: • pneumothorax • pulmonary oedema • collapse or consolidation • widening of the mediastinum (aortic dissection).

Myocardial infarction (MI)   Urgent transfer to a CCU is indicated. Give analgesia (usually diamorphine, 5 mg iv with prochlorperazine 12.5 mg), oxygen and (if breathless) iv furosemide (frusemide) (40 mg) before transfer and make sure that the patient has an intravenous cannula in place before he/she leaves the general ward or A&E department. If no bed is available on the CCU, arrange a bed-side cardiac monitor and ask the nursing staff to check pulse and BP every half hour. Treatment with a thrombolytic agent or with inotropic drugs (dobutamine, adrenaline (epinephrine)) may need to be considered: for this and other reasons you should inform the duty medical SHO or registrar.

Rapid tachycardia (over 140 per min)   This may be a compensatory reaction to the volume depletion but a tachyarrhythmia should also be considered, so look at the ECG and, if in doubt, ask for help with interpretation. If you are sure that the rhythm is an SVT then, provided the patient does not have asthma and there is no heart block, it would be reasonable to attach the patient to a cardiac monitor and to give iv adenosine, 3 mg rapidly (less if the patient has had a heart transplant or is taking dipyridamole); if this is unsuccessful, follow up with a dose of 6 mg, then 12 mg if required. If the patient is not at risk of heart failure and has not recently received a β-blocker, an alternative would be verapamil, 5–10 mg iv over 2 min, repeated if necessary.

Large pulmonary embolism (PE) → p 437 above.

Dissection of the thoracic aorta Give analgesia and, if the patient is distressed, a sedative. Contact your SHO or registrar urgently: he or she should speak to the duty surgical registrar at your nearest cardiac surgical centre.

Fall in systemic vascular resistance (SVR)

Fluid replacement The patient with an abnormally low SVR of whatever cause is, in effect, fluid depleted, so give fluid in the form of colloid solutions, i.e. Gelofusin, Haemaccel or hetastarch.

Septicaemia → p 450 above.

Pancreatitis → p 441 above.

Perforation of a viscus Arrange chest and abdominal X-rays. The patient may need urgent surgery or re-operation (if the problem arises postoperatively).

Miscellaneous

Tension pneumothorax Attach a large-bore needle to a syringe partially filled with normal saline. Insert the needle into the second intercostal space in the mid-clavicular line, remove the plunger from the syringe and allow the air to escape through the saline. This often results in a dramatic improvement in the patient's clinical condition. You should then insert a chest drain (→ p 488).

Adrenal insufficiency If you are really stuck for an explanation for the hypotension, consider this: take a blood sample to be stored for later estimation of serum cortisol and give iv hydrocortisone, 100–200 mg stat (depending on the size of the patient) then 100 mg every 6 hours, together with intravenous 0.9% saline.

ACUTE RENAL FAILURE

Science basics This condition, generally characterized by oliguria (<15 ml urine/hour) or anuria with a rising serum creatinine and potassium, is common and frequently reversible with appropriate therapy. Occasionally urine output may be normal despite deteriorating renal function.

Aetiology Causes are traditionally divided into three groups:

Pre-renal: due to volume depletion secondary to dehydration and haemorrhage or reduced cardiac output. It is characterized by oliguria and a high specific gravity (>1.020) and low urinary sodium (<10 mmol/l) if diuretics have not been used. If the underlying insult is prolonged acute tubular necrosis (ATN) develops, typified by oliguria with urine of low specific gravity (<1.010).

Intrinsic: due to renovascular disease, acute glomerulonephritis, malignant hypertension, myoglobinuria, sepsis, toxins, eg paracetamol, carbon tetrachloride, radiographic contrast, aminoglycosides, NSAIDs.

Post-renal: due to outlet obstruction in the renal tract, eg prostatic hypertrophy, ureteric stones, bladder or pelvic tumours. N.B. ARF is often multifactorial, eg toxins and infection on background of dehydration, also acute on chronic renal failure is very common.

Clinical features

Symptoms: nausea, vomiting, dehydration, confusion.

Signs: dehydration (JVP not visible, postural hypotension, absence of oedema, dry mucosae), 'fluid overload' (hypertension, raised JVP, pulmonary oedema +/– hypoxia, peripheral oedema), pallor, rash, pericardial rub, bruising.

Investigations

Laboratory: • serum urea, creatinine and potassium • FBC and clotting • ABG if hypoxic/hyperventilating • cardiac enzymes looking for elevated CK in rhabdomyolysis • serum calcium, raised in myeloma and primary hyperparathyroidism (cause of stones) • liver function tests abnormal in hepatorenal syndrome • serum amylase • blood cultures • immunology including ANF (raised in most connective-tissue diseases), ANCA, anti GBM, complement, serum and urine electrophoresis • urine dipstick and microscopy (blood, protein and casts) • MSU (pyelonephritis) • ECG looking for recent MI or tented T waves in hyperkalaemia.

Radiology: • US to look for obstruction and assess renal size (nephrostomy and urology referral if obstruction demonstrated) • CXR (pulmonary oedema) • plain abdomen film if stones suspected • IVU and renal angiography best avoided in acute setting because of risks of contrast nephropathy.

Management box

▸ This is aimed at reversing life-threatening complications and identifying the underlying cause. The initial management should be:

  – assessment and correction of ECF abnormalities: electrolyte solution in dehydration, blood in haemorrhage, inotropes if →

> > hypotension persists after ECF correction and trial of diuretics
> > in severe overload, up to 250 mg furosemide (frusemide)
> > (maximum 4 mg/minute).
> ▸ Fluid replacement in oliguric patient needs to be done with care
>   with frequent reassessments and if doubt, CVP monitoring.
> ▸ US to exclude postrenal renal failure.
> ▸ Dipstick analysis of urine. Significant blood and protein are
>   indicative of intrinsic renal disease if UTI excluded.
> ▸ Management should be discussed with more senior member
>   of team. If urgent dialysis is indicated (see below) the patient
>   should be discussed with local Renal Unit urgently. If kidney
>   size normal on US and urinalysis suggestive, renal biopsy may
>   be indicated.

Indications for urgent dialysis:
- Life-threatening hyperkalaemia (K >6.5, unmanageable by
  medical therapy ($\rightarrow$ p 409)). If patient passing urine and/or
  dehydrated, hyperkalaemia may be managed with insulin and
  dextrose infusion, iv calcium gluconate (stabilize cardiac
  conduction tissue), 1.26% sodium bicarbonate infusions
  (promotes urinary K loss), nebulized salbutamol (promotes
  cellular uptake), calcium resonium.
- Life-threatening pulmonary oedema unmanageable by medical
  therapy, ie diuretics, oxygen and nitrates (saturations <90% on
  O_2).
- Pericarditis/pericardial friction rub.
- Uraemia.
- Acidosis in a critically ill patient (usually in ITU setting).
- **N.B.** The threshold for dialysis is lower if the patient is
  oligoanuric without dehydration.

Ongoing management:
- *Daily* monitoring of U&E/fluid balance/body weight +/–CVP.
- Optimization of fluid balance/correction of hypovolaemia.
- Control of infection.
- Avoidance of nephrotoxic drugs especially NSAIDs, ACE
  inhibitors if suspicious of renovascular disease, caution with
  radiocontrast.
- Immunosupression, prednisolone and cyclophosphamide +/–
  plasma exchange for vasculitis.
- Angiography if patient dialysis-dependent and history
  suggestive.

Fluid replacement in renal failure – guiding principles:
- If the patient is oliguric she/he needs repeated clinical
  reassessments of fluid status.
- CVP line may help, but is not infallible.

- Meticulous assessment of input/output is vital.
- Fluid replacement volume of hourly urine output +20–30 ml/hour will maintain neutral fluid balance.
- If the patient is dehydrated hourly urine output +50–60 ml/ hour will lead to progressive rehydration of 750 ml/day (only matching urine output leads to progressive dehydration).
- Urine output + 30 ml/hour is safe in massive polyuria after relieving obstruction or recovering ATN.
- If the patient is acidotic alternate sodium bicarbonate 1.26% and dextrose (5 or 10%) is appropriate, otherwise use normal saline and dextrose.
- Do not use diuretics unless the patient is clearly volume-replete.
- **N.B**. Insensible losses are about 500 ml per day. These will be greater if the patient is febrile/has diarrhoea/vomiting/bowel obstruction/burns etc.

Section 4:
Practical
procedures

18

Practical procedures

SITING AN INTRAVENOUS CANNULA

Equipment
- Cannula (17 G or 18 G)
- Tourniquet
- Cannula dressing
- Cotton-wool balls
- Dressing pack
- Skin-cleansing solution
- Razor (in men)
- Bag of iv fluid attached to giving set and run-through
- 2-ml syringe containing 0.9% saline.

Procedure
1. Place the tourniquet on the upper forearm or above.
2. Inspect the arm for engorged veins: the best access-point is usually the cephalic vein over the distal radius (Fig. 18.1). Alternatives would include more proximal branches of the cephalic vein or the median forearm vein.

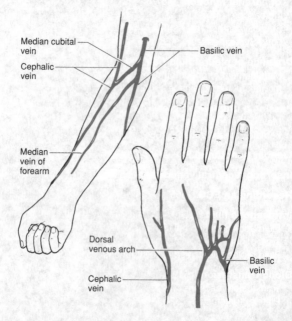

Fig. 18.1   Veins of the forearm.

3. Clean the skin well, then dry it with a cotton-wool ball or gauze. In men with hairy arms, shave the hair over a large enough area to allow the dressing to be sited onto hair-free skin.
4. Identify an entry-point, preferably where two tributaries of the vein join. Puncture the skin about 1 cm distal to the point where you plan to enter the vein.
5. Advance the needle and cannula slowly until you feel a 'give' as the needle enters the vein and until you see blood flash back into the hub of the needle.
6. Hold the hub of the needle with one hand and advance the cannula into the vein with the other.
7. If the cannula is to be used immediately for an iv infusion, press on the vein just proximal to the innermost end of the cannula, withdraw the needle completely and connect up the iv-giving set. Secure the cannula in place with the dressing.
8. If the cannula is not going to be used immediately, press on the vein just proximal to the innermost end of the cannula, withdraw the needle completely and screw the screw-cap over the end of the cannula. Secure the cannula in place with the dressing. Flush the cannula with saline via the side-arm.

Poor veins: place the patient's forearm in a bowl of warm water, leave for 10 minutes and try again. Alternatively, inflate a sphygmomanometer cuff on the arm to above systolic pressure and leave it in place for 2 minutes. After the cuff is released the lactic acid which has accumulated will cause reflex vasodilatation.

Fat arm: try the back of the hand, a smaller cannula may be necessary.

Fragile veins: use a smaller cannula, eg pink 20 G.

Rapid infusion: if a patient needs to be given a large volume of fluid (or blood) quickly, try to insert a larger cannula, eg grey, 16 G.

For an iv infusion, insert the cannula in the patient's non-dominant arm if possible. Do not keep on trying repeatedly if you fail to insert a cannula: two or three attempts are the most that you should allow yourself. Repeated unsuccessful attempts are distressing for the patient and may ruin those few accessible veins which the patient has. Ask someone else to do it.

Running an iv infusion through
It is very frustrating to try to set up an iv infusion if the line is full of air bubbles. Try to observe the following precautions when you run an infusion through:

1. Most iv-giving sets are packed with the valve open, so as soon as you unpack the set, close the valve completely.
2. Remove the seal on the bag of iv fluid and pierce it with the needle attached to the giving set. Hang the bag on a drip stand.

3. Squeeze the drip chamber to bring a quantity of fluid into it (until it is about half full).
4. Hold the giving set with the far end pointing upwards and held about 6 inches below the level of the bag. Open the valve slowly and allow fluid to flow along the tube until it reaches the end.

GIVING INJECTIONS

Intradermal injections

You are unlikely to need to use this technique except for Mantoux tests and other sensitivity tests.

Method Use a 1 ml syringe and a 25-G (brown or orange) needle, or an insulin syringe with a fixed needle. Stretch the skin between the thumb and forefinger of one hand. Holding the syringe in the other hand and with your index finger on the top of the needle hub, insert the needle at an angle of about 10° to the skin surface to a depth of about 2 mm (so that the bevel is just covered). A raised, blanched bleb showing the tips of the hair follicles is a sign that the injection has been given correctly (Note: considerable resistance is felt to a correctly given intradermal injection. If there is little or no resistance to the injection, the needle is too deep and you should withdraw it and try again.)

Subcutaneous injections

Method Use a small syringe and a 25- or 27-G needle. Pinch up the tissues with the thumb and forefinger of one hand and insert the needle at right angles to the skin; push the needle in up to its hilt or for a distance of 5–6 mm, whichever is the less.

Intramuscular injections

Method Use a syringe of appropriate size for the volume of drug and a 21-G (green) needle. The injection may be given into one of three sites:

• the deltoid muscle
• middle two-thirds, lateral aspect of the thigh
• the upper, outer quadrant of the buttock (Fig. 18.2); it is important not to use other parts of the buttock because of the danger of injury to the sciatic nerve.

Giving a local anaesthetic

Local anaesthesia is extremely effective provided that you give enough into the correct site and that you allow enough time for it to work before starting the procedure.

Method

1. Draw up 1% or 2% lidocaine (lignocaine) into a 5 ml or 10 ml syringe (according to the procedure) using a luer filler

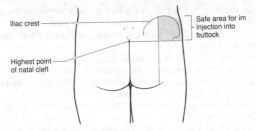

Fig. 18.2 Site for safe im injection in the buttock.

or a 21-G (green) needle. Change to a 25-G (orange) needle and expel any air.

2. Clean the skin thoroughly. Give a small dose of lidocaine (lignocaine) intradermally by holding the syringe with your index finger on the top of the needle hub and inserting the needle at an angle of about 10° to the skin surface to a depth of about 2 mm. A raised, blanched bleb showing the tips of the hair follicles is a sign that the injection has been given correctly. If you need to anaesthetize a large area of skin remove the needle and repeat the procedure a few millimetres away.

3. Change the needle to a 21-G (green) one. Insert the needle, at right angles to the skin, through the centre of the bleb and draw back on the piston. If no blood comes back, inject 0.1–0.2 ml of lidocaine (lignocaine), then advance the needle about half a centimetre, draw back again and inject another 0.1–0.2 ml. Repeat this process until you have reached the required depth. If you are going right down to bone (eg for a LP or chest-drain insertion) try to catch the needle tip on the periosteum and inject a small volume of lidocaine (lignocaine) under the periosteum. Remember that it is an extremely pain-sensitive structure.

4. Allow at least 3 minutes for the local anaesthetic to work before you go on. Before you proceed, test the area with a fine needle to check that anaesthesia has been successful. If not, give some more lidocaine (lignocaine).

Giving intravenous injections

Many drugs for intravenous administration do not come ready made up in solution but are provided in powder form, either with their own diluent or for dilution in sterile water. The bottle containing the drug is usually airtight with a rubber seal. This makes getting the diluent into the bottle (and the drug out) difficult. The following technique is recommended:

1. Draw up the required volume of diluent or water into a syringe by means of a 19-G (white) or 21-G (green) needle.

2. Put the drug bottle flat on the bench and remove the metal cap. Clean the rubber cap with an alcohol swab. Insert a 23-G (blue) or 25-G (orange) needle through the cap; this will act as an air vent.

3. Holding the bottle in one hand, insert the needle of the diluent syringe and inject the diluent. Do *not* inject too quickly as this may cause the solution to froth and to start coming out through the air vent.

4. Remove both needles from the bottle and shake the bottle to dissolve the drug.

5. Draw about 3 ml of air into the syringe, invert the drug bottle and introduce the needle. Inject the air into the bottle and draw up the solution. If you start to feel resistance, pull hard, then release the piston and continue drawing up.

6. When you have drawn up all the drug, draw a couple of millilitres of air into the syringe, tip it back and forth to pick up all the little bubbles, then expel the air via the needle.

7. Check the prescription sheet to ensure that it is the right patient, the right drug and the right dose. Give the injection slowly. If special care is needed about the speed of injection, use a watch to time yourself. If you are giving a cytotoxic drug, watch the area around the cannula entry-site carefully to make sure that the drug is not 'tissuing'.

8. Inject 1 ml of sterile saline into the cannula so as to keep it patent for the next time.

TAKING BLOOD FOR CULTURE

Blood cultures need to be taken with considerable care so as to give the best possible chance of successfully isolating a pathogen and of avoiding contamination with skin commensals. Try to take the blood for culture while the patient is actually febrile.

Equipment
- Set of blood-culture bottles (use resin bottles if the patient is already on antibiotics)
- 5-ml or 10-ml syringe
- 2 needles (21 G)
- Alcohol wipes
- 'Sharps' bin.

Procedure
1. Locate a suitable vein and swab the skin over it with two or three alcohol wipes. Allow the alcohol to dry. *Do not* touch the skin again unless you are wearing sterile gloves.

2. Withdraw a suitable volume of blood (as specified on the labels of the culture bottles).

3. Change the needle and add the correct volume of blood to each bottle. *Do not overfill*. Dispose of needles in 'sharps' bin.
4. Label the bottles and have them transported to the laboratory or (out of working hours) to an incubator. *Do not put them in the fridge.*

ARTERIAL BLOOD GASES (ABG)

Equipment
- 21-G (green) needle
- Pre-heparinized syringe (if pre-packed syringes are not available you can prepare one by taking a 2-ml syringe and drawing up 0.5 ml of heparin solution, 1000 u/ml. With the heparin in the syringe and the syringe/needle pointing vertically upwards, pull the piston down to the bottom of its travel, then push it up again and expel the air. Point the needle into the sink and expel the heparin.)
- Syringe cap
- Cotton-wool balls
- Drinking glass or paper cup containing ice
- 'Sharps' bin.

Procedure
Write out the request card before you start. You do not want to waste time doing it after you have got the sample.

Radial artery
1. Lay the patient's arm comfortably on the bed or a bed-table.
2. Check that the ulnar artery is patent by compressing both radial and ulnar arteries with your fingers. Ask the patient to open and close the fist several times. Release the ulnar artery and check that the hand flushes pink.
3. Palpate the radial artery between your first and second fingers. Try to gauge both the depth and the course of the artery.
4. Keeping one finger on the artery (but *not* compressing it!) advance the needle through the skin at an angle of 45°. Do *not* hold on to the piston of the syringe.
5. Continue advancing the syringe and needle slowly until blood flows spontaneously into the syringe. If this happens you can be sure that you have entered the artery and not a vein. If blood begins to enter the syringe but comes in very slowly, it is reasonable to apply *very gentle* traction to the piston. If the needle has gone into a depth of 5 mm or more but no blood has been obtained, withdraw the needle to just below the skin and advance it once again at a slightly different angle or in a slightly different direction.
6. Once you have 1–2 ml blood in the syringe withdraw the needle from the artery and apply firm pressure over the

puncture site with cotton-wool. Ask an assistant to maintain the pressure for at least 3 minutes.

7. Remove the needle and put the syringe cap on. Place the syringe in the cup of ice and label the cup or the base of the syringe with the patient's name and details. Arrange immediate transport to the laboratory.

8. Dispose of needle in 'sharps' bin.

Femoral artery

1. Lay the patient flat so that the hip is in full extension.
2. Palpate the artery between your first and second fingers. Try to gauge both the depth and the course of the artery. If the pulse is difficult to feel, ask the patient to bend the knee and externally rotate the thigh.
3. Advance the needle between your fingers and through the skin at right angles to the artery. Do *not* hold on to the piston of the syringe.
4. Steps 5–8 above (Radial artery).

Interpretation

Precise interpretation of the results of blood gases can be made by means of a Flenley diagram (Fig. 16.2). However, in case you do not have one or do not know how to use it, some simple pointers are given below.

Simple hypoxia (type 1 respiratory failure) The PO_2 is less than 8 kPa (60 mmHg) but the PCO_2 is normal. This commonly occurs in lobar pneumonia or other causes of lobar collapse or consolidation (eg PE); it may also occur in asthma (though in moderate asthma the PCO_2 is usually subnormal), pulmonary fibrosis, certain kinds of chronic obstructive airways disease (especially emphysema with superadded infection) or left ventricular failure.

Hypoxia with hypercapnia (type 2 respiratory failure) The PO_2 is low – less than 8 kPa (60 mmHg) – and the PCO_2 is raised (greater than 6.5 kPa; 49 mmHg). This occurs in patients with chronic bronchitis during acute exacerbations, in ARDS, severe pneumonia, severe left ventricular failure and in those with alveolar hypoventilation, eg Guillain-Barré syndrome.

Acidaemia (low pH) with a low PCO_2 and low plasma bicarbonate This represents a metabolic acidosis, eg aspirin poisoning, diabetic ketoacidosis.

Alkalaemia (raised pH) with high PCO_2 and normal or high bicarbonate This represents a metabolic alkalosis, eg prolonged vomiting.

Acidaemia with a high PCO_2, low PO_2 and high/normal or raised bicarbonate This is an acute respiratory acidosis and is the kind of pattern you would expect to see in someone with an exacerbation of chronic bronchitis who was sick.

Acidaemia with a high PCO₂, low PO₂ and normal bicarbonate
This is an acute respiratory acidosis and is the kind of pattern you would expect to see in someone with a severe respiratory illness but who had previously been well.

Normal pH with a low PO₂, raised PCO₂ and raised bicarbonate
This represents a compensated respiratory acidosis; you would see this in someone with chronic bronchitis (ie a 'blue bloater') when relatively well.

Alkalaemia with a normal PO₂, low PCO₂ and normal or high/ normal bicarbonate This is a respiratory alkalosis; the commonest cause is hyperventilation.

TETRACOSACTIDE (SYNACTHEN) TESTS FOR THE ASSESSMENT OF ADRENAL FUNCTION

INDICATIONS

- Exclusion of primary or secondary adrenal insufficiency (SHORT Synacthen test)
- Differentiation of primary from secondary adrenal insufficiency (LONG Synacthen test)

SHORT SYNACTHEN TEST

The patient does not need to fast for the test, which may be carried out at any time of day. If he/she has been taking hydrocortisone this should be stopped for 24–48 hours before the test; if steroid cover is felt necessary the patient should be given dexamethasone, 0.5 mg bd.

Equipment
- Alcohol wipes
- Cannula (Venflon or similar)
- Dressing for cannula
- 5 ml syringe containing normal saline
- 2 × 10-ml syringe
- 2 × 2-ml syringe
- Green needle for im injection
- 250 mcg of plain tetracosactrin
- 2 × plain serum tubes
- 'Sharps' bin.

Procedure
- Clean skin with alcohol and insert cannula. Secure with dressing. Dispose of needle in 'sharps' bin.
- Withdraw 10 ml blood into plain serum tube (0 min sample).

- Instil 1–2 ml saline into cannula and close-off with cap.
- Give 250 µg plain tetracosactide (Synacthen) im.
- At 30 mins, withdraw 2 ml blood from cannula and discard. Withdraw 10 ml for sample. The test is now complete.

Interpretation

A peak serum cortisol of >600 nmol/l, with a rise between 0 and 30 min of >330 nmol/l excludes primary or secondary adrenal insufficiency. If the result is abnormal, the patient should undergo a long tetracosactrin test.

LONG SYNACTHEN TEST

The patient does not need to fast for the test. If he/she has been taking hydrocortisone this should be stopped for 24–48 hours before the test; if steroid cover is felt necessary the patient should be given dexamethasone, 0.5 mg daily.

Equipment

- 3 × 10 ml syringes with venepuncture needles
- Green needle for im injection
- 1 mg of depot tetracosactide
- 3 × plain serum tubes

Procedure

- Take 10 ml blood into plain serum tube (0 min sample).
- Give 1 mg depot tetracosactide (Synacthen) im.
- At 8 hours take 10 ml blood sample.
- At 24 hours take 10 ml blood. Test is now completed.

Interpretation

A serum cortisol of >1000 nmol/l at 8 hours, together with a value >600 nmol/l at 24 hours, excludes primary adrenal insufficiency and indicates that the problem is at pituitary or hypothalamic level. Lesser responses suggest primary adrenal failure.

DRAINAGE OF PLEURAL FLUID/AIR

Symptomatic relief can often be achieved by aspirating a pleural effusion. You should observe the procedure on one or two occasions before doing it yourself and should be supervised during your first few attempts.

Equipment

- Minor dressing pack
- Gloves
- Antiseptic
- Lidocaine (Lignocaine)

- For local anaesthetic (if required): 10-ml syringe, 21-G needle (green) and 25-G needle (blue)
- Scalpel (if inserting a drain)
- For a diagnostic tap, 20-ml syringe and 19-G needle (white)
- For a therapeutic tap, 60 ml Luer-lock syringe, 3-way tap, 18-G cannula (Venflon, etc), drainage tube and a 2–l measuring jug to act as receiver (or one-piece 28-French (Fr) G drain, with trochar, and collecting bag if the effusion is to be drained slowly)
- Specimen bottles for biochemistry (protein content), microbiology and cytology
- Sutures
- 'Sharps' bin.

Procedure

1. Ask the patient to sit forward with the arms folded. The arms should be supported on a pillow which rests on a bed-table so that the weight of the patient's upper body is taken by the arms.
2. Percuss carefully and locate the upper limit of dullness. For a diagnostic aspiration, choose the intercostal space below this level and aim to enter it in the posterior mid-clavicular line; for a therapeutic drainage you can use the same entry site or, alternatively, a point in the 7th intercostal space mid-way between the mid-axillary and posterior axillary lines (this

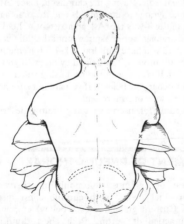

Fig. 18.3 Drainage of a pleural effusion. X marks the site for insertion of a chest drain, ie 7th intercostal space between the mid and posterior axillary lines.

represents the lowest level of the pleural reflection; see Fig 18.3). Remember that you must pass through the intercostal space *above* the rib which forms its lower limit, not below the rib which is its upper limit, as the intercostal nerves and vessels run just beneath each lower rib margin.

3. If you are inserting a drain give some iv analgesia such as 25–50 mg pethidine. If the patient is very anxious a small dose of iv sedation may also be desirable.

4. Wash your hands and put on gloves.

5. Clean the skin over the entry-site with antiseptic.

6. For a diagnostic tap, pass the needle through the chest wall, aspirating gently as you do so. Withdraw about 20 ml of fluid and note the colour. Remove the needle and put a dressing over the wound. Put the specimens into the respective bottles. Dispose of needles in the 'sharps' bin.

   Diagnostic aspirations should be done reasonably early in the day: fluid for cytology must be processed within a short time as the cells will degenerate if the specimen is kept in the fridge overnight.

7. For a therapeutic drainage, infiltrate the skin and subcutaneous tissues with lidocaine (lignocaine). If fluid has been drawn back while you are doing this, do not inject again as this could result in the seeding of tumour cells along the needle track in the case of malignant effusions.

8. Attach the cannula and 3-way tap to the syringe and introduce the needle with gentle aspiration. Once fluid is flowing freely, remove the needle, leaving the cannula in place. Attach the 3-way tap and syringe to the cannula and the drainage tube to the side-arm of the 3-way tap. Ask an assistant to hold the receiver under the drainage tube. Aspirate until the fluid ceases to flow freely or until you have withdrawn 1–1.5 l. Remember to send specimens for protein, culture and cytology. If you are leaving a drain in situ, this can be introduced using an enclosed needle or with a trochar (see below). If you are not sure how to use this, consult someone more senior.

9. The procedure for inserting a chest drain is described on pp 492–493.

MANAGEMENT OF PNEUMOTHORAX

Pneumothorax occurs most commonly in otherwise fit young adults or in older people with chronic chest disease, chiefly emphysema. Current guidelines (see below) emphasize that the traditional practice of putting in a chest drain whenever a pneumothorax needed to be drained can no longer be justified: many pneumothoraces can be drained very adequately by simple aspiration.

Patients without chronic chest disease

- If the pneumothorax is *small* (a small rim of air around the lung only), drainage is not necessary.
- If the pneumothorax is *moderate* in size (lung collapsed half way towards the heart border), drainage is not necessary unless there is significant dyspnoea.
- If the pneumothorax is *large* (complete collapse of the lung), a chest drain should be inserted (see below).
- Patients who do not require aspiration may be discharged from hospital but should be reviewed in the chest clinic 7–10 days later. If there is any deterioration in the condition, the patient should be told to return to hospital immediately. Air travel should be avoided until the X-ray changes have resolved.

Patients with chronic chest disease

- If the pneumothorax is *small* (a small rim of air around the lung only), drainage is not necessary unless the patient is significantly more breathless than normal. However, even if aspiration is not performed the patient should be observed in hospital overnight and the chest X-ray repeated the next day. If there is no deterioration clinically or radiologically the patient may be discharged but should be given an appointment for the chest clinic 7–10 days later. If there is any deterioration in the condition, the patient should be told to return to hospital immediately. Air travel should be avoided until the X-ray changes have resolved.
- If the pneumothorax is *moderate* in size (lung collapsed half way towards the heart border), aspiration should be undertaken.
- For a *large* pneumothorax (complete collapse of the lung) a chest drain should be inserted (see below).

Equipment for aspiration of air

- Minor dressing pack
- Gloves
- Antiseptic
- Lidocaine (Lignocaine)
- For local anaesthetic: 10-ml syringe, 21-G needle (green) and 25-G needle (blue)
- 50 ml Luer-lock syringe, 3-way tap, 16-G (or larger) cannula (Venflon, etc.), at least 3 cm long.
- 'Sharps' bin.

Procedure

1. Ask the patient to sit forward with the arms folded. The arms should be supported on a pillow which rests on a bed-table so that the weight of the patient's upper body is taken by the arms.
2. Identify the entry site, usually the second intercostal space in the mid-clavicular line (fifth space in the mid-axillary line is an alternative).

3. Wash your hands and put on gloves.
4. Clean the skin over the entry-site with antiseptic.
5. Infiltrate the skin and subcutaneous tissues with lidocaine (lignocaine); be sure to infiltrate down to the pleura.
6. Connect the 50-ml syringe and tap together. Pass the cannula/needle assembly into the pleural cavity. Remove the needle and connect the cannula to the 3-way tap.
7. Aspirate air, voiding through the side-arm of the tap. Discontinue if resistance is felt, if the patient coughs excessively or if more than 2.5 l of air have been withdrawn. Note that failure to aspirate sufficiently may be due to the cannula being inadvertently withdrawn from the pleural space or becoming kinked: if you suspect either of these, another attempt at aspiration should be considered.
8. Repeat CXR (departmental) in inspiration *only*. If the pneumothorax is very small or has resolved, no further drainage is required.

Once successful aspiration has been performed, a patient who was previously well can be discharged but should be asked to return to the chest clinic (see above). Patients who have had previous chest disease, however, should be observed overnight before discharge.

INTERCOSTAL TUBE DRAINAGE

If aspiration fails an intercostal tube drain should be inserted.

Equipment
- Minor dressing pack
- Gloves
- Antiseptic
- Lidocaine (Lignocaine)
- For local anaesthetic: 10-ml syringe, 21-G needle (green) and 25-G needle (blue)
- Scalpel
- 28-Fr G (adult) chest drain with trochar
- Underwater seal bottle containing sterile water
- Sutures
- 'Sharps' bin.

Procedure
1. Ask the patient to sit forward with the arms folded. The arms should be supported on a pillow which rests on a bed-table so that the weight of the patient's upper body is taken by the arms.
2. Identify the entry-site, usually the second intercostal space in the mid-clavicular line (fifth space in the mid-axillary line is an alternative, especially in young women as an anterior chest scar is unsightly).

3. Give some iv analgesia, such as 25–50 mg pethidine. If the patient is very anxious a small dose of iv sedation may also be desirable.

3. Wash your hands and put on gloves.

4. Clean the skin over the entry-site with antiseptic.

5. Put in the local anaesthetic to the skin (see above), then infiltrate down to the parietal pleura (this whole process will require at least 10 ml of lidocaine (lignocaine) solution). Aspirate intermittently – withdrawal of air will confirm entry to the pleural cavity.

6. Double-check the drain by dismantling and re-assembling it. Make sure that all tube connections fit correctly.

7. When the local anaesthetic has worked, make an incision in the skin and subcutaneous fat: this should be less than 2 cm long so as to ensure a tight fit. Insert two loose sutures across the incision for subsequent closure after removal of the drain.

8. Using blunt dissection with forceps make a wide track through the muscles down to and through the parietal pleura. Sweep your finger around inside the chest to clear away any adherent lung, then carefully insert the trochar and drain – *do not force it*.

   The point of a metal trochar is not sharp enough to penetrate the muscle and pleura easily but is sharp enough to cause damage to the lung if the trochar and drain are forced into the chest.

9. Once the trochar and drain are in the pleural space, withdraw the trochar about 5 cm and advance the drain in an apical direction. Remove the trochar and connect the drain to the underwater seal bottle.

10. Secure the drain firmly with a suture (one loop through the skin and multiple ties in at least four places on the tube itself). Loop the tube and secure it with plaster so that it cannot fall out or kink. Prescribe adequate analgesia (oral or im).

11. If the patient is to be moved and the drain needs to be disconnected from the bottle or bag, it should be connected instead to a Heimlich flutter valve or a bag with a flap valve. Chest drains should not, as a rule, be clamped.

Follow-up care of the intercostal drain

Re-X-ray the patient the next day

- If the lung has re-expanded and the drain has stopped bubbling, wait 24 hours, then remove the drain (see below). Repeat the X-ray once again: if the lung remains expanded the patient can be discharged with an appointment for the chest clinic. If, however, the lung has collapsed again, ask for help from a chest physician.

- If the lung re-expands after intubation but the drain continues to bubble, ask for help from a chest physician.
- If the lung fails to re-expand after intubation and the water in the bottle shows no bubbling or swinging, check to see if the tube has become blocked or kinked. If this has happened and the problem cannot be corrected by simple means, a new drain should be inserted through a clean incision.
- If the lung does not re-expand after intubation but there is bubbling or swinging in the bottle, ask for help from a chest physician.

If the underwater seal bottle is always kept below the level of the chest, clamping of the tube is unnecessary and potentially dangerous. As far as possible, have X-ray films taken in the department rather than on the ward; expiratory films are not necessary.

Removal of the drain

Bubbling of air should have stopped for at least 24 hours. Some patients find tube removal as traumatic as tube insertion, so consider premedication with atropine, 0.3–0.6 mg (to prevent a vasovagal reaction); if the patient is very anxious consider giving a small dose of intravenous midazolam (2 mg).

Equipment

- Gloves
- Stitch-cutter
- Disposable sterile forceps
- Gauze pads
- Collodion
- Adhesive tape (make sure the patient is not allergic to sticking plaster).

Procedure

1. Ask a nurse to help you (you will see why below).
2. Scrub up and put on gloves.
3. Remove the dressing from the drain site.
4. Cut the suture which holds the drain in place with the stitch cutter and remove the suture.
5. Patients should be asked to breathe in fully and perform a Valsalva manoeuvre while the drain is being removed; this will prevent air from being sucked back into the pleural cavity. Tie the two sutures to seal the wound.
6. Put some collodion on a piece of gauze, apply to the wound and secure in place with tape.

PASSING A URINARY CATHETER

Indications
- Monitoring urinary output, particularly peri- and post-operatively
- Acute urinary retention
- Chronic urinary retention
- Incontinence.

Catheterization of a female patient is usually performed by nursing staff, so your responsibility will usually be for male catheterization.

MALE CATHETERIZATION

Equipment
- Dressing pack
- Cleansing solution (eg Savlon)
- Gloves
- Drapes
- Gauze
- Lidocaine (Lignocaine) gel with sterile plastic nozzle
- Catheter (14 G)
- 20-ml syringe (Luer) containing 20 ml sterile water
- 50-ml catheter syringe
- Drainage bag.

Procedure
1. Lie the patient on his back, as flat as he can manage while remaining comfortable.
2. Wash your hands and put on gloves.
3. Ask an assistant to open the dressing pack and to pour some cleaning solution into the gallipot.
4. Put sterile drapes over the patient's legs and abdomen leaving the genital area exposed.
5. Open the lidocaine (lignocaine) gel pack and screw the nozzle onto the tube.
6. Hold the penis in your left hand using a gauze to avoid de-sterilizing your glove. Retract the prepuce fully.
7. Clean the urethral orifice and glans with antiseptic.
8. Introduce the lidocaine (lignocaine) gel into the urethra by inserting the nozzle and then squeezing in as much of the contents of the tube as possible.
9. Hold the catheter in your right hand and ask the assistant to pull the end of the plastic wrapper off. Hold the penis vertical and insert the catheter, gently advancing it for about 3 inches; as you do this, try to withdraw the plastic covering in stages so that the end of the cover does not touch the penis.

10. Lower the penis between the thighs and continue advancing the catheter until urine flows back down it or you have inserted about 6 inches of the catheter. *Do not* use force in advancing the catheter.
11. Once you think you are in the right place, inject about 10 ml water into the balloon via the smaller channel.
    If there is any resistance or if the patient complains of pain during inflation, deflate the balloon immediately.
12. Do not forget to bring the foreskin forward again!
    If urine does not flow straight away, it may be because the tip is blocked with gel. Gently aspirate the catheter using the 50 ml syringe. Alternatively, instil 20 ml sterile water into the catheter using the syringe, then gently re-aspirate.

Problems

Inability to insert Try a smaller catheter (12 G) or a Silastic catheter (which is firmer). If you are still not successful, ask for help.

Blood draining during insertion or soon after This is potentially a serious complication as it often means that a false passage has been created. Withdraw the catheter immediately and ask for help.

Relief of acute retention Rapid decompression of a grossly distended bladder may lead to mucosal haemorrhage, therefore you should clamp the catheter intermittently, releasing 200–300 ml every 30 minutes. Once the kidneys have been decompressed there may be a very brisk diuresis, so observe the patient's urine output carefully and be on the lookout for dehydration and hyponatraemia.

Catheter stops draining Ask the nursing staff to wash the catheter out with sterile water. If this does not solve the problem it is usually best to pass a new catheter.

Catheter 'bypassing' This term is used to describe the problem of urine flowing down the urethra past a catheter in an apparently adequate position. The most common cause is catheter blockage, so ask the nursing staff to wash it out with sterile water. If this does not solve the problem, pass a new catheter. Occasionally bypassing is caused by the catheter being too small: if bypassing occurs despite the fact that urine is draining through the catheter, replace the catheter with a larger one.

FEMALE CATHETERIZATION

You will occasionally be asked to do this if the nurses have been unsuccessful. The equipment needed is the same as for male patients. The procedure should preferably be carried out by a female. Males performing the procedure should always seek a chaperone.

Procedure

1. Ask the patient to lie flat on her back with the knees bent up, heels together and knees widely separated.
2. Place sterile towels over the abdomen and thighs and an absorbent ('incontinence') pad on the bed between the patient's legs.
3. Separate the labia minora with your left hand and clean the vulva with antiseptic.
4. Lubricate the tip of the catheter by dipping it into sterile water, then introduce the catheter.
5. If there is a problem in isolating the external urethral meatus, eg in a very obese patient, ask an assistant to elevate any dependent fat from the pubic area, place the index finger of your right hand in the vagina to elevate the anterior vulva and slide the catheter along your finger (using your left hand to guide it) into the urethra.

LUMBAR PUNCTURE (LP)

Indications

- To confirm or refute the diagnosis of:
  - subarachnoid haemorrhage
  - meningitis
  - Guillain-Barré syndrome
  - (rarely) neurosyphilis.
- To administer intrathecal drugs, especially chemotherapy.

Contraindications

- Focal neurological signs
- Papilloedema
- Suspicion of a space–occupying lesion within the skull
- Severe clotting defect (including heparin or warfarin therapy)
- Major spinal deformity
- Severe contamination of the back, eg with dirt, faeces.

Make sure that the indication is a sound one and that there are no contraindications. If an LP is considered desirable but there is a suspicion of raised intracranial pressure, the patient must have a CT scan of the brain before the LP; this condition also applies to almost all cases of suspected subarachnoid haemorrhage.

Procedure

You should watch several procedures before attempting LP yourself; make sure that you are well supervised when you perform your first one.

1. LP must be carried out as a full sterile procedure.
2. Position the patient in the left lateral position with maximum flexion (Fig. 18.4); the back should be as close as possible to the edge of the bed. Scrub up and put gloves on.
3. Put a sterile drape over the patient's hips and another over an incontinence pad which should be placed underneath the patient.
4. Clean the skin over the lumbar spine (and a wide area around) with iodine solution (check the patient is not allergic to iodine), chlorhexidine solution or other suitable skin-cleanser.
5. Feel for the highest point of the pelvic brim on the patient's right side and drop a perpendicular from here to the spine; this should bring you to the L3/L4 interspace.
6. Palpate this interspace with the end of a finger so that you are sure where to go in with the needle.
7. Draw up local anaesthetic (lidocaine (lignocaine) 1% or 2%) into a 10-ml syringe.
8. Fit a small (25-G) needle and inject the local anaesthetic into the skin over the planned point of entry of the LP needle. Change to a larger (21-G) needle and inject local anaesthetic into the deeper tissues.
9. Allow enough time for the local anaesthetic to work; when 3 or 4 minutes have elapsed test the skin with a needle to make sure that it is really anaesthetized.
10. Make sure that you have ready a 90-mm (18-G or 20-G) LP needle, 3-way tap, manometer, three plain sterile specimen bottles and a fluoride-oxalate (usually yellow) bottle such as is normally used for blood glucose estimation.
11. Palpate the intervertebral space again with your left hand, holding the LP needle in the right. Make sure that the stylet

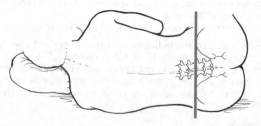

Fig. 18.4 Finding the correct site for a lumbar puncture. The line, a perpendicular from the highest part of the pelvic brim, should identify the L3/L4 interspace.

is fully home inside the needle and that the stud on the hub of the stylet is correctly located in the corresponding slot in the hub of the needle. Having located the correct site of entry, insert the needle with your right thumb over the end of the stylet. Advance the needle in the horizontal plane, aiming it towards the umbilicus (Fig. 18.5); if you hit bone or the needle seems reluctant to advance, withdraw the needle until the point is just beneath the skin and try again at a slightly different angle.

In most adult subjects you will need to advance the needle up to at least half its length before you reach the dura; when this happens you should feel a sudden 'give' as the needle goes through the ligamentum flavum. When you feel this, withdraw the stylet to see if fluid is flowing out; if not, fully re-insert the stylet, advance the needle a few more millimetres and try again.

12. If you have reached the subarachnoid space, CSF should flow out freely; in a healthy subject this will be perfectly clear (like distilled water). When you have a free flow, connect the three-way tap and manometer to the needle.
13. *Queckenstedt's test*: conscious patients able to cough should be asked to do so: the pressure should rise rapidly by a further 5–10 cm, then fall rapidly back to baseline. If the patient cannot cooperate, ask an assistant to compress the root of the neck just above the medial third of the clavicle. A similar rise and fall of CSF pressure should occur with compression and release.
14. Hold a specimen bottle under the lip of the drainage tube and turn the 3-way tap to allow 1–2 ml of fluid to flow into

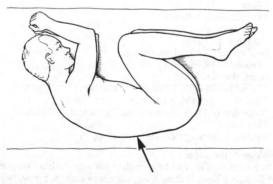

Fig. 18.5 Direction of approach for lumbar puncture. The needle is aimed towards the umbilicus.

the bottle. If the fluid is blood-stained, label this specimen as no 1 and collect two further specimens labelled 2 and 3. Finally, collect 1 ml or so of fluid into the fluoride-oxalate bottle. If the CSF pressure was very high, inject 10 ml of sterile normal saline into the needle after sampling.

15. Remove the 3-way tap and manometer and replace the stylet into the needle. Take a gauze pad in the left hand and withdraw the needle slowly with the right. Apply pressure to the puncture site with the gauze, cover with a cotton-wool ball or pad then secure the dressing with tape applied over the cotton-wool.

    If you suspect meningitis, you must take a blood sample for glucose measurement: the CSF glucose concentration is normally about two-thirds that of the blood but will be much lower if the patient has bacterial meningitis; a value below 50% of blood glucose is abnormal. Send CSF samples for microscopy, culture, protein and glucose estimation.

16. After the procedure the patient should be nursed flat for 24 hours, otherwise there is a high incidence of headache.

INSERTING A CENTRAL VENOUS LINE

You should not attempt to insert a central venous line unless you have watched the procedure being performed at least twice. Your first few procedures must be done under supervision.

Equipment
- Sterile drapes
- Gloves
- Skin-cleansing solution
- Dressing pack
- Cotton-wool balls
- 5-ml syringe for local anaesthetic
- 21-G and 25-G needles
- iv infusion set
- 500-ml bag of 0.9% saline or 5% glucose
- Central line set with guide-wire
- Ampoules of 1% or 2% lidocaine (lignocaine) solution
- Skin suture
- Occlusive dressing ('Opsite' or 'Tegaderm').

Position of the patient
The patient should be laid flat on the back with the head supported on a single pillow. If there is any reason to suspect hypovolaemia the patient should be tilted slightly head-down so as to cause engorgement of the subclavian and internal jugular veins.

Puncture site and procedure

A central vein can be entered by a subclavian, supraclavicular or internal jugular approach. It is a good idea to identify the site of entry and the approach before you scrub up.

Observe strict asepsis throughout Clean the skin and cover with sterile drapes. Identify the entry-point and infiltrate with local anaesthetic. While waiting for the local anaesthetic to work, unwrap the central line and make sure that you know what all the bits do and how they fit together. Identify the 'soft' end of the guide-wire. Make sure that the iv infusion is run-through and ready to connect to the central line.

Subclavian approach Palpate the ends of the right clavicle and identify a point 3 cm below the junction of the outer third and the inner two thirds (Fig. 18.6). Your aim will be to insert the needle at this point and to aim for the centre of the suprasternal notch. Attach the entry needle to a 10-ml syringe. Pass the needle through the skin and touch it gently against the clavicle. Direct the needle towards the suprasternal notch, keeping it in the horizontal plane and as close to the clavicle as you can, and apply gentle suction to the syringe as you advance. Once you enter the vein the blood should flow freely into the syringe. If you reach the hub of the needle without having drawn blood, you have gone too far. Withdraw the needle to just below the skin surface and advance again at a slightly different angle.

Supraclavicular approach Ask the patient to turn the head to the left. Palpate the junction of the sternomastoid muscle and the

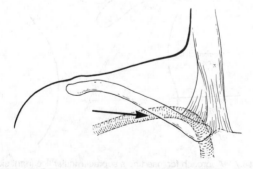

Fig. 18.6 Direction of approach for inserting a subclavian line. The needle is inserted under the midpoint of the clavicle, as close to the bone as possible, and aimed towards the middle of the suprasternal notch.

superior surface of the clavicle. If necessary, ask the patient to lift the head slightly off the pillow so as to make the muscle stand out. Place the middle joint of your left thumb over this junction and point the thumb backwards towards the right postero-lateral chest, bisecting the angle between the clavicle and the sternomastoid muscle (Fig. 18.7). The tip of your thumb will be over the entry point and you will be aiming to pass the needle in the horizontal plane, aiming for the centre of the manubrio-sternal joint. Attach the entry needle to a 10-ml syringe. Pass the needle through the skin and direct it, in the horizontal plane, to a point directly below the centre of the manubrio-sternal joint; apply gentle suction to the syringe as you advance. Once you enter the vein blood should flow freely into the syringe. If you reach the hub of the needle without having drawn blood, you have gone too far. Withdraw the needle to just below the skin surface and advance again at a slightly different angle.

Internal jugular approach   Define a point half-way between the mastoid process and the sternal notch (Fig. 18.8); the entry-point will be at this site, lateral to the carotid pulsation and medial to the medial border of the sternomastoid. Attach the entry needle to a 10-ml syringe. Pass the needle through the skin and direct it towards the

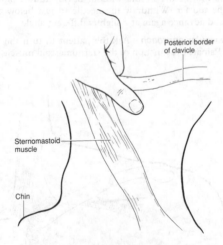

Posterior border
of clavicle

Sternomastoid
muscle

Chin

Fig. 18.7   Approach for inserting a supraclavicular line (right side). The operator stands at the patient's head and the patient looks to the left. The operator's left thumb is placed as shown, bisecting the angle between border of sternomastoid and clavicle. Tip of thumb marks the needle entry-point.

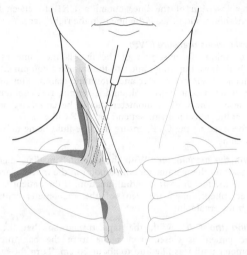

Fig. 18.8 Approach for inserting an internal jugular line (right side). The operator stands at the patient's head and the patient looks slightly to the left. The needle is inserted halfway between the mastoid process and the sternal notch. The operator aims towards the ipsilateral nipple, advancing under the border of sternomastoid until the vein is entered. (After Eaton, Essentials of Immediate Medical Care, Churchill Livingstone 1992).

ipsilateral nipple, advancing under the body of sternomastoid; apply gentle suction to the syringe as you advance. Once you enter the vein blood should flow freely into the syringe. If the needle goes into the tissues for more than 5 cm but you have not drawn blood, you have gone too far. Withdraw the needle to just below the skin surface and advance again at a slightly different angle.

Once you have a free flow of blood into the syringe, grip the hub of the needle in one hand, remove the syringe and insert the guide-wire, 'soft' end first. Advance the guide-wire but *do not force it*. Remove the needle and pass the central line over the guide-wire (with some central venous catheters you may need to nick the skin alongside the guide-wire before passing the central line). Remove the guide-wire and connect the syringe to the central line; aspirate to check that you are getting a free flow of blood from the line. Connect the iv-giving set to the central line and check the tightness of all connections. Secure the line in place with the skin suture and cover the wound with an occlusive dressing.

After insertion of the line, obtain a CXR to check for a pneumothorax and to see if the line is in the right place.

Central venous pressure (CVP)
The technique for insertion of the line is the same as that described above but, in addition to the standard equipment, you will need a CVP manometer and mounting clamp. This usually incorporates a centimetre scale and a zeroing rod containing a spirit level. The CVP manometer should be connected in-line between the infusion-giving set and the CVP catheter.

Before reading the CVP, ensure that the fluid being infused is 0.9% saline.

Zeroing the manometer With the patient lying flat, align the zero mark on the manometer with a point in the mid-axillary line opposite the fourth costochondral junction. If the patient is lying semirecumbent, align the zero of the manometer with the manubriosternal joint.

Reading the CVP With the taps turned so that the line to the patient is closed, run saline from the bag into the manometer until it is filled up to about 20 cm. Turn the taps so that the line to the bag is closed and that to the patient is open. The level of saline in the manometer should then fall freely until it reaches the level of the CVP. A normal CVP level would be: 1–8 cm measured with reference to the mid-axillary line –5 to +5 cm measured with reference to the manubriosternal joint.

Finally, remember to keep a very slow infusion of fluid going through the central line (of the order of 500 ml for 24 hours) in order to keep it open.

Problems with central lines

Fever If an unexplained fever develops in someone who has a central line in situ, it is wise to consider the line as the source of the fever. Take blood cultures both peripherally and from the line. If the patient is unwell the line should be removed and the tip sent for culture; a new line can be put in if required.

Blockage of the cannula If the line appears blocked, gently inject 10–20 ml of 0.9% saline. If this fails the line should be removed and a new one sited.

The line goes up into the neck This happens from time to time with a subclavian approach to CVP line insertion; it is much rarer with the supraclavicular approach. Lines in this position may still be usable for drug infusion but clearly are of no value for reading the CVP; if you need a CVP reading, ask someone else to manipulate the line or to site a new one.

RECORDING AN ECG

There is a wide range of ECG machines available, most of which now have 'intelligent' controls and a range of automatic or semi-automatic functions. Routine tracings will, of course, be recorded by a cardiographer but you should make sure that you are competent at recording an ECG as you may well be expected to do so during evenings and weekends and in an emergency. Try to get a cardiographer or an experienced nurse to show you how to operate the different types of ECG machine used in your hospital. In particular you need to know:

- whether the machine should be plugged into the mains during use
- into which sockets you should plug the mains lead and the patient cable
- what type of patient electrodes to use with a particular machine
- how to switch between leads
- how to re-centre the pen in the event of baseline 'drift' (especially important for the V leads).

Procedure

1. Explain to the patient what you are going to do and that the procedure is painless.
2. Check that you have the right types of electrodes and connectors.
3. If the machine is to be used on battery only, check that it is charged up.
4. Attach the limb electrodes to the patient. Try to attach to hairless areas of the limbs. The connecting wires are usually labelled and/or colour-coded, the most widely used convention for the colours being: *red* – right arm, *yellow* – left arm, *green* – left leg, *black* – right leg.
5. Palpate the intercostal spaces and attach the chest electrodes (Fig. 18.9) (in men with hairy chests you may have to shave the hair off the left side of the chest in order to get good electrical contact).
6. Check that the machine is set to **10 mm/mV** and to a paper speed of **25 mm/sec**.
7. Ensure that the patient is comfortable and is lying still. Set the paper in motion and mark a calibration mark.
8. Record the ECG, making sure to keep the tracing in the centre of the paper. If the patient has an arrhythmia, record a long rhythm strip (at least 10 complexes) in lead II or VI, depending on which is giving you the better signal.
9. Label each lead as soon as you have finished it and label the whole tracing with the patient's name and the date and time of recording: nothing is more frustrating than finding an ECG tracing lying around the notes trolley and not being

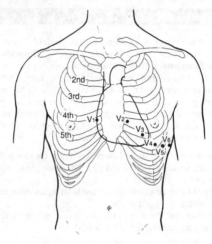

Fig. 18.9 Positions of the chest electrodes of the ECG. Note that V5 and V6 are in the same horizontal line as V4, not the same intercostal space.

    able to identify the patient to whom it relates or the date and time when it was recorded.
10. Remove the electrodes from the patient. Coil the cables up neatly and put them away.
11. Do not forget to tell the patient what the ECG has shown and to provide appropriate reassurance.

Common ECG patterns
Figures 18.10–18.21 illustrate the common rhythm disorders. Patterns for MI are shown in Figures 17.3–17.5 (→ pp 422, 423).

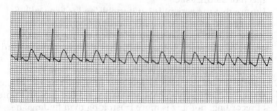

Fig. 18.10 Atrial flutter.

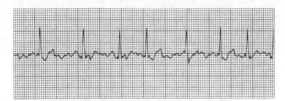

Fig. 18.11   Atrial fibrillation.

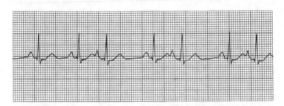

Fig. 18.12   Atrial ectopics.

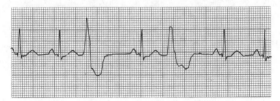

Fig. 18.13   Ventricular ectopics.

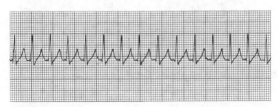

Fig. 18.14   Supraventricular tachycardia.

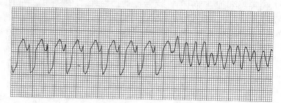

Fig. 18.15 Ventricular tachycardia and fibrillation.

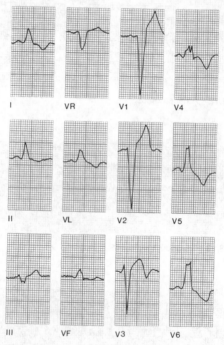

Fig. 18.16 Left bundle branch block.

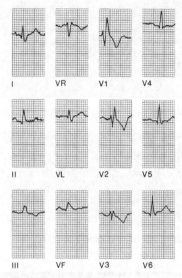

Fig. 18.17 Right bundle branch block.

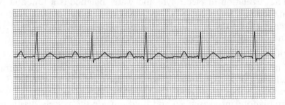

Fig. 18.18 First-degree heart block.

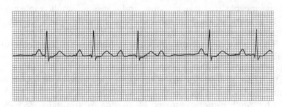

Fig. 18.19 Second-degree heart block (Mobitz type I or Wenckebach).

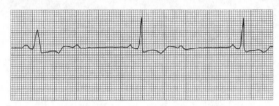

Fig. 18.20 Second-degree heart block (Mobitz type II)

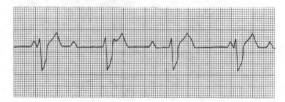

Fig. 18.21 Complete (third-degree) heart block.

INTRAVENOUS FLUIDS

The regulation of electrolyte and water balance is a function of the kidneys (with contributions from some other organs). Intravenous fluid therapy can be thought of as providing the kidneys and other vital organs with an adequate blood flow.

The normal distribution of body water and electrolytes

The body water is contained in two compartments, the intracellular fluid (ICF) and the extracellular fluid (ECF); the ECF is further subdivided into fluid within the blood vessels and circulation (intravascular) and fluid outside the vessels (tissue or interstitial fluid). The capillary endothelial membrane, which separates the intravascular fluid from the interstitial fluid, is permeable to water, ions and certain small molecules. The amount of fluid in the various compartments is shown in Fig. 18.22.

The term 'electrolytes' includes sodium, potassium, chloride and bicarbonate. Water can diffuse freely through all of the fluid compartments but electrolytes cannot move freely in and out of cells. The electrolytes make up the major solutes in the body fluids and account for most of the osmotic pressure.

The total osmotic activity of plasma is normally 285–295 mOsmol/kg water and most of this activity is provided by sodium and chloride, with a small amount from bicarbonate, potassium, urea, glucose, other minerals and proteins.

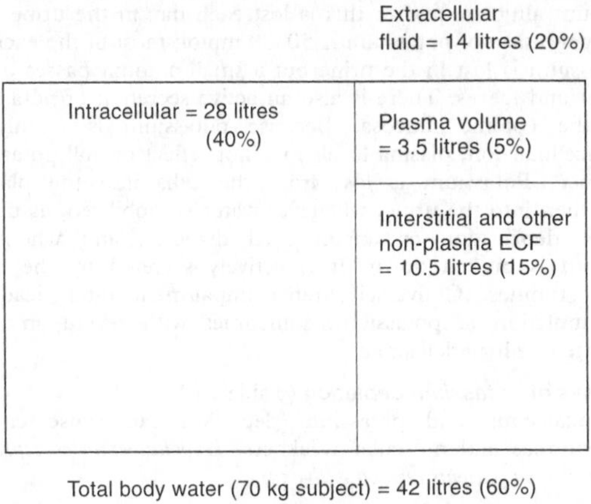

Fig. 18.22 Body fluid compartments. Volumes are for a 70 kg man; % figures are percentages of total body weight.

The osmotic pressure of the interstitial fluid differs from that of the plasma only by the contribution of plasma protein; this is about 1.5 mOsmol/kg and exerts a 'pull' which is roughly equivalent to a hydrostatic pressure of 25 mmHg.

Movements of fluid

Fluid moves because of a hydrostatic or osmotic gradient across a membrane. The plasma contains crystalloids (electrolytes, etc) which pass freely across the capillary membrane, and proteins to which the membrane is not freely permeable. Thus the plasma proteins, albumin and globulins, are in high concentration within the vascular compartment (60–80 g/l) whereas protein concentrations in the interstitial fluid are much lower (7–20 g/l). The osmotic pressure produced by proteins is called the colloid osmotic pressure (COP); about 75% of the COP of plasma is due to albumin (MW 69 000), the rest to globulins.

Thus fluid flow across capillary membranes depends on:

- the filtration properties of the capillary wall
- the hydrostatic pressure inside the capillary and the COP of the plasma
- the hydrostatic pressure and the COP in the interstitial fluid.

The electrolytes (sodium and potassium)

Sodium is maintained largely as an extracellular ion while potassium is mainly intracellular. The average daily intake of sodium in temperate climates is around 100–300 mmol; an amount almost equal to this is lost each day in the urine. The normal intake of potassium is 50–80 mmol; most of the excreted potassium is lost in the urine but a small amount passes out in sweat and faeces. There is also an active secretion of potassium by the colonic mucosa. Because potassium is mainly an intracellular ion, plasma levels may not reflect overall potassium balance. Potassium is lost from the cells into the plasma, and then into the urine, whenever water is mobilized, as during water deprivation or uncontrolled diabetes, and when cell protein is broken down. It is actively secreted by the distal renal tubules. Conversely, renal impairment often leads to accumulation of potassium, sometimes with severe and life-threatening hyperkalaemia.

Causes of potassium depletion (Table 18.1)
Hypokalaemia and potassium depletion can cause cardiac arrhythmias and muscular weakness. *Hypokalaemia is especially dangerous in patients receiving digoxin.*

Fluids available for replacement
Fluid can be given in the form of crystalloids, colloids or blood. Crystalloids can pass freely through the capillary membrane, ie between the circulation and the interstitial fluid. Colloids contain high-molecular-weight substances which cannot escape from the plasma (unless it is flowing through damaged capillaries), so they are chiefly retained in the circulation.

Water balance (Table 18.2)
The alimentary tract secretes a substantial volume of fluid (some 8 l) into its lumen each day (Table 18.3).

The changes in the volume of fluid are important in patients with GI disease or paralytic ileus.

Table 18.1
Causes of potassium depletion

Losses in the urine	Diuretic therapy, osmotic diuresis of diabetes, primary renal disease (occasionally)
Drugs other than diuretics	Steroids, salbutamol, insulin (during acute treatment of diabetic emergencies)
GI losses	Vomiting, pyloric stenosis, chronic diarrhoea (eg ulcerative colitis), excessive use of purgatives, malabsorption syndromes, villous adenoma of the rectum

Table 18.2
The daily water balance

Output (ml)	Intake (ml)
Lungs 500	Oral fluid 1700
Skin 900	Food 1000
Faeces 100	Metabolic water 300
Urine 1500	
Total 3000	Total 3000

Table 18.3
Volume of fluid secreted by alimentary tract

Saliva	1.5 l
Gastric juice	2.5 l
Small intestinal fluid	3.0 l
Bile	0.5 l
Pancreatic juice	0.7 l

The crystalloids

The contents of each litre of solution are summarized in Table 18.4.

Colloids

These solutions are used to support the circulation in hypovolaemic shock before blood is available or when it is not needed. They can also be used to 'bulk up' red cell concentrates, which may have as little as 40 ml of the original

Table 18.4
Contents of 1 litre of crystalloid solution

	Normal saline	5% Glucose	Glucose/ saline	Hartmann's
Sodium	150 mmol		30 mmol	135 mmol
Chloride	150 mmol		30 mmol	
Glucose		50 g	40 g	
Osmolality = 300 mmol/l for all the above				

Potassium chloride is usually added at 2 g/l (27 mmol/l of potassium)

plasma per unit. Albumin solution is the natural colloid which one might think of using but it is expensive and should only be used in carefully selected cases (see below). In most cases when a colloid is needed, one uses gelatins (Gelofusine, Haemaccel), synthetic colloids such as dextrans (eg Dextran 70, Macrodex, Lomodex) or modified starch such as hetastarch (Hespan). The properties of these colloid solutions are summarized in Table 18.5.

Table 18.5
Properties of colloid solutions

Dextran 70

Half-life in circulation	12 hours
Maximum dose	20 ml/kg
Osmolality	325 mOsm/kg
Special features	Has an anticoagulant effect but interferes with blood cross-matching, so a sample must be taken for this before beginning treatment with Dextran 70

Haemaccel

Half-life in circulation	5 hours
Maximum dose	30 ml/kg
Osmolality	290 mOsm/kg
Special features	Contains much more calcium than Gelofusine. This may cause clotting in warming coils when Haemaccel is mixed with citrated blood or FFP

Gelofusine

Half-life in circulation	4 hours
Maximum dose	30 ml/kg
Osmolality	274 mOsm/kg
Special features	Useful for rapid fluid volume replacement ($\rightarrow$ below)

Hespan

Half-life in circulation	17 days
Maximum dose	33 ml/kg
Osmolality	310 mOsm/kg
Special features	Very slowly eliminated from the body. It is a good deal more expensive than other colloid solutions!

FLUID ADMINISTRATION

The amount of fluid administered will depend on:

- projected fluid needs over the next 12–24 hours
- whether the patient is fluid overloaded, dehydrated or in balance.

As mentioned above (→ p 513), a subject who is adequately hydrated will lose 2500–3000 ml per day (ie 100–125 ml per hour) as the result of urinary losses (1500 ml), respiratory losses (500 ml) and evaporation from the skin (500–1000 ml). This is therefore the basic fluid requirement of a subject who cannot take any food or fluid orally. There may be additional losses due to fever, diarrhoea, GI fistulae, intestinal obstruction, etc.

Assessment of state of hydration This is based on clinical and biochemical evidence. Examination of skin turgor (over the chest wall, not the arm) can be misleading in the elderly or where there has been weight-loss. Early evidence of hypovolaemia is provided by peripheral vasoconstriction, ie pale, cool extremities and empty peripheral veins. Another useful sign is postural hypotension: if the systolic BP drops by 10 mm or more when the patient sits up from a lying position, or if it falls below 90 mm, then hypovolaemia is probably present. In young adults, however, there may be no helpful physical signs because of sympathetic compensatory mechanisms.

Evidence of volume depletion This usually takes the form of a rise in blood urea and haematocrit, though care must be taken to allow for pre-existing renal disease or anaemia. As regards urinary measurements, the most helpful information is related to urine volumes per unit time and to urine specific gravity. If possible, body weight should be measured daily since, in the short term, changes in body weight are a good guide to net gain or loss of fluid. If clinical or biochemical evidence of volume depletion is present then there is probably a deficit of at least 5% of total weight (ie 3–4 1). These observations do not always quantify the deficit but they do give essential information against which to control replacement.

Deficit corrections How fast the deficit is corrected depends on its severity: hypovolaemia resulting in oliguria must be rapidly corrected, with hourly assessments of progress. Aim for a urine output of 30 ml/hour or more.

In the absence of oliguria it is sensible to replace the fluid deficit over 12–24 hours (or even 48 hours in patients over 70). The main hazards of over-rapid rehydration are left ventricular failure, hyponatraemia and cerebral oedema. If a patient requires an urgent operation there are, nevertheless, usually 2–4 hours available in which to rehydrate the patient and stabilize his/her circulation; in such a situation the first litre of normal saline can be given in 30 minutes and a second in 60 minutes; subsequent infusion rates will depend on the clinical response and on the need for potassium (serum potassium levels below 3.5 mmol/l are not favoured by anaesthetists!).

Dangers of colloid solutions Many artificial colloid solutions contain substantial quantities of sodium which may cause problems in patients with cardiac or renal failure or with liver disease (see below).

Patients may display allergic reactions to colloid solutions; in the event of a serious reaction the infusion should be stopped and adrenaline (epinephrine), 0.5–1 ml of 1:1000 by im injection should be given immediately. Adrenaline (epinephrine) injections should be repeated every 15 minutes until improvement occurs. The patient should also be given hydrocortisone, 100–200 mg intravenously and, because of circulatory collapse, will need large volumes of crystalloid (1–2 l).

Prescribing iv fluids

All intravenous fluids must be prescribed and signed for. The prescription will state the volume, the nature of the fluid and the rate of infusion; this rate is usually controlled by an electro-mechanical automated infuser (IVAC, IMED or similar). If a manual infusion system is being used this will usually deliver 15 drops of fluid per ml infused. Thus an infusion rate of 1 l every 8 hours equates to a drip rate of 31 drops/min.

Fluid balance should be assessed each morning and the fluid requirements for the next 24 hours prescribed. This should be reassessed in the afternoon and adjusted on the basis of the measured fluid balance and laboratory results.

TYPE OF FLUID

The normal requirement of 2500 ml per day can be provided as 1000 ml of 'normal' (0.9%) saline and 1500 ml of 5% glucose or as 2500 ml of glucose saline (dextrose/saline); these fluids will also supply the required 75–100 mmol of sodium.

Supplementary potassium

Potassium chloride is added to the standard solutions at a concentration of 2 g/litre (27 mmol/l); thus 2.5 l will supply 68 mmol of potassium. Stronger infusions of potassium are sometimes indicated: in hypokalaemia infusion rates of up to 20 mmol per hour may be needed. At higher infusion rates (over 10 mmol per hour) you should consider ECG monitoring. Infusion at more than 20 mmol per hour is hazardous (risk of cardiac arrest) and should only be undertaken, if at all, with the agreement of a senior colleague. If a concentrated solution of potassium is to be infused, precautions *must* be taken to avoid over-rapid infusion, ie the infusion must be controlled by the use of an automatic, programmable infusor (eg an IVAC or IMED). When adding potassium chloride to a bag, remember that it is denser than the rest of the fluid and the bag must be shaken before use. An additive label must also be filled in and affixed to the bag before it is connected to the patient.

FLUID REPLACEMENT IN SPECIFIC SITUATIONS

Blood loss: upper GI haemorrhage, trauma or during surgery

Whole blood (group O, Rh-negative or grouped, uncross-matched in cases of extreme urgency) is clearly the fluid of choice (see Blood transfusion, below). While waiting for blood to arrive one can give a colloid solution. The gelatins (eg Haemaccel, Gelofusine) are effective short-term plasma substitutes and large volumes can be infused without impairing haemostasis. They have a short half-life so blood or plasma can be given soon after with less risk of fluid overload. Up to 1500 ml of blood-loss can be replaced by gelatin; between 1500 and 4000 ml blood-loss replacement should be with equal volumes of gelatin and blood. For losses over 4000 ml the ratio should be two parts blood to one part gelatin. The haematocrit should not be allowed to fall below 25%. Some patients with sepsis, severe trauma, liver disease or malignancy will have abnormalities of blood clotting such as DIC. If you are in any doubt about the integrity of the patient's clotting mechanisms, check platelet count, PT, KCCT/APTT and fibrinogen titre. If the clotting times are prolonged the patient may need FFP, vitamin K or platelet transfusion. Ask advice before giving these items.

Hypovolaemia and dehydration

Water and electrolyte deficiency   This may result from many causes, eg:

- diarrhoea and vomiting
- overdiuresis
- nausea and vomiting due to vestibular disease
- dysphagia due to oesophageal disease or cerebrovascular accident (CVA)
- septic shock
- burns.

As a general rule crystalloid (saline or glucose solution) should be used initially. A subject who is adequately hydrated will lose 2500–3000 ml/day (ie 100–125 ml/hour) as the result of urinary losses (1500 l), respiratory losses (500 ml) and evaporation from the skin (500–1000 ml). This is therefore the basic fluid requirement of a subject who cannot take any food or fluid orally. The dehydrated patient will need 1000–2000 ml of fluid/day over and above this basic requirement, ie a total of 3500–5000 ml/day (150–200 ml/hour). If, in order to restore normal hydration, more than 5 l are required, the addition of colloid may be beneficial. If the patient has cardiac or renal disease or is elderly it may be better to give fluid at the rate of 1500–2000 ml/day (60–80 ml/hour) or, if dehydrated, 2500–3000 ml/day (100–125 ml/hour).

Acute pancreatitis The mainstay of treatment is correction of hypovolaemia by replacement of fluid and electrolytes by infusion of crystalloids as above. Fluid sequestration in the first 48 hours may amount to 6 l, necessitating large positive fluid balances. In some cases blood or plasma may be needed.

Diabetic ketoacidosis and other diabetic emergencies (→ pp 452–454).

Fluid deficit in adult respiratory distress syndrome (ARDS) and anaphylaxis In these conditions, where plasma colloid osmotic pressure is low or the capillaries are leaky, a mixture of crystalloid and colloid (hetastarch) should be used in roughly equal amounts (for rates of fluid administration → p 515).

Use of albumin
Albumin is indicated in the treatment of severe hypoproteinaemia, especially when this is associated with a low plasma volume. Hypoproteinaemia of any cause tends to promote contraction of

Table 18.6
Albumin solutions

Plasma protein fraction (stable plasma protein solution)	
Albumin concentration	50 g/l
Colloid osmotic pressure	26–30 mOsm/kg
Sodium concentration	140–160 mmol/l
Potassium concentration	Less than 2 mmol/l
Human albumin solution 5%	
Albumin concentration	40–50 g/l
Colloid osmotic pressure	26–30 mOsm/kg
Sodium concentration	140–160 mmol/l
Potassium concentration	Less than 2 mmol/l
Human albumin solution 20%	
Albumin concentration	200 g/l
Colloid osmotic pressure	100–120 mOsm/kg
Sodium concentration	140–160 mmol/l
Potassium concentration	Less than 10 mmol/l

the intravascular volume, which leads to compensatory retention of water and sodium. If a patient with hepatic cirrhosis is oliguric and hypoalbuminaemic, albumin infusion together with intravenous diuretics and an aldosterone antagonist will usually produce a diuresis. Albumin is not effective as parenteral nutrition. The available albumin solutions are summarized in Table 18.6. The use of albumin solution is controversial so consult your SHO or registrar before prescribing it.

BLOOD TRANSFUSION

→ also Chapter 10, p 232

Indications for whole blood transfusion
Whole blood should be given to patients who are actively bleeding or who have recently lost blood.

Procedure

1. Take blood for FBC, serum iron or ferritin, B_{12} and folate and cross-match *before* giving any blood. *Take great care* over labelling the sample on the cross-match form. Mistakes in this area are potentially fatal.
   If a patient has already been transfused more than 72 hours before the time when you wish to transfuse them, a fresh sample of blood will need to be taken for cross-matching because of the possible development of antibodies. Thus, if prior transfusion has taken place within 3–14 days, the sample should be taken 24 hours or less before transfusion; if within 14–28 days the sample should be taken 72 hours or less before transfusion; if 28 days to 3 months, the sample should be taken within 1 week before transfusion.
2. If the patient is severly shocked, ask for group O, Rh-negative blood, which you can give to the patient before the cross-match has been completed (O Rh-positive blood is also acceptable in men or in post-menopausal women). If the patient needs blood quickly but is not actually shocked (eg someone who has had a large haematemesis but who is maintaining a systolic BP of >100 mmHg), ask for grouped, uncross-matched blood (grouping takes far less time than a full cross-match).
3. Give the blood at a rate of one unit every half an hour unless the patient's clinical state indicates a need to give blood more rapidly. During transfusion the patient's temperature, pulse and BP should be checked every half hour.

Practical points about blood transfusion
- Use a large-bore cannula wherever possible.
- When setting up the iv infusion, begin by infusing a small amount of normal saline to make sure that the line is flowing freely; do not use dextrose as it will cause the line to clog.

- Give whole blood, or blood plus gelatin, for the treatment of acute haemorrhage; packed cells for the treatment of anaemia.
- Give each unit over 4 hours, or more rapidly if the patient is actively bleeding or hypotensive. If the patient is shocked and especially if he/she is cold, consider giving the blood via a warming coil in a water bath.
- Consider giving 40 mg of furosemide (frusemide) orally or iv with the second unit and then with every alternate unit (especially in the elderly).
- If possible, start the transfusion early in the day: patients need frequent observations during a transfusion and if this is given overnight the patient will not get much sleep.
- Check the haemoglobin 24–48 hours after transfusion.

Indications for transfusion of packed red cells

Packed cells are given for the correction of anaemia. Only in very rare circumstances is it justifiable to transfuse someone whose anaemia has not been investigated ($\rightarrow$ p 399); transfusion may, however, be undertaken while the results of tests are awaited. Transfusion is usually carried out if the haemoglobin concentration is less than 7 g/dl or the patient is very symptomatic. As a general rule, each unit of packed cells will raise the haemoglobin concentration by about 1–1.5 g per dl.

Procedure

1. Take blood for FBC, serum iron or ferritin, B_{12} and folate and cross-match *before* giving any blood. *Take great care* over labelling the sample on the cross-match form. Mistakes in this area are potentially fatal.
   If a patient has already been transfused more than 72 hours before the time when you wish to transfuse them, a fresh sample of blood will need to be taken for cross-matching because of the possible development of antibodies. Thus, if prior transfusion has taken place within 3–14 days, the sample should be taken 24 hours or less before transfusion; if within 14–28 days the sample should be taken 72 hours or less before transfusion; if 28 days to 3 months, the sample should be taken within 1 week before transfusion.
2. Give blood at the rate of one unit every 3–4 hours. Do not give routine transfusions after 10 pm. The frequent nursing observations which the patients will require mean that they will get very little sleep.

If the patient is elderly or has a history of heart disease, transfusion should be performed under diuretic cover: give 40 mg of furosemide (frusemide) orally or iv with every alternate unit.

TRANSFUSION REACTIONS

A low-grade fever (less than 39°C) is relatively common in a patient receiving a transfusion and, if the patient is otherwise well, is not a cause for concern. However, if during a transfusion the patient develops one or more of the following:

- high fever (> 39°C) ± rigors
- urticarial rash
- agitation
- chest or abdominal pain
- hypotension
- wheezing
- severe back pain

  then it is likely that you are dealing with a transfusion reaction. In that case you should:

1. stop the transfusion and return the rest of the unit to the laboratory
2. give 100 mg of hydrocortisone and 10 mg of chlorphenamine (chlorpheniramine) iv
3. if the patient is unwell or is getting worse *inform your SHO or registrar urgently*
4. ask the laboratory to re-check the cross-match between the patient's and the donor's blood
5. monitor urine output carefully (if necessary, catheterize the patient). There is a risk of acute renal failure.

Other complications of blood transfusion

- Transmission of infection, eg hepatitis.
- Hyperkalaemia (stored red cells tend to leak potassium into the fluid phase).
- Hypocalcaemia due to the action of the anticoagulant; this may be a practical problem if the volume transfused has been particularly large (more than 8 units).
- Thrombocytopenia: platelets do not survive for long in stored blood. This rarely causes a practical problem except in patients whose platelet count is already low (eg those with leukaemia or aplastic anaemia).
- Clotting factor depletion: this rarely causes a clinical problem except in those whose clotting was already severely impaired (eg severe liver disease). Clotting factor replacement should *not* be undertaken routinely just because the patient has had a large-volume blood transfusion, but may be required if laboratory measures show a severe coagulation defect.

PLATELET TRANSFUSIONS

These may be required in patients who have severe

thrombocytopenia, eg those with leukaemia or aplastic anaemia. The level of the platelet count is, on the whole, *not* a good guide to the need for a platelet transfusion, but transfusion is indicated if any of the following apply:

- There is spontaneous bruising/bleeding into the skin or optic fundi, from venepuncture sites, etc.
- The platelet count is less than 20×10^9/litre.
- The patient requires surgery and the platelet count is less than 50×10^9/litre.

If you do decide to give platelets, give 4 or (preferably) 6 units as a rapid infusion.

Fresh frozen plasma (FFP)

This is given to correct deficiencies in clotting factors. The major indications are:

- warfarin overdosage with moderate or severe bleeding (INR usually greater than 5)
- liver disease with coagulation disorder (both clinical and on laboratory tests)
- DIC.

If you do give FFP, give either 2 or 4 units as a rapid infusion. FFP is expensive and carries all the hazards of blood transfusion. It should not be used simply as a source of plasma proteins or as a volume expander.

Section 5:
Drug usage

19

Drug usage

526

INTRODUCTION

The range of drugs available to doctors is very large and continues to grow; no attempt will be made, therefore, to describe them all here. Before prescribing any drug with which you are unfamiliar, you are strongly advised to consult the current edition of the BNF or the manufacturer's data sheet. It is especially important that you do this before prescribing anything for a patient who is already on several drugs, for a pregnant or nursing mother or for someone with liver or renal disease.

DRUGS FOR ACUTE PAIN

ANALGESICS

An analgesic is given to relieve pain and also to keep pain at bay. Therefore, if a patient requires painkillers, on an 'as required' basis, more often than twice in a day, consider the following questions:

- Are you confident that you understand the cause of the pain?
- Should the patient have regular analgesia (every 4 or 6 hours, say) rather than prn (as required) treatment?

Aspirin and paracetamol
These are the drugs that should almost always be used first; most patients know which drug suits them best.

Dose Adults aspirin, 600 mg every 4–6 hours
paracetamol, 1 g every 4–6 hours.

Codeine and dihydrocodeine
These are more powerful than the above but have a higher incidence of side-effects, especially constipation, drowsiness and respiratory depression and, in the case of dihydrocodeine, nausea and vomiting.

Dose Adults 30–60 mg 4–6 hourly. In some instances it is useful to combine a small dose of codeine with paracetamol, using a combined preparation of co-codamol 30/500 (paracetamol 500 mg plus codeine phosphate 30 mg, eg Tylex) or co-codamol 8/500 (paracetamol 500 mg plus codeine phosphate 8 mg); the dose is 1–2 tablets or capsules every 4–6 hours (maximum 8 per day).

Non-steroidal anti-inflammatory drugs (NSAIDs)
Ibuprofen is the mildest; diclofenac, naproxen, ketoprofen, etc, are of medium strength; indometacin is the most powerful. These are useful drugs for such things as muscular, joint or skeletal pain

and also for pericarditis. Increased potency goes hand-in-hand with increased side-effects, notably dyspepsia and frank peptic ulceration (+/– perforation or bleeding). It is sometimes useful to apply the NSAID topically as a gel, for example in pain localized to a single joint or to the back. NSAIDs should be used with great caution in the elderly as they can cause fluid retention (thereby precipitating heart failure) and because of an increased incidence of side-effects. NSAIDs are contra-indicated in patients known to have peptic ulcer disease.

Dose	*Adults*	ibuprofen	400–600 mg 3 times daily or, for the modified-release form, 1600 mg once daily
		diclofenac	75–150 mg daily in 2–3 divided doses; 100 mg by suppository
		naproxen	500–1000 mg daily, usually in divided doses; in ACUTE GOUT the dosage is 750 mg initially, then 250 mg 8 hourly until the attack has passed
		indometacin	50–200 mg daily in divided doses.

Buprenorphine (Temgesic)

This drug, given sublingually, is an effective and relatively safe form of pain relief. It causes less respiratory depression than morphine but its effects are only partly reversed by naloxone. It commonly gives rise to nausea or vomiting.

Dose *Adults* 200 µg 8 hourly, increased to a maximum of 400 µg 6 hourly.

Pethidine

Given by injection, pethidine is an effective but short-acting opiate analgesic.

Dose *Adults* 25–100 mg; may be repeated after 4 hours.

Nefopam

This is said to be an effective analgesic for some patients with moderate pain which doesn't respond to other simple analgesics. It is contra-indicated in patients with epilepsy. Side-effects include nausea, nervousness, urinary retention, dry mouth and light-headedness.

Dose *Adults* 30–90 mg tid; lower doses are recommended in the elderly.

Morphine sulphate

This drug can be very useful in acute pain and, in short-term use, does not cause serious problems with dependence. It can be given in liquid form (eg Oramorph) and by suppository. Nausea, drowsiness, constipation and psychological disturbance are common side-effects. Modified-release formulations such as MST Continus are *not* suitable for acute pain relief.

Dose   Adults   10–20 mg every 4 hours if given by mouth or by sc or im injection; for iv use, 5–10 mg doses should be used. In patients with chronic or severe pain requiring frequent morphine one can often switch the patient to an equivalent dose of slow-release morphine 12 hourly (see below).

Diamorphine

This is the drug of choice for severe pain, eg in MI or aortic dissection. Nausea is very common and diamorphine is routinely given along with an anti-emetic such as prochlorperazine (12.5 mg) or metoclopramide (10 mg). Diamorphine is usually given by sc, im or iv injection or infusion.

Dose   Adults   5 mg every 4 hours (occasionally 10 mg in larger subjects). In MI, give a further 2.5 mg if the initial dose has not been effective after 15–20 minutes. Diamorphine can also be given by continuous sc infusion, with an anti-emetic, for patients who are terminally ill or who have severe intractable pain for other reasons – see below.

THE 'ANALGESIC LADDER'

Doctors are fairly successful at treating acute pain but are often criticized by patients with chronic pain for prescribing drugs which are too weak and for prescribing them too infrequently, often because of misplaced fears of dependency or addiction. Therefore, if you are treating a patient with chronic pain, do not continue with a particular analgesic for more than 48 hours unless it is successfully controlling the pain; if not, move up to the next step on the 'analgesic ladder' (Table 19.1) and consider combinations of drugs with different modes of action (eg a mild opiate plus an NSAID). The basic principles of treating chronic pain can be summarized briefly as follows:

Table 19.1
The 'analgesic ladder'

Step 1	Aspirin, paracetamol
Step 2	Mild opiates (codeine, dihydrocodeine)
Step 3	NSAIDs
Step 4	Strong opiates (morphine, diamorphine, etc.)

- Give an analgesic which fully suppresses the pain, wherever possible.
- Give analgesics orally wherever possible.
- In terminal illness, be prepared to give very large doses of opiates if that is what is needed to control pain.
- Give analgesics frequently enough to prevent pain re-emerging: it is easier to keep the patient comfortable if pain is suppressed rather than if one has to treat repeated episodes of 'breakthrough' pain.
- If the patient is needing frequent doses of oral morphine, especially in malignant disease, consider using a modified-release morphine tablet such as MST Continus. For example, if someone has needed 120 mg of oral morphine in the last 24 hours, this could be given as one 60 mg tablet every 12 hours.

  Modified-release morphine *must not* be given more frequently than every 12 hours.
- If the patient cannot take oral treatments, an iv or sc continuous infusion of analgesic is kinder and more effective than intermittent injections. One can also combine the analgesic with an anti-emetic in the same syringe: thus one can combine diamorphine 10–20 mg with hyoscine (Buscopan) 800 µg or levomepromazine (methotrimeprazine, Nozinan) 50 mg, in a small volume (10–20 ml) of 0.9% saline and infuse the mixture sc over 24 hours; the dose of either component can be increased if needed.
- Remember other forms of treatment for pain such as radio-therapy (for bone metastases), steroids (for liver metastases), transcutaneous electrical nerve stimulation, local heat.
- If you or a nurse can find time to talk to patients about pain and their illness generally, this will ease a lot of the distress associated with the pain.
- Many hospitals have staff with expertise in managing severe or persistent pain such as anaesthetists who run pain clinics or, in the case of malignant disease, Macmillan nurses. Do not feel reluctant to refer your patient to one of these specialist services.

PRESCRIBING OF CONTROLLED DRUGS

The law on the prescribing of controlled drugs for use outside hospital is very strict. So, for example, if you are prescribing a controlled drug on a TTO prescription, you *must* observe the following rules:

- The entire prescription, including the patient's name and address, must be in the doctor's own handwriting.
- The form of the drug (tablet or elixir) must be stated, together with the strength.

- The total amount of the drug to be dispensed must be stated in *words and figures*.
- The prescription must be signed and *dated* in the doctor's own handwriting.

Controlled drugs regulations apply to all opiate analgesics except codeine and dihydrocodeine, and also to many barbiturates, notably amobarbital, butobarbital, secobarbital and, in a slightly less severe form, phenobarbital. If in doubt, check with the BNF.

DRUGS FOR CARDIOVASCULAR DISEASE

ANTI-ANGINAL DRUGS

Nitrates

Glyceryl trinitrate This is a safe and effective drug for the acute relief of anginal pain. It can be given as a sublingual tablet or as a buccal spray: the tablets, once the bottle is opened, have a limited life (8 weeks); the spray has a longer life but is more expensive. Nitrates frequently cause headache and can, in large doses, cause faintness.

Dose Acute attack 1–2 sublingual tablets or doses of spray, repeated as required.

Glyceryl trinitrate can also be given in sustained-release forms, including a buccal tablet (held between the gum and upper lip) such as Suscard; a patch form for transdermal administration is also available. These long-acting forms are useful for preventing angina but must not be given continuously: a break in therapy of 6–8 hours in 24 is necessary to sustain clinical benefit.

Dose Suscard Buccal 1–5 mg tid nitrate patch
5–10 mg once daily.

In severe angina, glyceryl trinitrate can be given intravenously (see below).

Long-acting oral nitrates These are effective in preventing angina. There are a wide variety of preparations available, with differing lengths of action, and it is best to become familiar with one or two of them. Both isosorbide dinitrate and mononitrate are marketed; choice is largely a matter of personal preference, though current fashion seems to be in favour of the mononitrate. These drugs should not be given continuously throughout the 24 hours: a break in therapy of 6–8 hours is necessary to sustain clinical benefit. For this reason, if one is giving the drug bd, the second dose should be given in the early afternoon.

Dose Isosorbide mononitrate: 10 mg bd for 3 days, then 20 mg bd, increased as necessary. Maximum 120 mg per day. (Mononitrate of this form, given bd, is quite a lot cheaper than modified-release nitrates given once a day)

Isosorbide mononitrate (modified release): 30–60 mg once daily, increased to 120 mg once daily if needed.

In unstable or severe angina, nitrates can be given *intravenously* in the form of glyceryl trinitrate (eg Nitronal) or isosorbide dinitrate (eg Cedocard IV or Isoket).

All intravenous nitrates should be given using glass or poly-ethylene apparatus: loss of potency will occur if polyvinylchloride (PVC) is used.

Headache and hypotension are important side-effects of iv nitrates, so begin with a small dose (1–2 mg/hour, depending on the size of the patient) and increase the dose every half hour until either the pain is fully controlled or the systolic BP falls below 100 mmHg. Maximum dose 12 mg per hour (GTN) or 20 mg/hour (isosorbide dinitrate).

β-blockers

These are highly effective anti-anginal drugs but there are many side-effects and contraindications. There are a large number of β-blockers on the market so try to become familiar with just two or three of them.

Absolute contraindications These include: known hyper-sensitivity to these drugs; a history of asthma; heart block; bradycardia; hypotension.

Relative contraindications These include: peripheral vascular disease; chronic liver or renal disease (depending on the drug); late pregnancy heart failure.

Side-effects These include: breathlessness (due either to bronchospasm or to heart failure); bradycardia; hypotension; lethargy; nightmares, GI disturbances; impotence.

Dose

atenolol	25–100 mg daily
metoprolol	50–100 mg 2–3 times daily
oxprenolol	80–160 mg/day in 2–3 divided doses, maximum 320 mg/day
labetalol	50–100 mg twice daily initially, increased to 400 mg twice daily or to a maximum of 2.4 gm daily in 3–4 doses
bisoprolol	5–10 mg once daily; occasionally 20 mg daily

Calcium channel blockers

These drugs are effective anti-anginal agents with a better adverse-effect profile than β-blockers, though they tend to be more expensive. The number of drugs and formulations continues to increase, so try to become familiar with two or three of them.

Absolute contraindications These include: known hypersensitivity; advanced aortic stenosis; pregnancy. Verapamil and diltiazem are also contraindicated in the presence of bradycardia, sick-sinus syndrome, any degree of heart block, cardiogenic shock or a history of heart failure.

Relative contraindications These include: hepatic or renal impairment; abrupt worsening of angina after starting therapy. Verapamil is usually contraindicated in the acute phase after MI because of the risk of precipitating heart failure.

Side-effects These include: constipation; nausea and vomiting; flushing; headache; fatigue; ankle oedema; hypotension; bradycardia; heart failure; depression.

Dose   For acute anginal attacks:
nifedipine 5–10 mg (the patient should bite into the capsule and then swallow it)
For angina prophylaxis:

nifedipine retard	10–40 mg bd
verapamil	80–120 mg tid
verapamil sustained release	360–480 mg once daily
diltiazem	60–120 mg tid
diltiazem sustained release	90–180 mg once or twice daily or up to 300 mg once daily
amlodipine	5–10 mg daily

Nicorandil
This is a useful addition to anti-anginal therapy if a patient's pain is not adequately controlled despite several other drugs.

Absolute contraindications These include: cardiogenic shock, hypotension.

Side-effects These include: headache (usually transient), flushing, nausea, vomiting and dizziness.

Dose   10 mg bd, increased to 20 mg or 30 mg bd if needed

Aspirin
This may also be a useful addition to anti-anginal therapy if a patient's pain is not adequately controlled by other drugs.

Absolute contraindications These include: known hypersensitivity; peptic ulceration; bleeding disorders.

Relative contraindications These include: asthma; uncontrolled hypertension; recent stroke (if patient has not had a CT scan).

Side-effects These are uncommon at low dosage but can include bronchospasm, dyspepsia, GI haemorrhage. Clopidogrel may be used in people who are allergic to aspirin, but this drug also carries a risk of GI haemorrhage.

Table 19.2
Summary of treatment of unstable angina

Bed rest
β-blockade (unless contraindicated)
Aspirin
iv nitrate
Calcium antagonist
Heparin
Consider early exercise testing and/or coronary angiography

Dose 75–300 mg once daily

Heparin and low-molecular-weight heparinoids

Heparin can be added to the treatment of patients with unstable angina who are not responding well to other treatment. It should be given intravenously in conventional anticoagulating doses (p 572). As an alternative one can give a LMW heparinoid such as enoxaparin (Clexane) – the dose is 1 mg/kg every 12 hours.

Summary (Table 19.2)

Left ventricular failure (LVF) (manifested by pulmonary oedema) may be present without audible crackles in the chest and vice versa. A common catch is the fact that in people over 70 basal lung crackles are very common without there being any pulmonary oedema at all. Therefore if you are in any doubt about the need for anti-failure treatment it is wise to arrange a CXR.

HEART FAILURE

Diuretics

For mild heart failure a thiazide diuretic such as bendro-flumethiazide (bendrofluazide) or hydrochlorothiazide may be adequate. More severe degrees of heart failure will require loop diuretics such as furosemide (frusemide) or bumetanide; in the most severe cases the loop diuretics will be best given intravenously. In chronic heart failure of moderate or severe degree, metolazone (a very powerful drug, especially if combined with furosemide (frusemide)) may be useful, sometimes on an intermittent basis (alternate days or even once a week).

Potassium supplements or potassium-sparing drugs need not be given routinely with thiazides: a slight fall in serum potassium (to between 3.0 and 3.5 mmol/l) is usually clinically insignificant. Hypokalaemia is, however, dangerous in people with severe coronary atherosclerosis or a history of ventricular arrhythmias and in patients taking digoxin. Many patients taking loop diuretics will require potassium replacement but in any case such patients should be having regular measurements of serum potassium. For medium to long-term use, combined tablets containing a diuretic together with a potassium-sparing drug are often useful; examples would include Moduretic and Dyazide (thiazide plus potassium-retaining drug), Frumil, Frusene, Burinex A and Aldactide (loop diuretic plus potassium sparing drug).

Thiazides

Contraindications These include: pregnancy, hyperuricaemia.

Side-effects These include: hypokalaemia; impotence, hyponatraemia; hypomagnesaemia; hyperuricaemia; hyperglycaemia.

Doses	bendroflumethiazide (bendrofluazide)	5–10 mg daily
	hydrochlorothiazide	25–100 mg daily
	co-amilozide	between one tablet of co-amilozide 2.5/25 daily and 2 tablets of co-amilozide 5/40 tid
	dyazide	1–3 tablets daily

Co-amilozide (Moduretic) users have a high incidence of hyponatraemia, sometimes severe.

Loop diuretics

Absolute contraindications These include: known hypersensitivity; severe liver failure or cirrhosis.

Relative contraindications These include: pregnancy; diabetes mellitus; gout; severe liver disease.

Side-effects These include: hypokalaemia; hyponatraemia; hypotension; nausea; muscle cramps; glucose intolerance; hyperuricaemia; (in large doses) tinnitus or deafness – these ototoxic effects are a particular risk if iv preparations are given too quickly.

Dose	Oral furosemide (frusemide)	40 mg once daily to 80 mg bd; higher doses in renal failure
	bumetanide	1–2 mg daily; up to 5 mg daily in resistant cases
	metolazone	5 mg once a week to once daily, usually as an adjunct to a loop diuretic; higher doses needed occasionally.

If you are giving someone more than 80 mg per day of furosemide (frusemide) (or 2 mg daily of bumetanide) for heart failure, you should consider changing the patient to an ACE inhibitor, either alone or in combination with a diuretic.

Dose	Combined oral preparations	
	co-amilofruse 5/40	1–2 tablets daily or bd
	Burinex A	1–2 tablets daily
	Intravenous furosemide	20–50 mg as initial treatment in an

(frusemide)	emergency; dose should be given over 5 minutes (may also be given as an iv infusion at 1–4 mg/hour)
	40–160 mg daily in subacute or chronic severe heart failure
bumetanide	1–2 mg as initial treatment in an emergency
	1–4 mg daily in subacute or chronic heart failure.

Angiotensin converting enzyme (ACE) inhibitors

There is increasing evidence that ACE inhibitors are effective treatments for heart failure, not simply in relieving symptoms but also in improving cardiac performance and survival. These drugs are therefore being introduced at an earlier stage in the management of heart failure than they used to be. There are now eight ACE inhibitors available in the UK and the number may increase further, so try to become familiar with just two or three drugs.

Absolute contraindications   These include: known hypersensitivity; known or suspected renal artery stenosis; aortic stenosis or outflow tract obstruction; pregnancy; severe hypotension.

Relative contraindications   These include: renal failure; recent high-dose diuretic therapy.

Side-effects   These include: angioneurotic oedema; dizziness; persistent dry cough; nausea; fatigue; loss of taste; sore throat; hypotension; hyperkalaemia; proteinuria; rashes; worsening renal impairment (especially in patients with diabetes); neutropenia or thrombocytopenia; liver damage.

If a patient is being treated with a diuretic together with an ACE inhibitor, it is not usually necessary to give supplements of potassium or a potassium-retaining drug.

Dose   Initiation of ACE inhibitor therapy is best done in hospital if the patient is on large doses of diuretics, is hyponatraemic (serum sodium less than 130 mmol/l), has renal impairment (serum creatinine above 150), is elderly or has a low BP (less than 100 mmHg systolic). If the patient is on a large dose of diuretic (more than 80 mg furosemide (frusemide) or 2 mg bumetanide per day) this should, if possible, be stopped for 24 hours before introducing an ACE inhibitor. To initiate therapy, give a single dose of 6.25 mg captopril while the patient is lying down. Ask the nurses to measure the BP every $\frac{1}{4}$ hour for 2 hours, then $\frac{1}{2}$ hourly for 2 hours, then hourly. If the systolic pressure remains above 90 mmHg and the patient has no symptoms of faintness, ACE inhibition can be safely continued.

Maintenance treatment should consist of captopril, 12.5 mg bd, increased to 25–50 mg bd; enalapril 5 mg bd increased to 10 mg bd or lisinopril 5 mg daily increased to 20 mg daily.

Note: if patients are to derive maximum benefit from ACE inhibitor therapy the dose should be worked up gradually until one has reached quite a high dose (20 mg or more of lisinopril) or the patient has begun to notice side-effects.

Renal function must be closely monitored during the early stages of ACE inhibitor therapy.

Angiotensin II receptor antagonists (SARTANS)

These are useful where ACE inhibitors are not tolerated, particularly because of cough. Overall these drugs have a very good side-effect profile. Use of these drugs for the treatment of heart failure is outside the licence – this does not mean that such use is illegal but you should not initiate treatment with a sartan in heart failure unless you have discussed it with a more senior member of the team.

Absolute contraindications   Known hypersensitivity; pregnancy; renal artery stenosis.

Relative contraindications   These include: dehydration (risk of hypotension); liver failure or severe liver disease; renal failure.

Side-effects   These include: angioneurotic oedema; dizziness; rash; myalgia; diarrhoea; hypotension; hyperkalaemia; worsening renal impairment.

Dose   Losartan   50–100 mg daily (start with 25 mg in the elderly)

Valsartan   80–160 mg daily (start with 40 mg in the elderly).

Vasodilators

These may be useful in the treatment of heart failure where ACE inhibitors are contraindicated, are not tolerated or are insufficient.

Nitrates

These have a useful effect in heart failure. There are a wide variety of preparations available, with differing lengths of action, and it is best to become familiar with one or two of them. Both isosorbide dinitrate and mononitrate are marketed; choice is largely a matter of personal preference, though current fashion seems to be in favour of the mononitrate. Another alternative is glyceryl trinitrate, which may be given as a buccal tablet (Suscard Buccal). These drugs should *not* be given continuously throughout the 24 hours: a break in therapy of 6–8 hours is necessary to sustain clinical benefit. For this reason, if one is giving the drug bd, the second dose should be given in the early afternoon.

Dose Oral isosorbide mononitrate 10 mg bd for 3 days, then 20 mg bd, increased as necessary. Maximum 120 mg/day
isosorbide mononitrate (modified release) 30–60 mg once daily, increased to 120 mg once daily if needed.

In severe heart failure nitrates can be given iv, either in the form of glyceryl trinitrate (e.g. Nitronal) or isosorbide dinitrate (e.g. Cedocard iv or Isoket).

All intravenous nitrates should be given using glass or polyethylene apparatus: loss of potency will occur if PVC is used.

Side-effects of iv nitrates The most important are headache and hypotension.

Dose Begin with a small dose (1–2 mg/hour, depending on the size of the patient) and increase the dose every half hour until either the failure is fully controlled or the systolic BP falls below 90 mmHg. Maximum dose 10 mg/hour.

Hydralazine
This drug is only effective if given together with a diuretic.

Absolute contraindications These include: systemic lupus erythematosus; severe tachycardia; cor pulmonale; aortic stenosis or outflow tract obstruction; dissecting aortic aneurysm; recent MI; porphyria.

Relative contraindications These include: renal impairment; coronary artery disease; cerebrovascular disease; pregnancy or breast feeding.

Side-effects These include: tachycardia; fluid retention; nausea; headache; SLE-like syndrome; hypotension.

Dose *Adults* 25 mg bd increased if necessary to 50 mg bd.

Digoxin
The beneficial effects of digoxin in heart failure are comparatively weak. It should only be used after consultation with your seniors.

Inotropic agents
Intravenous inotropes are useful in certain patients with acute, severe cardiovascular disease associated with hypotension, eg cardiogenic shock. You should *not* initiate treatment with an inotrope without consulting a more senior colleague.

Dobutamine
This drug is effective but its use may be limited by tachycardia: a ventricular rate above 140/min reduces cardiac filling and tends to cancel out the benefit of the positive inotropic action. The drug is given in *diluted form* and the manufacturers supply a 'ready reckoner' chart to help you work out the dose.

Make sure that both you and the nurse supervising the infusion understand the chart.

Dose   Adults   2.5–10 µg/kg/minute; occasionally doses up to 20 µg may be used.

Dobutamine should not be discontinued abruptly; the dose should be reduced gradually over 24-48 hours.

Enoximone

This drug works by a different mechanism from that associated with dobutamine. There are no absolute contraindications to enoximone.

Relative contraindications   These include: hypertrophic obstructive cardiomyopathy; outflow tract obstruction; renal impairment.

Side-effects   These include: ectopic beats or other arrhythmias; hypotension; headaches; insomnia; nausea and vomiting, diarrhoea. Platelet count and liver enzymes should be monitored during treatment with enoximone.

It is important to avoid extravasation of enoximone; it must always be infused into a central vein.

Dose   Adults   90 µg/kg/min initially, followed by 5–20 µg/kg/min
Total dose in 24 hours should not exceed 24 mg/kg.

ANTIHYPERTENSIVE DRUGS (→ pp 47, 432)

See also details of individual drugs above.

SUPRAVENTRICULAR TACHYCARDIAS (SVT)

There is no ideal drug for treating SVT, particularly paroxysmal SVT. The choice of drug will depend on safety, side-effects and the preferences of your superiors.

Digoxin

This is the drug of choice for the control of tachycardia in atrial fibrillation. It has many potential toxic effects and a narrow 'therapeutic window' (ie the effective dose is close to the toxic dose).

Absolute contraindications   These include: severe hypokalaemia; Wolf-Parkinson-White syndrome.

Relative contraindications   These include: hypokalaemia; renal failure; hypertrophic obstructive cardiomyopathy; hypothyroidism.

Side-effects   These include: anorexia; nausea and vomiting; diarrhoea; confusion; ventricular arrhythmias; heart block. Side-effects are more likely in the elderly and in patients who are hypokalaemic or who have pre-existing myocardial or conducting-system disease.

Dose   Adults   Oral – for urgent digitalization, 1–1.5 mg in divided doses over 24 hours; less urgent cases, 250–750 µg initially, followed by 250 µg 6 hours later; maintenance dose 62.5–500 µg per day, in 1 or 2 doses

iv–750–1000 µg diluted in 50 ml of 5% glucose and infused over 2 hours, followed by maintenance doses as above. An alternative is to give half of the digitalizing dose over 10–20 min, then a further fraction 4–8 hours later (also over 10–20 min), then a third fraction again 4–8 hours later.

Digoxin levels in blood   Blood for digoxin assay must be taken 6 or more hours after the last dose. Levels cannot be used to fine-tune the dose of digoxin which a patient needs, nor does a level within the 'therapeutic range' exclude the possibility of digoxin toxicity. A very low level suggests that the patient may not be taking digoxin consistently, while a level at or above the top of the range indicates a high risk of toxicity.

Patients who are seriously ill due to digoxin toxicity should be treated with digoxin monoclonal antibodies (Digibind). The dosage is complex and depends on the blood level of digoxin, so consult the manufacturer's data sheet.

Verapamil

This drug is very effective, given intravenously, for the acute termination of SVT. It is less satisfactory for chronic oral use as its effectiveness tends to wane with the passage of time. It is sometimes useful, as an adjunct to digoxin, for the control of rapid atrial fibrillation.

Absolute contraindications   These include: hypotension; bradycardia; second-and third-degree AV block; sick sinus syndrome; history of heart failure or left ventricular (LV) dysfunction; recent or concomitant β-blocker therapy; Wolf-Parkinson-White syndrome.

Relative contraindications   These include: hepatic impairment; pregnancy; acute MI. You should not give verapamil to someone with a broad-complex arrhythmia unless you are quite sure that it is not ventricular tachycardia. Patients taking verapamil should not drink grapefruit juice as it may affect the metabolism of the drug.

Side-effects   These are uncommon with acute iv use, more common with oral use. They can include: heart failure; hypotension; heart block; constipation, ankle oedema; nausea and vomiting; flushing; headache.

Dose   iv with ECG monitoring, 5–10 mg given slowly; a further 5 mg may be given 10 min later if required.

Disopyramide

This drug is effective, both intravenously and orally. It impairs myocardial contractility but probably less so than verapamil.

Absolute contraindications These include: second- and third-degree heart block; sinus node disease; severe heart failure.

Relative contraindications These include: glaucoma; prostatic enlargement; liver or renal impairment; moderate heart failure; pregnancy; old age.

Side-effects These include: ventricular tachycardia, VF or torsade de pointes; myocardial depression: hypotension; atrioventricular block; dry mouth; blurred vision; urinary retention.

Dose Oral 100 mg tid, increased to 200 mg qid if needed. May also be given in modified-release form (Dirthymin SA or Rythmodan Retard) every 12 hours.

iv with ECG monitoring 2 mg/kg slowly over 5 min, to a maximum of 150 mg, followed immediately by 200 mg orally, then 200 mg every 8 hours; may also be given by iv infusion at a rate of 0.4 mg/kg/hour to a maximum of 300 mg in the first hour.

Esmolol (β-blocker)

Esmolol, a very short-acting β-blocker, is useful for the acute treatment of SVT.

Absolute contraindications These include: asthma; obstructive airways disease; heart failure; cardiogenic shock; sick sinus syndrome.

Relative contraindications These include: late pregnancy; liver disease; renal disease; peripheral vascular disease.

Dose Adults 50–200 µg/kg/min by iv infusion. Consult data sheet.

Sotalol (β-blocker)

Sotalol is useful for the treatment of SVT because it possesses class III anti-arrhythmic properties as well as its β-blocking action. Contraindications are the same as for esmolol; there is also a risk of ventricular arrhythmias so it is **particularly important to avoid hypokalaemia**.

Side-effects These include: breathlessness (due either to bronchospasm or to heart failure); bradychardia; hypotension; lethargy; nightmares; GI disturbances; impotence.

Dose Adults 20–240 mg daily, in 1 or 2 doses.

Amiodarone

This is an extremely effective anti-arrhythmic drug. It does not cause as much myocardial depression as other anti-arrhythmic drugs. It can be used for both supraventricular and ventricular arrhythmias. It has many potential toxic effects.

Absolute contraindications These include: sinus bradycardia; sinus node or sino-atrial disease; pregnancy and breast feeding;

thyroid dysfunction; iodine sensitivity. Contraindications to iv use: severe respiratory failure; severe hypotension; severe cardiac failure.

Relative contraindications These include: renal impairment; cardiac failure; old age.

Side-effects These are numerous and sometimes serious. They include: peripheral neuropathy; myopathy; bradycardia; potentiation of the effects of digoxin (which should be stopped or reduced when amiodarone is being given); potentiation of warfarin; photosensitivity; hypo- or hyperthyroidism; pulmonary alveolitis; hepatitis; headache.

Patients taking warfarin who are started on amiodarone should have their warfarin dose reduced and closely monitored.

Dose Oral   200 mg 3 tid for a week, then 200 mg bd for a week, then 100–200 mg daily

iv   1200 mg by infusion over 24 hours. The initial dose is usually 5 mg/kg, given over 30 min followed by the remainder of the 1200 mg over the succeeding 23½ hours.

Amiodarone infusion must always be given via a central venous catheter.

Flecainide

This drug is useful for 'medical cardioversion' of atrial fibrillation, provided that there is no risk of heart failure. It is much more likely to be successful in AF of recent onset, eg for terminating an episode in someone with paroxysmal AF. Flecainide can also be used to prevent attacks of paroxysmal AF.

Absolute contraindications These include: previous ventricular arrhythmias following MI; actual or incipient heart failure; haemodynamically significant valvular disease.

Relative contraindications These include: presence of a pacemaker (threshold may rise considerably); sinus node dysfunction; conduction defects; AF following heart surgery; elderly; hepatic and renal impairment.

Side-effects These include: dizziness; visual disturbances; arrhythmias; nausea and vomiting.

Dose iv   2 mg/kg over 10–30 min, to a maximum of 150 mg. In occasional cases a follow-on infusion of 1.5 mg/kg/hour is used Oral   50–150 mg bd (lower doses in the elderly.)

Adenosine

This is a short-acting drug which can be used in several types of SVT, including those associated with Wolff-Parkinson-White syndrome. It can also be used in a diagnostic test for broad-complex tachycardias (those which respond are supraventricular in origin).

Absolute contraindications These include sick sinus syndrome; second- or third-degree atrioventricular (AV) block; asthma.

Relative contraindications These include: atrial flutter or fibrillation in patients with an accessory pathway; cardiac transplant.

Side-effects These include: facial flushing; chest pain; dyspnoea; bronchospasm; choking sensation; nausea; light headedness; severe bradycardia (requiring pacing).

Dose Adults Given into a large peripheral vein by rapid injection – 3 mg over 2 seconds, followed if necessary by 6 mg 1–2 min later and by 12 mg after a further 1–2 min. If high-level AV block develops dose increments should NOT be made. If the patient is taking dipyridamole, initial dose should be reduced to 0.5–1 mg.

Propafenone

This is a relatively new drug which has some β-blocking activity. It may be useful as a second-line drug in paroxysmal atrial flutter or fibrillation and paroxysmal re-entrant tachycardias.

Absolute contraindications These include: severe hypotension; severe obstructive airways disease; congestive heart failure; cardiogenic shock; severe bradycardia; sinus node disease; myasthenia gravis; second- or third-degree AV block or bundle branch block (BBB).

Relative contraindications These include: heart failure; hepatic or renal impairment; the elderly; pregnancy; obstrucive airways disease.

Side-effects These include: constipation; blurred vision; dry mouth; dizziness; nausea and vomiting; fatigue; diarrhoea; headache; allergic skin reactions.

Dose Adults 150 mg tid, increased after 3 days to 300 mg bd and then 300 mg tid if needed.

Lower doses in the elderly and in patients weighing less than 70 kg.

Quinidine

This is a rather old-fashioned drug but it is effective, particularly in paroxysmal SVT. There are, however, a number of potential side-effects.

Absolute contraindication Heart block.

Side-effects These include: nausea; diarrhoea, rashes; myocardial depression; heart failure; thrombocytopenia; ventricular arrhythmias; haemolytic anaemia.

Dose Adults 200 mg test dose to detect hypersensitivity, then 500 mg every 12 hours, given as a modified-release preparation (Kinidin Durules).

VENTRICULAR TACHYCARDIAS (VT)

Ventricular ectopic beats rarely require treatment: although they have been claimed to predict more serious arrhythmias there is no evidence that treatment of ectopics improves survival, no matter how 'serious' they look on the ECG monitor. Drug treatment is therefore restricted to ventricular tachycardia (VT); the diagnosis and the management of VT can be very difficult so you are advised to consult your SHO or registrar.

Lidocaine (lignocaine)
This is the first-line drug for the suppression of VT.

Absolute contraindications   Theses include: sino-atrial or atrio-ventricular block; severe heart failure; porphyria.

Relative contraindications   These include: congestive cardiac failure; liver failure; following cardiac surgery.

Side-effects   These include: dizziness; drowsiness; confusion; respiratory depression; convulsions; hypotension; bradycardia.

Dose   Adults   100 mg intravenously over 2–3 min (50 mg in lighter subjects) followed by 4 mg/min by iv infusion for 30 mins, 2 mg/min for 2 hours, then 1 mg/min.

Amiodarone
This is an extremely effective anti-arrhythmic drug. It does not cause as much myocardial depression as other anti-arrhythmic drugs. It can be used for both supraventricular and ventricular arrhythmias. It has many potential toxic effects.

Absolute contraindications   These include: sinus node or sino-atrial disease; pregnancy and breast feeding; (for i.v. use) severe respiratory failure; severe hypotension; severe cardiac failure; thyroid dysfunction; iodine sensitivity.

Relative contraindications   These include: renal impairment; cardiac failure; old age.

Side-effects   These are numerous and sometimes serious. They include: peripheral neuropathy; myopathy; bradycardia; potentiation of the effects of digoxin (which should be stopped or reduced when amiodarone is being given); phototoxicity; hypo- or hyperthyroidism; pulmonary alveolitis; hepatitis; headache.

Dose   Oral   200 mg tid for a week, then 200 mg bd for a week, then 100–200 mg daily.
iv   1200 mg by infusion over 24 hours. The initial dose is usually 5 mg/kg, given over 30 min followed by the remainder of the 1200 mg over the succeeding $23\frac{1}{2}$ hours.

Amiodarone infusion must always be given via a central venous catheter.

Mexiletine

This drug is similar in its actions to lidocaine (lignocaine) and can also be given by mouth. Effective dosing is often limited by side-effects, especially nausea and vomiting.

Absolute contraindications Bradycardia; cardiogenic shock; high degree AV block.

Relative contraindication Hepatic impairment.

Side-effects These include: nausea and vomiting; constipation; hypotension; bradycardia; confusion; convulsions; atrial fibrillation; psychiatric disturbances; nystagmus; tremor, jaundice.

Dose Oral 400 mg initially, then 200 mg 2 hours later, then 200–250 mg 3 to 4 times daily
iv 100–250 mg at a rate of 25 mg/min, then by infusion of 250 mg as 0.1% solution over 1 hour, then 250 mg over 2 hours then 0.5 mg/min.

Propafenone

This is a relatively new drug. It has some β-blocking activity.

Absolute contraindications These include: severe hypotension; severe obstructive airways disease; congestive heart failure; cardiogenic shock; severe bradycardia; sinus node disease; myasthenia gravis; second- or third-degree AV block or bundle branch block (BBB).

Relative contraindications These include: heart failure; hepatic or renal impairment; the elderly; pregnancy; obstructive airways disease.

Side-effects These include: constipation; blurred vision; dry mouth; dizziness; nausea and vomiting; fatigue; diarrhoea; headache; allergic skin reactions.

Dose *Adults* 150 mg tid, increased after 3 days to 300 mg bd and then 300 mg tid if needed.
Lower doses in the elderly and in patients weighing less than 70 kg.

DRUGS ACTING ON THE CENTRAL NERVOUS SYSTEM (CNS)

HYPNOTICS

These drugs are still over-used and alternatives to hypnotics should be considered, such as a dose of analgesic at bed-time. Their use is, however, justified in some patients who are anxious about being in hospital. There is a danger of dependence so prescription should be limited to a week.

Benzodiazepines

Temazepam, loprazolam and lormetazepam are short-acting, nitrazepam, flurazepam and diazepam are longer-acting, with a consequently greater risk of drowsiness.

Absolute contraindications These include: respiratory depression; severe lung disease; severe hepatic impairment; sleep apnoea syndrome; myasthenia gravis; phobic or obsessional states.

Relative contraindications These include: chronic lung disease; personality disorders; muscle weakness; pregnancy and breast feeding; old age; hepatic or renal impairment.

Side-effects These include: drowsiness and light-headedness the next day; confusion; dependence.

Dose	Loprazolam	1–2 mg at night (elderly 0.5–1 mg)
	Lormetazepam	0.5–1.5 mg at night (elderly 0.5 mg)
	Nitrazepam	5–10 mg at night (elderly 2.5–5 mg)
	Temazepam	10–30 mg at night (elderly 5–15 mg)
	Diazepam	5–15 mg at night.

Chloral

The only drugs in this group which are worth considering are triclofos and cloral betaine (Welldorm); it is said to cause less respiratory depression than benzodiazepines.

Absolute contraindications These include: cardiac disease; gastritis; liver or renal impairment; pregnancy and breast feeding.

Relative contraindications These include: respiratory disease; history of drug or alcohol abuse; severe personality disorder; old age.

Side-effects These include: drowsiness the next day; gastric irritation; abdominal distension and flatulence; vertigo; ataxia; staggering gait; rashes.

Dose *Adults*	triclofos 10–20 ml
	cloral betaine 1–2 tablets, with water
	or 5–20 ml of mixture, with water.

Clomethiazole

This causes less hangover than other drugs and may sometimes, therefore, be useful in the elderly. It is absolutely contraindicated in respiratory failure.

Relative contraindications These include: cardiac and respiratory disease; a history of drug abuse; personality disorder; pregnancy and breast feeding; liver or renal impairment.

Side-effects These include: nasal irritation and congestion; conjunctival irritation; headache; paradoxical excitement; confusion; dependence; gastrointestinal disturbances.

Dose *Adults* 1–2 capsules or 5–10 ml syrup.

Zopiclone

This is a relatively new drug. It is said to have a lower potential for dependence and abuse than benzodiazepines, though this remains to be proven.

Absolute contraindications These include: myasthenia gravis, respiratory failure; severe sleep apnoea; severe liver impairment; pregnancy and breast feeding.

Relative contraindications These include: liver and renal disease; old age; a history of drug abuse; psychiatric illness. Not for prolonged use.

Side effects These include: abnormal taste; GI disturbances including nausea and vomiting; dry mouth; drowsiness the next day; irritability; confusion; depressed mood; dizziness; light-headness; headache.

Dose *Adults* 7.5–15 mg at bed-time; elderly 3.75 mg.

ANTICONVULSANTS (→ also p 447)

For the emergency treatment of a fit, give Diazemuls, 10–20 mg intravenously slowly (5 mg/min) or 30 mg of diazepam rectally. If fits recur after two doses of iv or rectal diazepam you should start the patient on an infusion of phenytoin (→ p 450).

For maintenance treatment of epilepsy, single anticonvulsants are to be preferred wherever possible. The choice of drug should normally be made by a more senior member of your team.

Carbamazepine

This is useful in a wide variety of different forms of epilepsy.

Absolute contraindications These include: various forms of AV conduction disorders; history of bone marrow depression.

Relative contraindications These include: hepatic or renal impairment; possibility of pregnancy or pregnant state up to 13 weeks' gestation (risk of neural tube defects); cardiac disease; history of haematological reactions to other drugs; glaucoma.

Side-effects These are common, especially with higher doses. They include: nausea and vomiting; dizziness; blurred vision; drowsiness; headache; ataxia; confusion; agitation; constipation or diarrhoea; anorexia; generalized rash; blood dyscrasias.

Dose Adults 100–200 mg bd, increased gradually to between 800 mg and 1.2 g daily in divided doses. Careful dose timing and the use of modified-release tablets may help to reduce side-effects.

Plasma levels, taken together with clinical effects, can provide some guidance as to dosage requirement. Therapeutic range 4–12 mg/l (20–50 μmol/l).

Phenytoin

This drug is widely used for both tonic-clonic and partial epilepsy. There are no absolute contraindications but side-effects are common and the drug has a narrow therapeutic window (ie the effective dose is close to the toxic dose). Small increases in dosage can result in large increases in blood levels.

Relative contraindications These include: liver disease; pregnancy up to 13 weeks (risk of neural tube defects); porphyria.

Side-effects These are numerous and include: nausea and vomiting; confusion; dizziness; headache; tremor; nystagmus; ataxia; rashes; facial coarsening; hirsutism; megaloblastic anaemia.

Dose Adults Oral – 150–300 mg daily initially, increased to 500 mg/day if needed; doses higher than 300 mg/day should be divided in two.
iv (→ p 450).

Blood levels are very helpful in adjusting the dose of phenytoin, though clinical effect must also be considered. Therapeutic range 10–20 mg/l (40–80 μmol/l).

Sodium valproate

This is a very useful drug for tonic-clonic seizures and is a drug of choice for primary generalized epilepsy, generalized absences and myoclonic epilepsy.

Absolute contraindications These include: moderate or severe liver disease.

Relative contraindications These include: possibility of pregnancy or pregnant state up to 13 weeks' gestation (risk of neural tube defects); risk of significant liver disease.

Side-effects These are numerous and include: gastric irritation; nausea; tremor; weight-gain; hepatic disturbance; transient hair loss; oedema; thrombocytopaenia and impaired platelet function; amenorrhoea.

Dose Adults 300 mg bd, increased gradually if necessary to between 1 g and 2 g daily; maximum 2.5 g daily. Sustained-release tablets available (Epilim Chrono).

Blood levels of valproate, though easy to measure, are a poor guide to dosage requirement. The only value of measuring blood levels is to make sure that the patient is actually taking the tablets.

Ethosuximide

This is the drug of choice for simple absence seizures and may be used in patients with some other kinds of seizures as well.

Cautions Possible hepatic or renal impairment. Pregnancy or breast feeding are relative contra-indications.

Side-effects These are numerous and include: gastro-intestinal disturbances; weight loss; drowsiness; dizziness; ataxia; dyskinesia; hiccough; photophobia; headache; depression. Avoid sudden withdrawal.

Dose Adults 250 mg daily initially, increased gradually to between 1 g and 1.5 g daily; maximum 2 g daily.

Clonazepam

This is a useful drug for all forms of epilepsy, including myoclonic epilepsy.

Absolute contraindications Respiratory depression; acute pulmonary insufficiency.

Relative contraindications These include: respiratory disease, hepatic and renal impairment; elderly and debilitated; pregnancy and breast feeding; porphyria. Avoid sudden withdrawal.

Side-effects These include: drowsiness; fatigue; dizziness; muscle hypotonia; inco-ordination; paradoxical irritability; mental changes.

Dose Adults 1 mg at night for four nights, increased gradually to between 4 and 8 mg daily in divided doses. Use 500 mcg initially in the elderly.

Phenobarbital

This drug is effective for both tonic-clonic and partial seizures but often causes sedation. It is rarely used as monotherapy but may be useful, in combination with another anticonvulsant, in difficult cases. There are many possible interactions with other drugs.

Relative contraindications These include: debilitated patients; impaired liver or renal function; old age; respiratory depression (to be avoided if severe); pregnancy; porphyria.

Side-effects These include: drowsiness; lethargy; depression; ataxia; allergic skin reactions; restlessness and confusion; megaloblastic anaemia. Avoid sudden withdrawal.

Dose Adults Oral 60–180 mg at night

im 50–200 mg repeated after 6 hours if necessary.

Lamotrigine

This is a very new drug which appears to have great potential in patients with difficult epilepsy.

Absolute contraindications   Hepatic impairment.

Cautions   Patients require close monitoring, especially of liver and renal function and clotting; the drug should be withdrawn if rash, fever, 'flu-like symptoms, drowsiness or worsening seizure control develop. A serious skin rash has also been reported.

Side-effects   These are numerous and include: rashes; fever; malaise; hepatic disturbance; neutropaenia and thrombocytopaenia; angioedema; photosensitivity. Avoid sudden withdrawal.

Dose   Dosage schedules are complex and depend on whether the drug is being given as monotherapy or in combination – see BNF.

Gabapentin

This is a new drug which is used as an adjunct in the treatment of partial seizures.

Relative contraindications   Elderly patients; renal impairment; pregnancy and breast feeding.

Side-effects   These include: somnolence; dizziness; ataxia; fatigue; nystagmus; headache; tremor; diplopia; nausea and vomiting. Avoid sudden withdrawal.

Dose   300 mg on first day, then 300 mg bd on second day, then 300 mg tid, then increased as needed, up to 1.2 gm daily.

DRUGS FOR PARKINSONISM

Levodopa

This is the drug of choice for patients with disability due to idiopathic Parkinson's disease. It is much less valuable in older than in younger patients (older patients are more likely to have arteriosclerotic Parkinsonism) and in those with long-standing disease. It is best given with a peripheral decarboxylase inhibitor so as to reduce the incidence of non-CNS side-effects. Low doses should be used initially and dose increases should be gradual. It should not be used in drug-induced Parkinsonism.

Absolute contraindications   Closed-angle glaucoma; severe psychosis.

Relative contraindications   These include: lung disease; peptic ulceration; cardiovascular disease; osteomalacia; skin melanoma; psychiatric illness; open-angle glaucoma.

Side-effects These include: anorexia and vomiting; insomnia; agitation; postural hypotension; dizziness; tachycardia; arrhythmias; involuntary movements; hypomania or psychosis.

| **Dose** | Sinemet Plus | 1 tablet tid, increased gradually. Higher doses may be given as Sinemet or Sinemet CR instead of Sinemet Plus. |
| | Madopar 62.5 | 1 capsule bd (for heavier patients, start with Madopar 125). Higher doses may be given as Madopar 250 or Madopar CR. |

Bromocriptine

This drug acts as a dopamine agonist but has few advantages over levodopa. You should not initiate treatment with bromocriptine except with the advice of a senior colleague.

Selegiline

This drug is helpful, as an adjunct to levodopa, in patients with end-of-dose deterioration in symptoms. Some neurologists also believe that it slows the progression of Parkinson's disease, though this remains unproven. Selegiline interacts with levodopa, the dosage of which may need to be reduced by 20–50% when selegiline is added.

Absolute contraindications Severe psychosis.

Relative contraindications These include: peptic ulceration; uncontrolled hypertension; arrhythmias; angina.

Side-effects These include: hypotension; nausea and vomiting; confusion; agitation; dry mouth; altered liver enzymes; sleep disturbances.

Dose 10 mg daily, in the morning, or 5 mg at breakfast and at mid-day.

Lisuride, pergolide, cabergoline, ropinirole

These are recently introduced dopamine agonists whose place in treatment is not fully defined. They should not be used outside specialist units.

Antimuscarinic drugs

These are weaker than levodopa but are useful for patients with milder symptoms, especially tremor and rigidity. They are also of value in the treatment of drug-induced Parkinsonism and can be given by injection.

Trihexyphenidyl (benzhexol), orphenadrine and procyclidine are the most widely used drugs.

Absolute contraindications These include: urinary retention; closed-angle glaucoma; GI obstruction.

Relative contraindications These include: cardiovascular disease; hepatic or renal impairment; elderly patients.

Side-effects These include: dry mouth; blurred vision; dizziness; GI disturbances; urinary retention; nervousness; confusion; psychiatric disturbances. Avoid abrupt withdrawal.

Dose

Oral	Trihexyphenidyl (benzhexol)	1 mg daily, increased gradually to 5–15 mg/day in 3–4 doses
	orphenadrine	150 mg daily in divided doses, gradually increased; maximum 400 mg/day
	procyclidine	2.5 mg tid, gradually increased; maximum 30 mg/day.
im	procyclidine	5–10 mg, repeated if necessary after 20 min; maximum 20 mg/day
iv	procyclidine	5 mg (usually effective within 5 min), occasionally 10 mg needed.

Benzatropine

This is similar to trihexyphenidyl (benzhexol) but it tends to cause sedation rather than stimulation. It can be given by injection.

Dose Oral 0.5–1 mg daily at bed-time, increased gradually to 1–4 mg daily; maximum 6 mg daily

im or iv 1–2 mg, repeated if symptoms recur.

DRUGS FOR MIGRAINE

The first-line of treatment should be a simple analgesic such as aspirin (900 mg) or paracetamol (1 g), combined with an anti-emetic such as domperidone or metoclopramide. Opiates are often used but carry certain risks such as rebound headache with prolonged use, and are probably best avoided.

5HT$_1$ AGONISTS

This group includes sumatriptan, zolmitriptan and naratriptan. Sumatriptan is poorly absorbed by mouth; better oral availability is reported for the other two. Sumatriptan is also available as an sc injection and a nasal spray.

Sumatriptan

Absolute contraindications Ischaemic heart disease; previous myocardial infarction; coronary vasospasm; uncontrolled hypertension.

Relative contraindications These include: conditions predisposing to ischaemic heart disease; renal or hepatic impairment; pregnancy and breast feeding; should not be taken within 24 hours of any ergotamine preparation.

Side-effects These include: sensation of heat; tingling; heaviness, pressure or tightness of any part of the body; flushing; dizziness; fatigue; transient increases in BP.

Dose Oral 50–100 mg at onset of attack. Dose may be repeated if attack, having settled, then recurs but repeat dose should not be taken during the same attack. Maximum 300 mg in 24 hours.

sc 6 mg as soon as possible after start of attack. May be repeated 1 hour more later if migraine recurs. Maximum 12 mg in 24 hours.

Nasal spray 20 mg into one nostril, as soon as possible after onset of attack. Dose may be repeated after not less than 2 hours if migraine recurs. Maximum 40 mg in 24 hours.

Zolmitriptan

Dose 2.5 mg as soon as possible after onset of attack, repeated after 2 hours if necessary. Maximum 15 mg in 24 hours.

Naratriptan

Dose 2.5 mg as soon as possible after onset of attack, repeated after 4 hours if migraine returns. Maximum 5 mg in 24 hours.

PROPHYLAXIS OF MIGRAINE

β-blockers, pizotifen and amitriptyline all have a place in the prophylaxis of migraine in appropriate subjects. β-blockers such as propranolol, atenolol, metoprolol or timolol are the drugs of choice unless contraindicated (→ p 532). Calcium channel blockers have also been reported to be useful in some cases. Prophylactic anti-migraine drugs should not usually be taken for more than 6 months; their use should then be reviewed.

Pizotifen

Relative contraindications These include: urinary retention; closed-angle galucoma; renal impairment; pregnancy and breast feeding.

Side-effects These include: antimuscarinic effects; drowsiness; increased appetite and weight gain; dizziness.

Dose 500 µg nocte, increased gradually to up to 3 mg nocte.

DRUGS ACTING ON THE GASTROINTESTINAL (GI) TRACT

INDIGESTION

Symptomatic remedies are undoubtedly valuable for short-term use and in this context simple antacids should be used first: do not go straight to more powerful drugs such as H_2-receptor antagonists or proton pump inhibitors. If symptoms persist, further investigation by endoscopy or X-ray studies is usually necessary. There are many preparations on the market, so try to become familiar with just two or three of them.

ANTACIDS

Magnesium trisilicate mixture

This is widely used and generally well tolerated. It is contraindicated in patients with hypophosphataemia and should be used with caution or avoided in those at risk of cardiac, hepatic or renal failure as it contains significant amounts of sodium (6 mmol/10 ml). It can cause diarrhoea.

Dose   Suspension   10 mg tid.
Tablets (also contain aluminium hydroxide) 1–2 as required.

Co-magaldrox (Maalox and Maalox TC)

This is a suitable alternative to magnesium trisilicate. It is very low in sodium and is available both as a tablet and as a suspension. Maalox is more expensive than magnesium trisilicate.

Dose   Tablets   1–2 tablets, chewed, 20 minutes after meals and at bed-time
Suspension   5–10 ml 3–4 times daily as required (usually after meals and at bed-time).

Alginate-containing antacids

These are preferred by some patients, particularly those with reflux oesophagitis. Gastrocote and Gaviscon are the most widely prescribed brands; Gastrocote is slightly lower in sodium than Gaviscon.

Dose   Tablets   1–2 tablets (chewed and followed by water) up to qid
Liquid   10–20 ml qid.

In either case the preparation is usually given after meals and at bed-time.

H_2-RECEPTOR ANTAGONISTS

These drugs are useful in the treatment of peptic ulceration and in reflux oesophagitis. They also promote healing in ulceration associated with NSAIDs. There is little evidence that newer (and more expensive) drugs are better than older ones, although famotidine and nizatidine are said to relieve peptic oesophagitis better than cimetidine and ranitidine. There is no evidence that H_2-receptor antagonists are of value in the treatment of acute haemorrhage from peptic ulcers and it is, therefore, *rarely (if ever)* necessary to give them by injection.

Cimetidine

This is the best-known and cheapest H_2-receptor antagonist available.

Relative contraindications These include: renal impairment; breast feeding; old age (unless gastric cancer has been definitely excluded).

Side-effects These are rare but include: dizziness; diarrhoea; headache; altered liver function tests; rashes; tiredness. There are also significant drug interactions with warfarin, phenytoin and theophyllines.

Dose 400 mg bd or 800 mg at night
Maintenance 400 mg once or twice daily.

Ranitidine

This is more expensive than cimetidine but has fewer side-effects and does not interact with other drugs. It is probably more suitable for the elderly because it is less likely to cause confusion.

Dose 150–300 mg bd or 300 mg at night. Occasionally 300 mg bd.

Nizatitidine

This is more expensive than cimetidine and ranitidine. It may be more effective than the older drugs in the treatment of peptic oesophagitis.

Side-effects. These are rare but include: dizziness; sweating; diarrhoea; headache; altered liver function tests; rashes; tiredness.

Dose 150–300 mg bd or 300 mg at night.

PROTON PUMP INHIBITORS

Omeprazole, lanzoprazole and pantoprazole are powerful inhibitors of gastric acid secretion. Their main use is in the treatment of severe, ulcerative oesophagitis and in the eradication of *Helicobacter pylori* infection (pp 106–107). They should *not* be used as first-line treatment for dyspepsia (there are much cheaper alternatives), nor in patients who have not been investigated.

Omeprazole

Relative contraindications These include: pregnancy and breast feeding: liver disease.

Side-effects These include: urticaria; nausea; abdominal pain; constipation; dizziness; skin reactions; photosensitivity; muscle and joint pain; oedema.

Dose 20 mg daily for 4 weeks; in severe cases 40 mg daily for up to 8 weeks.

HELICOBACTER ERADICATION REGIMENS

These are used for patients with *gastric or duodenal ulcer* who have been shown to be *Helicobacter*-positive for recent infection (eg a positive CLO test). Their use in *H. pylori*-positive subjects with non-specific dyspepsia or other GI symptoms is controversial. Eradication regimens are usually given for 7 days and consist of omeprazole, 40 mg daily, plus two antibiotics. The following combinations are commonly used:

clarithromycin, 250 mg bd plus metronidazole 400 mg bd
amoxicillin 1 g bd plus clarithromycin 500 mg bd
amoxicillin 500 mg tid plus metronidazole 400 mg tid
Note that the antibiotic doses used vary according to the combinations in which they are included.

LAXATIVES

These drugs should only be used if you are satisfied that the patient has true constipation (not just infrequent bowel actions) and after intestinal obstruction has been excluded.

Bulk laxatives

These may take several days to be effective. They should be taken with adequate fluid.

Side-effects These are rare except for nausea, which may limit their use. Some patients also report troublesome flatulence.

Dose *Adults* Trifyba 1 sachet, added to food, 2–3 times daily
Fybogel $\frac{1}{2}$ –1 sachet once or twice daily
Regulan $\frac{1}{2}$ –1 sachet once or twice daily.

Osmotic laxatives

These are effective and safe but frequently produce diarrhoea if given in large doses or for too long.

Dose Lactulose 15 ml bd, adjusted as needed.

Stimulant laxatives

Senna

This is generally safe if used appropriately. It is very economical.

Dose *Adults* 2–4 tablets at night.

Docusate sodium (Dioctyl; Docusol)

This is preferred by some physicians as it acts both as a stool softener and a stimulant. It can be given either as a tablet or a liquid.

Dose Adults up to 5 tablets or 50 ml of solution daily, in divided doses.

Co-danthramer and Co-danthrusate

These are frowned upon because of a possible risk of carcinogenesis (suggested by animal studies). They are, however, useful in terminal care, as an adjunct to potent analgesics.

Side-effects These include red discoloration of the urine (warn the patient) and skin irritation or excoriation (in the incontinent).

Dose Adults 1–3 capsules or 5–15 ml of suspension at bed-time.

Rectal preparations

Glycerin suppositories

These are useful in patients who are constipated for some short-term reason such as immobilization.

Enemas

These are of use in patients with constipation or faecal impaction who cannot swallow. Sodium citrate enemas (eg Micralax) or phosphate enemas (eg Fletchers' Phosphate Enema) are milder; arachis oil enemas are more potent and are more effective as stool softeners.

DRUGS FOR NAUSEA AND VOMITING
(→ also p 370)

Prochlorperazine (stemetil)

This is a good anti-emetic which can be given both orally and by injection. It has many potential side-effects.

Absolute contraindications These are few but include bone-marrow depression.

Relative contraindications These include: cardiovascular disease; cerebrovascular disease; epilepsy (lowers the fit threshold); pregnancy and breast feeding; parkinsonism; renal and hepatic disease; a history of jaundice.

Side-effects These include: involuntary movements (especially in children and young adults); extrapyramidal symptoms; dry mouth; hypothermia; hypotension; tachycardia; arrhythmias; alteration in liver function (including frank jaundice).

Dose   Adults – oral 20 mg initially, then 10 mg after 2 hours. For prophylaxis 5–10 mg 2–3 times daily.
– deep im 12.5 mg as required. The same dose is commonly given iv, for example in coronary care units when patients are receiving diamorphine. This is, however, an unlicensed use: check with your superiors or a senior nurse.
– buccal 1–2 tablets bd.

Metoclopramide

This is again a very effective drug. There is, however, a high incidence of dystonic reactions in young people, so this drug should not be given to those under 20 except with specialist advice.

Relative contraindications   These include: hepatic and renal impairment; elderly; pregnancy (though the dangers of this have probably been overstated); breast feeding; recent GI surgery (best avoided).

Side-effects   These include: dystonic and other extrapyramidal reactions; hyperprolactinaemia; drowsiness; diarrhoea; depression; neuroleptic malignant syndrome.

Dose   Adults   oral, im or iv 10 mg up to 4 times daily. Chemotherapy by continuous iv infusion 2–4 mg per kg over 15–20 min then 3–5 mg per kg over 8–12 hours (maximum over 24 hours, 10 mg per kg).

Domperidone

This drug does not cross the blood-brain barrier except in small amounts, so it is unsuitable for the treatment of nausea due to vestibular or CNS disease. It is particularly useful if the nausea is due to oesophageal or gastric causes, including reflux. It cannot be given by injection.

Relative contraindications   These include: renal impairment; pregnancy and breast feeding. Not recommended for chronic administration.

Side-effects   These are uncommon but include: rashes and other allergic reactions; acute dystonic reactions are reported.

Dose   Adults   oral 10–20 mg every 4–8 hours
rectal 30–60 mg every 4–8 hours.

Ondansetron and granisetron

These drugs are used primarily for the prevention and treatment of vomiting associated with chemotherapy for malignant disease. They may in certain circumstances be combined with dexamethasone. Ondansetron and granisetron are also licenced for the prevention and treatment of post-operative nausea and vomiting.

Ondansetron

Relative contraindications These include: pregnancy and breast feeding: hepatic impairment (more than mild).

Side-effects These include: constipation; headache; sense of heat or flushing; hiccoughs; altered liver function tests; transient visual disturbances; involuntary movements; seizures; chest pain.

Dose Post-operative (prevention) oral 16 mg 1 hour before anaesthesia or 8 mg 1 hour before anaesthesia plus 8 mg at 8-hour intervals for two further doses

Post-operative (treatment) 4 mg by im or slow iv injection.

Chemotherapy: for dosage schedules, consult a senior member of your team or the BNF.

Granisetron

Relative contraindications Pregnancy and breast feeding.

Side-effects These include: constipation; headache; rash; altered liver function tests.

Dose Post-operative (prevention and treatment): 1 mg before induction of anaesthesia, given diluted to 5 ml and injected over 30 sec or 1 mg given as required. Maximum 2 mg in 24 hours.

Chemotherapy: for dosage schedules, consult a senior member of your team or the BNF.

ANTIDIARRHOEAL AGENTS (→ also pp 376–377)

It is usually unnecessary to treat diarrhoea specifically, as it is often self-limiting. If diarrhoea is due to infection the use of anti-diarrhoeal drugs or antibiotics will often prolong it. Where symptomatic treatment is required, use loperamide or codeine phosphate. 5-aminosalicylic acid derivatives such as mesalazine or sulfasalazine are used in the treatment of colitis due to inflammatory bowel disease.

Codeine phosphate
This drug is generally safe in adults, but should not be given to children.

Absolute contraindications Acute ulcerative colitis; antibiotic-induced colitis.

Relative contraindications Renal impairment.

Side-effects The commonest, not surprisingly, is constipation. Nausea and vomiting are a problem for some patients.

Dose Oral 30–60 mg 3–4 times daily.

Loperamide

This drug has similar properties to codeine (see above) but is a little more powerful. It may cause abdominal cramps and skin reactions, including urticaria.

Dose Adults 4 mg initially then 2 mg after each loose stool for up to 5 days. Usual dose 6–8 mg/day, maximum 16 mg/day.

Mesalazine

Absolute contraindications Salicylate hypersensitivity; moderate or severe renal impairment; severe liver disease; blood clotting abnormalities (see below).

Relative contraindications Pregnancy and breast feeding.

Side-effects These include: diarrhoea; nausea; headache; abdominal pain; hypersensitivity reactions, eg rashes, allergic lung reactions, allergic myocarditis; blood dyscrasias.

It is recommended that patients taking aminosalycilates should report any unexplained bleeding, bruising, purpura, sore throat, fever or malaise. A blood count should be performed and the drug stopped immediately if there is any suspicion of a blood dyscrasia.

Dose Oral   acute attack of colitis: 6 × 400 mg daily, in divided doses; maintenance of remission: 3–6 tabs of 400 mg/day, in divided doses.

Foam enema   1–2 g daily for 4–6 weeks.

Suppositories   3–6 suppositories of 250 mg daily, in divided doses; last dose at bed-time.

Sulfasalazine

Absolute contraindications Salicylate hypersensitivity; sulphonamide hypersensitivity; moderate or severe renal impairment; severe liver disease; blood clotting abnormalities (see below).

Relative contraindications These include: pregnancy and breast feeding; hepatic and renal impairment; G6PD deficiency; porphyria.

Side-effects These are very numerous and include: diarrhoea; nausea; headache; loss of appetite; hypersensitivity reactions, eg rashes, photosensitization, anaphylaxis; blood dyscrasias.

It is recommended that patients taking sulfasalazine should report any unexplained bleeding, bruising, purpura, sore throat, fever or malaise. A blood count should be performed and the drug stopped immediately if there is any suspicion of a blood dyscrasia. When the drug is first started, routine blood counts and LFTs should be performed monthly for the first 3 months and function tests should be performed regularly.

Dose Oral   acute attack of colitis, 1–2 g qid
Maintenance of remission   500 mg qid
Enema   3 g at night, retained for at least an hour
Suppositories   0.5–1 g morning and night, after a bowel movement.

DRUGS FOR CHEST DISEASES

β-ADRENERGIC AGONISTS

The treatment of acute asthma depends crucially on the use of nebulized β-adrenergic agonists, chiefly salbutamol and terbutaline (→ p 434). If you are treating asthma the nebulizer should be driven by *oxygen*; if, however, the patient has chronic bronchitis or any past history of carbon dioxide retention, it should be driven by *air* with simultaneous administration of oxygen via nasal cannulae at 1–2 l/min.

Salbutamol
This drug is extremely effective and usually well-tolerated.

Cautions Hyperthyroidism; severe ischaemic heart disease; history of cardiac arrhythmias; hypertension.

Side-effects The commonest is tremor if the drug is given in large doses. Other side-effects include: headache; palpitations; hypokalaemia (which can be severe–see below); hypersensitivity reactions.

Dose By nebulizer   2.5–5 mg every 4–6 hours. Nebulized salbutamol should be mixed in normal saline, not water

iv   5 µg/min initially, adjusted as necessary (according to response and to heart rate) within the range 3–20 µg/min.

If you are giving intravenous salbutamol to a patient with diabetes, monitor the blood glucose carefully; loss of diabetic control, and even ketoacidosis, have been reported.

Remember to monitor the serum potassium closely when treating severe asthma.

Once the patient is well enough not to need salbutamol by nebulizer it can be given by inhaler. A metered-dose aerosol is effective if used properly but fails in many cases because the patient cannot coordinate breathing with pressing the inhaler button; in such cases a volume spacer (Volumatic) may be helpful. Alternatively, a different form of inhaler may be suitable such as a breath-actuated device (Ventolin Easi-breathe; Aerolin Auto-haler) or a dry powder device (Ventolin Rota-haler).

Metered dose inhaler   100–200 µg 3–4 times daily
Dry powder inhaler   200–400 µg 3–4 times daily.

If a patient is having problems using inhalers, ask the pharmacist or physiotherapist to display a range of inhalers so that a choice can be made.

Tablets   8–16 mg every 12 hours. Oral salbutamol is of very little value but some patients with chronic bronchitis like it, particularly to help them with sleep.

Terbutaline

This is very similar in its properties and usage to salbutamol. Some patients prefer the dry powder form of this drug (Bricanyl Turbo-haler) to the corresponding form of salbutamol.

Dose   Nebulizer   5–10 mg every 6 hours
iv   1.5–5 µg per minute (occasionally more for short periods)
Inhaler   500 µg 2–4 times daily.

Salmeterol

This drug is longer acting than salbutamol or terbutaline and is used in patients who have troublesome or 'difficult' asthma. Such patients should also be taking an inhaled steroid or cromoglycate. Salmeterol should *not* be used for the immediate relief of acute attacks of bronchospasm.

Side-effects   These are similar to those of salbutamol. There is a significant incidence of paradoxical bronchoconstriction with this drug.

Dose   Inhaler   50–100 µg (2 to 4 puffs) every 12 hours.

ANTIMUSCARINIC DRUGS

These drugs may be a useful adjunct to treatment with β-agonists, particularly in patients with chronic bronchitis.

Ipratropium bromide (Atrovent)

This drug is relatively safe with few serious side-effects, though dry mouth occurs occasionally. High doses are potentially risky in patients with glaucoma.

Dose   Nebulizer   100–500 µg qid
Inhaler   20–80 µg 3–4 times daily.

Oxitropium bromide (Oxivent)

This drug is relatively safe with few serious side-effects, though dry mouth or blurring of vision occur occasionally. High doses are potentially risky in patients with glaucoma.

Dose   Inhaler   200 µg (2 puffs) 2–3 times daily.

Combined salbutamol plus ipratropium bromide (Combivent)
Combinations of this sort are frowned upon by pharmacological purists but are liked by patients and by some physicians because of their convenience.

Dose Nebulizer 1 vial 3–4 times daily
Inhaler 2 puffs qid.

THEOPHYLLINES

These drugs provide relief of bronchial constriction and may be useful in both asthma and chronic bronchitis, particularly the latter. They may have an additive effect when combined with β-agonists; however, such combinations may increase the risk of side-effects, including hypokalaemia. They have a narrow margin between therapeutic and toxic dose and there are differences in bioavailability between brands, so it is now recommended that prescribers should specify which brand of theophylline is to be used.

Cautions Heart disease; hypertension; hyperthyroidism; epilepsy; peptic ulcer; liver disease; pregnancy and breast feeding; elderly.

Side-effects These include: nausea; tachycardia: palpitations; GI disturbances; headache; insomnia; convulsions; cardiac arrhythmias (including ventricular fibrillation); hypokalaemia.

Theophyllines display a number of important interactions with other drugs: clearance of theophylline is *inhibited* by (amongst others) carbimazole, ciprofloxacin, clarithromycin, erythromycin, cimetidine, diltiazem, fluconazole and oral contraceptives; it is *enhanced* by smoking and heavy drinking and by enzyme-inducing drugs such as phenytoin, carbamazepine, rifampicin and barbiturates.

Safe use of theophyllines is greatly enhanced by *monitoring of plasma levels*, which should be maintained within the range 10–20 mg/l (55–110 μmol/l).

Dose Oral Nuelin SA   175–500 mg every 12 hours
Slo-Phyllin   250–500 mg every 12 hours
Phyllocontin   225–450 mg every 12 hours
Theo-Dur   300 mg every 12 hours
Uniphyllin   200–400 mg every 12 hours.

It may be appropriate to give a larger dose of theophylline in the evening than in the morning in order to relieve symptoms of nocturnal bronchospasm.

Intravenous aminophylline
Great caution required if the patient has been taking an oral theophylline.

This may be given by very slow bolus injection (250 mg over 20 mins) or by infusion but you should not do this without advice and instruction from your SHO or registrar. For advice on the use of aminophylline by infusion, → p 435.

INHALED STEROIDS

Any patient with asthma, or chronic bronchitis with some reversibility, must be thought of as a potential candidate for inhaled corticosteroids; the only exception would be someone with very mild asthma whose symptoms are easily controlled with inhaled β-adrenergic agonists needed infrequently.

It is *essential* that patients understand that inhaled steroids do not relieve acute breathlessness and that they must be used continuously.

Side-effects These are few, but if used in high doses they can show effects similar to those of oral steroids, notably bone thinning and adrenal suppression. Inhaled steroids may also cause sore throat and oropharyngeal thrush. The possibility of paradoxical bronchospasm should also be borne in mind.

As with β-adrenergic agonists, inhaled steroids will only provide benefit if used correctly. Metered-dose aerosols are unsuitable for many patients because they cannot coordinate breathing with pressing the inhaler button; in such cases a volume spacer (Volumatic or Nebu-haler) may be helpful. Alternatively one can use a different form of inhaler such as a breath-actuated device (Becotide Easi-Breathe) or a dry powder inhaler (Becotide Rota-haler, Pulmicort Turbo-haler, Flixotide Accuhaler). Steroids may also be given by nebulizer.

Patients using steroid aerosols, especially in high doses, should be advised to rinse the mouth out with water after using the inhaler – this will reduce the risk of oral thrush.

Dose	Inhaler	Becotide Aerobec	100–200 μg 3–4 times daily or 200–400 μg bd
		Flixotide	100–250 μg bd
	Dry powder inhaler	Becotide Rotacaps	200 μg 3–4 times daily or 400 μg bd
		Flixotide Accuhaler	100–250 μg bd
	High-dose inhaler	Becloforte AeroBec Forte	500 μg bd or 250 μg qid
	Dry powder inhaler	Pulmicort Turbo-haler	200 μg bd
		Flixotide Accuhaler	0.5–1 mg bd
	Nebulizer	Pulmicort Respules	1–2 mg bd, diluted if necessary 0.9% saline.

SODIUM CROMOGLICATE

This drug can reduce the incidence of attacks of asthma, particularly in children and young adults. It is also useful for the prophylaxis of exercise-induced asthma, being taken half an hour before exercise. Some patients find the dry powder form causes bronchospasm, in which case a β-agonist inhaler should be used a few minutes before the cromoglicate. It is *essential* that patients understand that cromoglicate is of no value in relieving acute bronchospasm and that it only works if taken continuously. The use of compound inhalers which contain isoprenaline and cromoglicate (Aerocrom) is not recommended as neither drug is being used to optimal effect.

Side-effects   Coughing; transient bronchospasm.

Dose   Inhaler   10 mg (2 puffs) qid, increased in severe cases to 6–8 times daily

Dry powder inhaler   20 mg (1 Spincap) qid, increased in severe cases to 8 times daily

Nebulized   20 mg qid, increased if needed to 6 times daily.

It is difficult to predict which patients with asthma will respond to cromoglicate. A 4-week trial is reasonable: if the patient has shown no response in this time, cromoglicate should be stopped and an inhaled corticosteroid considered instead.

LEUKOTRIENE RECEPTOR ANTAGONISTS

These drugs, represented currently by montelukast (Singulair) and zafirlukast (Accolate) belong to a new class of anti-asthma compounds. Their place in the management of asthma is still being evaluated. Montelukast is currently licensed only for mild to moderate asthma, though it is used, outside its licence, in more severe cases. Zafirlukast is licensed for asthma treatment without reference to grade.

Montelukast

Cautions   Pregnancy and breast feeding.

Side-effects   Abdominal pain; headache; diarrhoea; upper respiratory tract infection; dizziness; asthenia.

Dose   Oral   10 mg daily at bed-time.

OXYGEN

Oxygen should be regarded as a drug and should be prescribed on the routine prescription sheet. It can be given either by face mask or nasal cannulae. Patients' reactions to oxygen adminis-

Table 19.3
Flow rates for oxygen delivery ('Lifecare' mask system)

24% – 2 l/min
28% – 4 l/min
35% – 8 l/min
40% – 8 l/min
60% – 12 l/min

tration vary: some find it comforting and seem to get as much psychological as physiological benefit from it, while others find the face mask claustrophobic. On the whole it is unwise to use oxygen as a placebo. Patients should be encouraged not to rely on oxygen alone instead of obtaining medical help when their breathing deteriorates.

The aim of oxygen therapy should be to maintain the patient's arterial PO_2 within the range 10–14 kPa (75–105 mmHg). The amount of oxygen delivered to the patient depends on the type of mask used and the flow-rate: many hospitals use a range of masks or mask adaptors which contain a venturi type of delivery system (eg Venti-mask); these are often colour-coded. Make sure that you understand which mask is which and what flow-rate is recommended (Table 19.3).

Oxygen concentration For primary hypoxic illnesses such as pneumonia, pulmonary embolism, pulmonary fibrosis and also for acute LVF, give the highest flow-rate that the patient can comfortably tolerate, ie 40–60%. If a bed-side pulse oximeter is available, aim to keep the saturation level above 90%. After an hour or so, re-check the blood gases to ensure that the PaO_2 is within the required range. High concentrations of oxygen (60%) should not be used for long periods without the advice of a more senior member of the firm.

In chronic bronchitis, give 28% oxygen initially, then recheck the blood gases after half an hour to make sure that the $PaCO_2$ is not rising. You may need to reduce the oxygen concentration to 24% or even discontinue it (see below).

In asthma, give 60% oxygen initially. However, it is particularly important to watch out for CO_2 retention, so *be sure to recheck the blood gases* 1–2 hours after starting oxygen.

If you cannot maintain the PaO_2 above 8 kPa then the patient is in respiratory failure and may need respiratory stimulants or mechanical ventilation: consult your SHO or registrar. If the $PaCO_2$ rises above 8.0 kPa (6.0 kPa in the case of acute asthma) the situation is again one of respiratory failure and is potentially dangerous. The patient may need respiratory stimulants or mechanical ventilation: consult your SHO or registrar.

DOXAPRAM

This drug is a respiratory stimulant which acts on the respiratory centre. It is not a substitute for bronchodilators, antibiotics, chest physiotherapy, etc, but can be a useful adjunct to these measures in getting people, particularly those with chronic chest disease, over a crisis without the need for mechanical ventilation.

Contraindications These include: severe hypertension; status asthmaticus; coronary artery disease; thyrotoxicosis; epilepsy.

Relative contraindications These include: impaired cardiac reserve; liver disease; pregnancy (avoid if possible).

Dose iv infusion 1.5–4 mg/min given concurrently with oxygen and adjusted according to the results of blood gas measurements.

CORTICOSTEROIDS

Steroids have a wide variety of uses. You are most likely to be asked to prescribe them for asthma, inflammatory bowel disease, rheumatic diseases (mainly polymyalgia rheumatica and SLE), cerebral oedema or, occasionally, for people with adrenal insufficiency.

Steroids are of no value in patients with septicaemia, even if shocked. Their role in rheumatoid arthritis is very limited, being confined essentially to intra-articular injection. You should not prescribe systemic steroids in rheumatoid arthritis except under the supervision of a specialist rheumatologist.

Prednisolone

This is the most widely used systemic steroid. It is very potent but has many potential side-effects.

Contraindications Systemic infections, unless specific antimicrobial treatment is given. Avoid live virus vaccines in those receiving immunosuppressive doses.

Relative contraindications These include: diabetes mellitus; peptic ulceration; osteoporosis; psychiatric disease; undiagnosed fever.

Side-effects These are many and include: glucose intolerance (provoking latent diabetes or worsening the control of existing diabetes); mental disturbances including euphoria, paranoid psychosis; dyspepsia or peptic ulceration; candidiasis; suppression of signs of infection (allowing it to spread unnoticed). Adrenal suppression is not usually a problem if courses of steroids last for 3 weeks or less. In long-term use steroids can cause osteoporosis;

avascular necrosis of the femoral head; skin atrophy; tendon rupture; muscle wasting; adrenal suppression; Cushing's syndrome.

Patients taking steroids for more than a few weeks should carry a steroid card; these are obtainable from hospital pharmacies or Health Authorities. The patient should also be warned of the danger of a severe attack of chickenpox if they should be exposed to someone with the disease.

Side-effects are unlikely if the dose of prednisolone is 5 mg per day or less, though there is still a possibility of adrenal suppression. Adverse effects are further reduced if maintenance prednisolone is given on alternate days rather than daily. Where possible, prednisolone should be given once daily in the morning; it is only necessary to divide up the dose if this makes tablet taking more convenient.

Dose	*Adults*	asthma	30–60 mg/day
		polymyalgia rheumatica	15–20 mg/day
		cranial arteritis	60–80 mg/day
		inflammatory bowel disease	30–60 mg/day orally (or hydrocortisone 100 mg 6-hourly iv) together with steroid enemas
		SLE	40–60 mg/day
		polymyositis	1 mg/kg/day.

Dexamethasone

This is the steroid of choice for the treatment of cerebral oedema. Its side-effects are the same as those of prednisolone; however, it is rarely necessary to give dexamethasone long-term.

Dose	*Adults*	oral	4 mg 6 hourly, reduced after a few days to 2–4 mg 2 to 3 times daily
		im	10 mg initially, then 4 mg qid
		iv	(slow injection or infusion) 10 mg initially, then 4 mg qid.

Hydrocortisone

This is the compound of choice for steroid replacement in people with adrenal insufficiency or hypopituitarism. It is also used for urgent treatment in asthma, inflammatory bowel disease, etc, and in patients with adrenal insufficiency who cannot take their treatment orally. Hydrocortisone has mineralocorticoid activity and is more likely than other steroids to cause fluid retention and hypertension. Side-effects do *not* occur when hydrocortisone is given in appropriate replacement doses; if side-effects are, apparently, occurring then the 'replacement' dose being given is too high.

Dose   Oral   for adrenal replacement: 10 mg on waking, plus 5 mg at lunch-time and again at tea-time. Occasionally patients may need higher doses.

im or iv   100–200 mg every 6 hours (use the succinate ester).

Patients on long-term steroids who develop any intercurrent illness (infection, fracture, MI, etc) should have the steroid dose increased to *at least double the normal* amount during the acute phase of the illness. In patients who cannot swallow, hydrocortisone should be given by injection in a dose of 100–200 mg 3–4 times daily.

ANTICOAGULANTS AND THROMBOLYTIC AGENTS

The only commonly used oral anticoagulant is warfarin. This is an effective and generally safe drug, the main adverse effect being bleeding. Warfarin is also teratogenic and its use in pregnancy is very restricted. Warfarin also interacts with very many other drugs (Table 19.4).

Rapid anticoagulation can be achieved using intravenous heparin; however, for many applications it is now better to use a low-molecular-weight (LMW) heparinoid such as tinzaparin, dalteparin, enoxaparin, etc. These drugs can be given subcutaneously and do not require laboratory monitoring.

Warfarin

This is used short-term for the treatment of DVT and PE and long-term for the prevention of thromboembolism in those with valvular heart disease (especially where a prosthetic valve is present), patients with atrial fibrillation and people with a history of recurrent DVT or PE.

Contraindications Pregnancy, peptic ulcer, severe hypertension, infective endocarditis (risk of embolization), poor compliance or intellectual impairment, alcohol abuse (breast feeding is not a contraindication).

Relative contraindications These include: hepatic or renal disease; recent surgery.

Side-effects Haemorrhage (including gastrointestinal, cerebral, cutaneous, optic fundi, etc); hypersensitivity; rash; diarrhoea; skin necrosis; jaundice; hepatic dysfunction.

Drug interactions Table 19.4

Dose Table 19.5

Heparin

This is used to achieve rapid anticoagulation and is given by intravenous infusion. It has been superseded in many conditions by low-molecular-weight (LMW) heparins – see below. Unfractionated heparin is still indicated, however, for severe pulmonary embolism, for acute peripheral arterial occlusion and to maintain patency in coronary arteries after certain forms of thrombolysis. It is also used in some units for the treatment of unstable angina.

Table 19.4
Drugs which interact with warfarin

Potentiate warfarin
Alcohol
Non-steroidal anti-inflammatory drugs
Paracetamol (prolonged use)
Amiodarone
Propafenone
Quinidine (possibly)
Antibiotics, especially broad-spectrum agents, ciprofloxacin,
  erythromycin, metronidazole, numerous others
Antidepressants of the SSRI group (possibly)
Glibenclamide and similar antidiabetic drugs
Sodium valproate
Fluconazole and similar antifungals
Aspirin
Cisapride
Danazol
Tamoxifen
Fibrates
Simvastatin
Thyroxine
Cimetidine
Omeprazole
Phenytoin (sometimes)
Numerous others

Reduce action of warfarin
Rifampicin
Carbamazepine
Phenytoin (sometimes)
Griseofulvin
Oestrogens and progestogens (include oral contraceptives)
Vitamin K

Contraindications Haemorrhagic disorders, severe hypertension, thrombocytopaenia, peptic ulcer, recent cerebral haemorrhage, severe liver disease, recent surgery (especially to eye or CNS), certain cases of renal failure.

Side-effects Haemorrhage (including gastrointestinal, cerebral, cutaneous, optic fundi, etc); skin necrosis; thrombocytopaenia; hypersensitivity reactions (including angioedema and anaphylaxis); osteoporosis (after prolonged use).

Dose Table 19.6.

Table 19.5
Warfarin schedule*

Day	International normalized ratio (INR) (9–11 am)	Warfarin dose (mg) given at 5–7 pm
1	< 1.4	10
2	< 1.8	10
	1.8	1
	> 1.8	0.5
3	< 2.0	10
	2.0–2.1	5
	2.2–2.3	4.5
	2.4–2.5	4
	2.6–2.7	3.5
	2.8–2.9	3
	3.0–3.1	2.5
	3.2–3.3	2
	3.4	1.5
	3.5	1
	3.6–4.0	0.5
	> 4.0	0
		Predicted maintenance dose
	< 1.4	>8
	1.4	8
	1.5	7.5
	1.6–1.7	7
	1.8	6.5
	1.9	6
	2.0–2.1	5.5
4	2.2–2.3	5
	2.4–2.6	4.5
	2.7–3.0	4
	3.1–3.5	3.5
	3.6–4.0	3
	4.1–4.5	Miss out next day's dose, then give 2 mg
	> 4.5	Miss out 2 days' doses, then give 1 mg

*Suggested warfarin schedule based on INR. Modified from Fennerty et al *BMJ* 1988; 297: 1285–1288

Table 19.6
Heparin infusion schedule

Loading dose	5000 iu iv over 5 min
Initial infusion rate	25 000 iu heparin made up in saline to 50 ml gives a final concentration of 500 iu/ml, to be started at 2.8 ml/hour (1400 iu/hour)

Check APTT at 6 hours. Adjust according to APTT ratio(APTT:control) as follows:

APTT ratio	Infusion rate change
>7	stop for 30 min to 1 hour and reduce by 500 iu/hour
5.1–7.0	reduce by 500 iu/hour
4.1–5.0	reduce by 300 iu/hour
3.1–4.0	reduce by 100 iu/hour
2.6–3.0	reduce by 50 iu/hour
1.5–2.5	no change
1.2–1.4	increase by 200 iu/hour
< 1.2	increase by 400 iu/hour

Low-molecular-weight heparins (LMWH)

These compounds act like heparin but have the advantage that they can be given by sc injection and do not require laboratory monitoring. They are as effective as heparin in the treatment of DVT and pulmonary embolism and are as safe or possibly safer. Certain LMWHs are licensed for the treatment of unstable angina. The three most widely used compounds are dalteparin (Fragmin), enoxaparin (Clexane) and tinzaparin (Innohep).

Contraindications Haemorrhagic disorders, severe hypertension, thrombocytopaenia, peptic ulcer, recent cerebral haemorrhage, severe liver disease, recent surgery (especially to eye or CNS), certain cases of renal failure.

Side-effects Haemorrhage (including gastrointestinal, cerebral, cutaneous, optic fundi, etc); skin necrosis; thrombocytopenia; hypersensitivity reactions (including angioedema and anaphylaxis); osteoporosis (after prolonged use). Preservative in tinzaparin causes increased risk of hypersensitivity reactions in patients with asthma.

Dose → Table 19.7.

Thrombolytic agents

Streptokinase, anistreplase, alteplase and reteplase are widely used in the treatment of myocardial infarction (→ p 424). Thrombolytic agents are also used, in some cases, for the treatment of DVT

Table 19.7
LMWH dosages

Dalteparin dosage for prophylaxis against DVT
  surgery, moderate risk = 2500 u 1–2 hours before surgery,
    then 2500 u daily
  surgery, high risk = 2500 u 1–2 hours before surgery, then
    2500 u 8–12 hours later, then 5000 u daily
  immobility = 2500 u daily
Dalteparin dosage for treatment of DVT or PE
  200 u/kg daily (or 100 u bd if increased risk of haemorrhage),
    maximum 18 000 u/day
Dalteparin dosage for treatment of unstable angina
  120 u/kg every 12 hours, maximum 10 000 u bd
Enoxaparin dosage for prophylaxis against DVT
  surgery, moderate risk = 20 mg 2 hours before surgery, then
    20 mg daily
  high risk = 40 mg 12 hours before surgery, then 40 mg/day
  immobility = 20 mg daily
**Enoxaparin dosage for treatment of DVT, PE or unstable
angina**
  volume of solution required equals (body weight in kg) ÷ 100;
    this dose to be given every 12 hours
Tinzaparin dosage for prophylaxis against DVT
  general surgery = 3500 u 2 hours before surgery, then 3500 u
    daily
  orthopaedic surgery (high risk) = 50 u/kg 2 hours before
    surgery, then 50 u/kg/day
Tinzaparin dosage for treatment of DVT or PE
  volume of solution (20 000 u/ml) required according to body
    weight =

Weight (kg)	Volume of solution (ml)
40	0.35
45	0.40
50	0.45
55	0.50
60	0.55
65	0.55
70	0.60
75	0.65
80	0.70
85	0.75
90	0.80
95	0.85
100	0.90
105	0.90
110	0.95
115	1.00

Table 19.7
LMWH dosages (cont'd)

Weight (kg)	Volume of solution (ml)
120	1.05
125	1.10
130	1.15

Note: laboratory monitoring is not required with this treatment

and pulmonary embolism. Urokinase is used for thrombolysis in the eye and in arteriovenous shunts.

Contraindications   Recent trauma, haemorrhage or surgery; unconsciousness; haemorrhagic disorders; aortic dissection; severe hypertension; thrombocytopenia; peptic ulcer; history of cerebro-vascular disease, especially recent events; heavy vaginal bleeding; pulmonary disease with cavitation; acute pancreatitis; oesophageal varices; severe liver disease. Note that diabetic retinopathy is not a contraindication to thrombolysis after myocardial infarction unless there is preretinal haemorrhage or severe proliferative retinopathy.

Patients may form antibodies against streptokinase or anistreplase, therefore these drugs are contraindicated in people who have shown a previous allergic reaction to either substance. Streptokinase and urokinase should not be given between 4 days and 1 year after a previous dose.

Side-effects   These include: nausea and vomiting; haemorrhage (including gastrointestinal, cerebral, cutaneous, optic fundi, etc); allergic reactions, including acute anaphylaxis. In the treatment of acute myocardial infarction hypotension, bradycardia or other 'reperfusion arrhythmias' may be seen.

Dose	Streptokinase	myocardial infarction 1.5 million units by iv infusion over 1 hour
		venous thrombo-embolism 250 000 units over 30 min, then 100 000 u/hour (see data sheet)
	Anistreplase	30 units over 4–5 min by iv injection
	Alteplase	myocardial infarction, within 6 hours 15 mg by iv injection followed by iv infusion; 50 mg over 30 min, then 35 mg over 60 mins (lower doses in patients less than 65 kg)
		myocardial infarction 6–12 hours 10 mg by iv injection; followed by iv infusion: 50 mg over 60 mins then 4

| | infusions each of 10 mg over 30 mins pulmonary embolism 10 mg by iv injection over 1–2 min, then iv infusion of 90 mg over 2 hours |
| Reteplase | myocardial infarction 10 units by iv injection over less than 2 mins, then a further 10 units after 30 mins. |

Note: in the case of myocardial infarction, patients who present less than 4 hours after an anterior infarct and are aged under 70, those who are allergic to streptokinase or anistreplase or those who have had streptokinase or anistreplase within the previous 12 months should be given alteplase as initial treatment. Other patients are usually given streptokinase or anistreplase.

DRUGS USED TO TREAT DIABETES

Oral hypoglycaemic agents – metformin, glibenclamide, tolbutamide, etc – are used in people with type 2 diabetes (formerly called maturity onset or non–insulin-dependent diabetes). Many type 2 patients eventually go on to insulin. Insulin is virtually always used in the young and in those with marked ketonuria, weight-loss, etc. Short-, intermediate- and long-acting insulins are available, as are a variety of short- and intermediate-acting insulins. Most insulin is now given using injection pens, either durable (refillable) or disposable.

Metformin
This drug is extremely useful as monotherapy in overweight patients. It does not cause weight-gain or hypoglycaemia. It may also be given as an adjunct to a sulphonylurea (glibenclamide, etc). It should not be given in renal failure or hepatic disease.

Contraindications Liver disease; renal failure (serum creatinine >150); intercurrent severe illness (risk of lactic acidosis); heart failure; dehydration; alcohol dependence; pregnancy or breast feeding.

Relative contraindications These include: milder versions of the above conditions; use of X-ray contrast media (increased risk of metformin toxicity).

Side-effects Anorexia, nausea, vomiting; diarrhoea; lactic acidosis; vitamin B_{12} deficiency (reduced absorption).

Dose 500 mg bd after food, increased as necessary to 850 mg tid (occasionally 1 g tid)

Sulphonylureas
These drugs (glibenclamide, tolbutamide, gliclazide, glipizide, chlorpropamide, etc) are used in patients whose diabetes is not

controlled after an adequate trial of diet. Their main adverse effects are weight-gain and hypoglycaemia. Some members of this group, notably glibenclamide and chlorpropamide, should not be given in renal failure. All sulphonylureas are hazardous in hepatic disease. Sulphonylureas should always be given before food.

Contraindications Liver disease; renal failure (less risk with tolbutamide, gliclazide or gliquidone); intercurrent severe illness; ketoacidosis; pregnancy or breast feeding; porphyria.

Relative contraindications These include: overweight patients; elderly (over 70), especially those living alone – caution with glibenclamide and chlorpropamide; renal or hepatic impairment.

Side-effects Hypoglycaemia (may be prolonged or severe with glibenclamide or chlorpropamide); weight-gain; gastrointestinal disturbances; headache; hypersensitivity reactions. Hyponatraemia may occasionally occur with chlorpropamide.

Dose	Glibenclamide	2.5 to 15 mg daily; higher doses divided (pre-breakfast and pre-lunch)
	Tolbutamide	500 mg to 2 g daily, in 2 or 3 divided doses
	Chlorpropamide	100–500 mg once daily in the morning
	Gliclazide	40–320 mg daily; higher doses divided
	Glipizide	2.5–40 mg daily; doses above 15 mg divided.

Insulin and insulin analogues

Insulin is given by injection, usually by means of an injection pen (NovoPen, B-D Pen, Humapen, etc). Its main side effect is hypoglycaemia, which is particularly dangerous in those who have lost warning symptoms of hypoglycaemia or people who live alone. Lipohypertrophy of injection sites may also occur if patients do not spread the injections sufficiently. Local allergic reactions are rare. Claims that some patients are intolerant of human-formula insulin and must have animal insulins seem to be based on anxiety or personality factors rather than any differences in pharmacology.

Short-acting (soluble) insulin (Actrapid, Humulin S, Hypurin Neutral, Velosulin) can be given alone or mixed with an intermediate-acting insulin; the injection should be given 15–20 min before a meal. Hypoglycaemia due to soluble insulin typically occurs 2–4 hours after injection. Soluble insulin is also given intravenously in acutely ill patients, for example those with diabetic ketoacidosis.

Insulin lispro (Humalog) is an insulin analogue with a very rapid onset of action. It is used like soluble insulin but is given immediately before meals; if necessary it can be given after eating. Insulin lispro is not licensed for use in pregnancy.

Isophane insulin (Humulin I, Insulatard, Hypurin Isophane) can be combined with soluble insulin in twice-daily injection regimes or can be used as a basal insulin and given at bed-time. Hypoglycaemia due to isophane insulin usually occurs 4–12 hours after injection.

IZS insulin (Humulin Lente, Monotard, Hypurin Lente) behaves very like isophane insulin but is preferred by some patients.

IZS crystalline insulin (Humulin Zn, Ultratard) is used as a basal insulin by some patients on basal/bolus regimes. It has a very variable action and a high risk of unpredictable hypoglycaemia and is best avoided.

Pre-mixed insulins (Mixtard 10, 20, 30, 40, 50; Humulin M2, M3, M5) contain varying proportions of soluble and isophane insulin. They are convenient and are liked by many patients, including children and older people; they are given twice daily, before breakfast and before the evening meal. The suffixes refer to the proportion of soluble insulin in the mixture, ie 10%, 20%, etc. The most popular mixture is 30% soluble/70% isophane (Mixtard 30; Humulin M3).

Humalog Mix 25 is a mixture of 25% insulin lispro and 75% isophane insulin lispro. It is used in the same way as other insulin mixtures but is injected immediately before meals.

ANTIBIOTICS

A full discussion of individual antibiotics is beyond the scope of this book. However, advice on the management of common infections is contained in Table 19.8 (see below).

Table 19.8
Antibiotics for common infections

Disease	Drugs recommended
Septicaemia	
Unknown source	Gentamicin IV + metronidazole + ampicillin *or* cefuroxime* iv (adjust according to possible primary focus of infection)
Neutropenia	Piperacillin + gentamicin (metronidazole should be added in cases of oral muscositis or perianal sepsis)
Meningitis	Benzylpenicillin or (if allergic) chloramphenicol
Gastrointestinal infection	
Diarrhoea	Nil (antibiotic rarely needed; consult microbiologist if in doubt)

Table 19.8
Antibiotics for common infections (*cont'd*)

Disease	Drugs recommended
Biliary tract infection	Cefuroxime* iv
Peritonitis	Gentamicin iv + metronidazole + ampicillin OR cefuroxime* iv
Bone and joint infection	
Osteomyelitis, septic arthritis (not prosthetic joint)	Flucloxacillin + sodium fusidate
Respiratory tract infection	
Acute tonsillitis or pharyngitis	Penicillin V or erythromycin (many episodes are viral and do not need antibiotics)
Acute otitis media	Amoxicillin or erythromycin
Epiglottitis	Chloramphenicol
Pneumonia – community acquired	Clarithromycin oral, OR, if severe or life-threatening, cefuroxime* iv + clarithromycin iv . Follow on with oral clarithromycin alone
Pneumonia – aspiration	Cefuroxime* iv + metronidazole
Exacerbation of COAD	Amoxicillin oral, OR, if severe or life-threatening, cefuroxime* iv or co-amoxiclav iv, follow on with oral cefaclor or co-amoxiclav)
Exacerbations of cystic fibrosis	Piperacillin + gentamicin
Skin and soft tissue infection	
Surgical wounds (lower GI or GU surgery)	Cefuroxime* iv + metronidazole OR ampicillin + flucloxacillin + metronidazole
Cellulitis	Benzylpenicillin iv + flucloxacillin OR clindamycin, follow on with amoxicillin + flucloxacillin orally
Bites	Co-amoxiclav
Urinary tract infection	
Uncomplicated UTI	Trimethoprim OR nitrofurantoin
Pyelonephritis	Gentamicin + ampicillin iv OR gentamicin + cefuroxime*
Prostatitis	Ciprofloxacin

*Oral therapy following intravenous cefuroxime should be with cephalexin (non-respiratory tract) or cefaclor (respiratory infection) unless proven resistance

ADVERSE DRUG REACTIONS AND DRUGS COMMONLY INVOLVED

SKIN
Urticaria
Aspirin
Penicillin
Sulphonamides

Erythema multiforme
Barbiturates
Chlorpropamide
Codeine
Phenytoin
Phenylbutazone
Sulphonamides
Tetracycline
Thiazides

Bullae
Allopurinol
Barbiturates
Penicillin
Phenylbutazone
Phenytoin
Sulphonamides

Dermatitis
Barbiturates
Gold
Penicillin
Phenylbutazone
Phenytoin
Quinidine

Fixed drug eruption
Barbiturates
Captopril
Phenolphthalein
Quinine
Salicylate
Sulphonamides

Non-specific rash
Allopurinol
Ampicillin
Barbiturates
Phenytoin

Hyperpigmentation
ACTH
Busulfan
Gold
Oral contraceptives
Phenothiazines
Amiodarone

Erythema nodosum
Oral contraceptives
Penicillin
Sulphonamides

HAEMATOLOGICAL

Agranulocytosis
Captopril
Carbimazole
Chloramphenicol
Cytotoxics
Gold
Indometacin
Phenylbutazone
Phenothiazines
Propylthiouracil
Sulphonamides
Tolbutamide
Tricyclic antidepressants

Aplastic anaemia
Chloramphenicol
Cytotoxics
Gold
Phenylbutazone
Phenytoin
Sulphonamides

Thrombocytopenia
Aspirin
Carbamazepine
Carbenacillin
Chlorpropamide
Chlortalidone
Digitoxin
Furosemide (Frusemide)
Indometacin
Methyldopa
Phenylbutazone

Phenytoin
Quinidine
Quinine
Thiazides

Megaloblastic anaemia
Cotrimoxazole
Folate antagonists
Oral contraceptives
Phenobarbital
Phenytoin
Primidone
Triameterene
Trimethoprim

Haemolytic anaemia
Aspirin
Cephalosporins
Chlorpromazine
Dapsone
Insulin
Isoniazid
Levodopa
Mefenamic acid
Methyldopa
Penicillin
Phenacetin
Procainamide
Quinidine
Rifampicin
Sulphonamides

Lymphadenopathy
Phenytoin
Primidone

CARDIOVASCULAR
Arrhythmias
Adriamycin
Anticholinesterases
Atropine
Clarithromycin or erythromycin in certain combinations (eg amiodarone)
Digitalis
Lithium
Phenothiazines
Propranolol
Procainamide

Quinidine
Sympathomimetics
Tricyclic antidepressants
Thyroxine
Verapamil

Hypotension
Citrated blood
Calcium antagonists
Diuretics
Levodopa
Morphine
Nitroglycerin
Phenothiazines

Hypertension
ACTH
Corticosteroids
MAOI + sympathomimetics
Oral contraceptives
Phenylbutazone
Sympathomimetics
Tricyclic antidepressants with sympathomimetics
β-blocker withdrawal
Ergotamine
Hydralazine
Methysergide
Oxytocin
Thyroxine
Vasopressin

Cardiomyopathy
Adriamycin
Daunorubicin
Lithium
Phenothiazines
Sulphonamides
Sympathomimetics

Pericarditis
Hydralazine
Methysergide
Procainamide

Thromboembolism
Oral contraceptives

Anaphylaxis
Dextran
Demeclocycline
Iodinated contrast media or drugs
Iron dextran
Insulin
Penicillin

RESPIRATORY
Asthma
Aspirin and other NSAIDs
β-blockers
Cholinergic drugs
Cephalosporins
Streptomycin

Respiratory depression
Aminoglycosides
Hypnotics
Opiates
Polymixins
Sedatives

Pulmonary oedema
Contrast media
Heroin
Hydrochlorthiazide
Methadone

Pulmonary infiltrates
Amiodarone
Bleomycin
BCNU
Busulfan
Cyclophosphamide
Melphalan
Methysergide
Nitrofurantoin
Procarbazine

GASTRO-ENTEROLOGY
Peptic ulcers
Aspirin and other NSAIDs
Etacrynic acid
Phenylbutazone
? steroids

Nausea and vomiting
Digitalis
Ferrous sulphate
Levodopa
Oestrogen
Opiates
Potassium chloride
Erythromycin
Metronidazole

Diarrhoea
Antibiotics (especially clindamycin and lincomycin)
Colchicine
Digitalis
Magnesium containing drugs
Methyldopa

Constipation
Aluminium containing drugs
Barium sulfate
Calcium carbonate
Ferrous sulphate
Ganglionic blockers
Ion exchange resins
Opiates
Phenothiazines
Tricyclic antidepressants

Malabsorption
Antibiotics
Ion exchange resins
Colchicine

Pancreatitis
Azathioprine
Corticosteroids
Ethacrynic acid
Furosemide (Frusemide)
Opiates
Oral contraceptives
Sulphonamides
Thiazides

HEPATIC
Cholestasis
Anabolic steroids
Androgens
Chlorpropamide

Erythromycin estolate
Gold
Oral contraceptives
Phenothiazines

Hepatitis
Allopurinol
Aminosalicylic acid
Erythromycin estolate
Halothane
Isoniazid
Ketoconazole
Methotrexate
Methoxyflurane
Methyldopa
Monoamine oxidase inhibitors
Nitrofurantoin
Phenytoin
Propylthiouracil
Rifampicin
Salicylates
Sulphonamides
Tetracycline
Valproate

RENAL
Urinary retention
Anticholinergics
Disopyramide
Monoamine oxidase inhibitors
Tricyclic antidepressants

Nephrotic syndrome
Captopril
Gold
Penicillamine
Probenecid

Tubular necrosis
Aminoglycosides
Amphotericin
Cephaloridine
Colistimethate sodium
Ciclosporin
Iodinated contrast media (increased toxicity of metformin)
Polymyxins
Sulphonamides
Tetracycline

NEUROLOGICAL
Extrapyramidal
Haloperidol
Levodopa
Methyldopa
Metoclopramide
Oral contraceptives
Phenothiazines
Reserpine
Tricyclic antidepressants

Peripheral neuropathy
Chlorpropamide
Chloroquine
Clofibrate
Demeclocycline
Disopyramide
Ethambutol
Hydralazine
Isoniazid
Metronidazole
Nitrofurantoin
Nalidixic acid
Perhexiline
Procarbazine
Phenytoin
Tolbutamide
Tricyclic antidepressants
Vincristine

Fits
Amfetamines
Isoniazid
Lithium
Lidocaine (Lignocaine)
Nalidixic acid
Penicillins
Phenothiazines
Physostigmine
Theophylline
Tricyclic antidepressants
Vincristine

MUSCULOSKELETAL
Osteoporosis
Corticosteroids
Heparin

Myopathy
Amphotericin B
Carbenoxolone
Chloroquine
Clofibrate
Corticosteroids
Oral contraceptives

METABOLIC
Hypercalcaemia
Antacids
Lithium
Thiazides
Vitamin D

Hyperglycaemia
Chlortalidone
Corticosteroids
Diazoxide
Etacrynic acid
Furosemide (Frusemide)
Growth hormone
Oral contraceptives

Hyponatraemia
Corticosteroids
Chlorpropamide
Cyclophosphamide
Diuretics
Tricyclic antidepressants and SSRIs
Vincristine

Hyperkalaemia
ACE inhibitors
Amiloride
Corticosteroid withdrawal
Cytotoxics
Lithium
Potassium salts
Succinylcholine
Spironolactone
Triamterene

Hypokalaemia
Amphotericin B
Corticosteroids
Diuretics
Insulin
Laxatives

SYSTEMIC

Gynaecomastia
Cimetidine
Digoxin
Isoniazid
Methyldopa
Oestrogens
Spironolactone
Testosterone

Fever
Amphotericin B
Antihistamines
Barbiturates
Bleomycin
Cephalosporins
Methyldopa
Penicillin
Phenytoin
Procainamide
Quinidine
Sulphonamides

Lupus-like syndrome
Acebutolol
Hydralazine
Isoniazid
Procainamide

MISCELLANEOUS

Cataracts
Busulfan
Chlorambucil
Corticosteroids
Phenothiazines

Deafness
Aminoglycosides
Aspirin
Bleomycin
Chloroquine
Etacrynic acid
Furosemide (Frusemide)
Quinine

Precipitate porphyria
Barbiturates
Chlordiazepoxide

Chlorpropamide
Oestrogens
Oral contraceptives
Sulphonamide

MECHANISMS OF DRUG INTERACTIONS

There are many mechanisms by which the effects of one drug can be altered by the prior or concurrent administration of a second drug:

- Opposing pharmacological effects
- Similar pharmacological effects
- Alteration of gastric absorption
- Alteration of pH
- Alteration of gastrointestinal motility
- Interference with metabolism: enzyme induction, enzyme inhibition
- Displacement from site of protein binding
- Interference with excretion.

Table 19.9 contains a list of possible drug interactions but is by no means exhaustive and the reader is referred to the BNF for more detailed information.

Body surface area may be calculated from Figure 19.1 to allow the dose of a particular drug to be calculated, eg cytotoxic drugs.

Table 19.9
Drug interactions

Affected drug	Interacting drug	Result of interaction
ACE inhibitors	Potassium-sparing diuretics	Hyperkalaemia
	Alcohol	Enhanced hypotension
Allopurinol	Thiazide diuretics	Enhanced toxicity
Aminoglycosides	Furosemide (frusemide)	Increased risk of ototoxicity
Aminophylline	Cimetidine, erythromycin	Decreased metabolism with enhanced toxicity
Amitriptyline	Alcohol	Increased sedation
	OCP	Reduced effect
Antihistamines	Alcohol	Increased sedation
Azathioprine	Allopurinol	Increased cytotoxicity

Table 19.9
Drug interactions *(cont'd)*

Affected drug	Interacting drug	Result of interaction
Barbiturates	Alcohol	Increased CNS depression
Benzodiazepines	Opioid analgesics, antidepressants, antihistamines, cimetidine	Enhanced sedation
β-blockers	Alcohol, sympathomimetics, verapamil	Enhanced hypotension
	Ergotamine	Enhanced vasoconstriction
Calcium-channel blockers	Amiodarone, quinidine	Increased bradycardia, hypotension
Carbamazepine	Erythromycin, isoniazid	Increased toxicity
Cephalosporins	Loop diuretics	Increased nephrotoxicity
	Alcohol	Disulfiram-like action
Clomethiazole	Cimetidine	Increased sedation
Cimetidine	Antacids	Reduced absorption
Contraceptive (OCP)	Rifampicin, tetracylines	Reduced contraceptive effect
Corticosteroids	Carbenoxolone	Hypokalaemia
	Aminoglutethamide	Enhanced metabolism
Co-trimoxazole	Ciclosporin	Increased nephrotoxicity
	Methotrexate	Increased antifolate effect
Digoxin	Diuretics	Toxicity increased by hypokalaemia
	Antacids	Reduced absorption
	Phenytoin, rifampicin	Increased metabolism
Erythromycin	Benzodiazepines	Increased sedation
Furosemide (frusemide)	Thiazides	Hypokalaemia
Heparin	Aspirin, dipyridamole	Increased anticoagulant effect

Table 19.9
Drug interactions *(cont'd)*

Affected drug	Interacting drug	Result of interaction
Iron	Antacids	Reduced absorption
L-DOPA	Phenothiazines	Antagonism
	Metoclopramide	Extra-pyramidal effects
Lithium salts	Diuretics	Sodium depletion
	Haloperidol	Extra-pyramidal effects
	Antidepressants	CNS toxicity
	Diltiazem, verapamil	Nephrotoxicity
MAOIs	Alcohol, tyramine	Hypertensive crisis
Methyldopa	NSAIDs, diuretics	Hypotension
	corticosteroids	Antagonism of hypotension
Metoclopramide	Lithium	Extra-pyramidal effects
Metronidazole	Alcohol	Disulfiram-like effect
Metformin	Alcohol	Lactic acidosis
Mianserin	Alcohol, anxiolytics	Enhanced effect
NSAIDs	Probenecid	Reduced excretion
	Antacids	Reduced absorption
	Haloperidol	Drowsiness
	Diuretics, ACE inhibitors	Nephrotoxicity
Opioid analgesics	Anxiolytics, cimetidine	Sedation
Penicillins	Antacids	Reduced absorption
	Probenecid	Reduced excretion
Phenothiazines	Alcohol	Sedation
	Rifampicin	Increased metabolism
	Metoclopramide	Extra-pyramidal effects
Phenytoin	Cimetidine, isoniazid, aspirin, amiodarone	Increased toxicity due to decreased metabolism
	Carbamazepine, alcohol	Increased metabolism
Sulphonylureas	Alcohol, β-blockers	Hypoglycaemia
	Rifampicin	Increased metabolism

Table 19.9
Drug interactions *(cont'd)*

Affected drug	Interacting drug	Result of interaction
Tetracylines	Antacids	Decreased absorption
	Phenytoin	Increased metabolism
Thyroxine	Phenytoin	Reduces thyroxine by increasing metabolism
Valsproate	Aspirin	Enhanced effect
	Antidepressants	Antagonism effect
	Other antiepileptics	Increased metabolism
Warfarin	Barbiturates, carbamazepine, rifampicin	Reduced anticoagulant effect due to increased metabolism
	Cimetidine, amiodarone, alcohol	Increased effect due to inhibition of coumarin metabolism
	Sulphonamides	Increased effect due to displaced protein binding

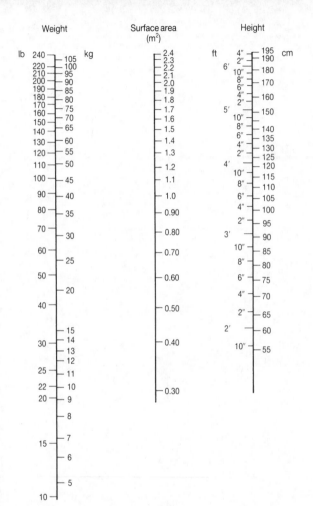

Fig. 19.1 A nomogram for surface area from height and weight.

Page numbers in **bold** refer to medical emergencies. Abbreviations used in the index are: ACE = angiotensin converting enzyme; ARDS = adult respiratory distress syndrome; ARF = acute renal failure; CCB = calcium channel blocker; CNS = central nervous system; COPD = chronic obstructive pulmonary disease; CRF = chronic renal failure; CSF = cerebrospinal fluid; DVT = deep vein thrombosis; EAA = extrinsic allergic alveolitis; GI = gastrointestinal; IBD = inflammatory bowel disease; IBS = irritable bowel syndrome; LVF = left ventricular failure; MI = myocardial infarction; PE = pulmonary embolism; RA = rheumatoid arthritis; SLE = systemic lupus erythematosus; TB = tuberculosis; URTI = upper respiratory tract infection; UTI = urinary tract infection.